www.harcourt-international.com

Bringing you products from all Harcourt Health Sciences companies including Baillière Tindall, Churchill Livingstone, Mosby and W.B. Saunders

- ▶ **Browse** for latest information on new books, journals and electronic products

- ▶ **Search** for information on over 20 000 published titles with full product information including tables of contents and sample chapters

- ▶ **Keep up to date** with our extensive publishing programme in your field by registering with eAlert or requesting postal updates

- ▶ **Secure online ordering** with prompt delivery, as well as full contact details to order by phone, fax or post

- ▶ **News** of special features and promotions

If you are based in the following countries, please visit the country-specific site to receive full details of product availability and local ordering information

USA: www.harcourthealth.com

Canada: www.harcourtcanada.com

Australia: www.harcourt.com.au

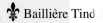
Baillière Tind

D0281394

Mosby's Color Atlas and Text of

Pediatrics and Child Health

Bill Chaudhry MRCP PhD
Fellow in Paediatric Intensive Care
Great Ormond Street Hospital for Sick Children
London
UK

David Harvey FRCPCH
Professor of Paediatrics and Neonatal Medicine
Imperial College School of Medicine
Hammersmith Hospital
London
UK

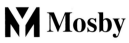 **Mosby**

EDINBURGH LONDON NEW YORK PHILADELPHIA ST LOUIS SYDNEY TORONTO 2001

MOSBY
An imprint of Harcourt Publishers Limited

© Mosby International Limited 2001

M is a registered trademark of Harcourt Publishers Limited

The right of David Harvey and Bill Chaudhry to be identified as authors
of this work has been asserted by them in accordance with the Copyright,
Designs and Patents Act 1988

First published 2001

ISBN 0 7234 2436 5

British Library Cataloguing in Publication Data
A catalogue record for this book is available from the British Library

Library of Congress Cataloging in Publication Data
A catalog record for this book is available from the Library of Congress

Note
Medical knowledge is constantly changing. As new information becomes
available, changes in treatment, procedures, equipment and the use of
drugs become necessary. The authors and the publishers have, as far as it is
possible, taken care to ensure that the information given in this text is
accurate and up-to-date. However, readers are strongly advised to confirm
that the information, especially with regard to drug usage, complies with
the latest legislation and standards of practice.

Commissioning Editor: Ellen Green
Project Development: Fiona Conn
Project Management: Frances Affleck
Design Direction: Judith Wright
Illustrations: MTG (Susan Tyler, Kate Nardoni)

The
publisher's
policy is to use
paper manufactured
from sustainable forests

Printed in China

Contents

Contents

Preface

This book has been written as an introduction to paediatrics and child health for undergraduates and those entering a career in the medical care of children.

Paediatrics is an exciting and rewarding field and we hope that it will continue to be so. One of us was told when he qualified over three decades ago that it was a dying speciality and he should not choose it. We can only reflect how misguided that advice was. The modern care of the newborn was only beginning and the care of disabled children in the community hardly existed. It was thought that children with organ disorders would be cared for by specialist adult physicians: what happened instead was the establishment of sub-specialities within paediatrics.

Since the 1970s, the improvement in the outlook for many disorders in childhood has been fantastic. Preterm babies at about 30 weeks used to die, but now survive intact. The mortality of leukaemia has shrunk. There have been many advances in prevention, particularly the introduction of new vaccines. The care in hospital of children and their families has greatly improved—it would be unthinkable today to forbid parents to stay in hospital with their children. We must not rest: many medical advances are needed to treat diseases which are still incurable, and we need to reduce the distress caused by investigations and treatment. Evidence on which to base treatment is still lacking in many areas. There is a darker side to paediatrics: we still see too many children who need protection from abuse. However, every day we are able to admire parents who bring up their children beautifully in adverse circumstances, particularly poverty.

The book was planned to include as many illustrations as possible and a relatively short text. We are grateful to our colleagues who have lent us pictures and to the children and their families who have allowed them to appear in the book. It is a privilege to work with children and we hope that they will continue to prevent us from becoming pompous. It is our hope that the readers of this book will improve the medical care of babies and children in the future.

BC and DH
2001

Acknowledgements

We are grateful to the following friends and colleagues who have contributed images and advised on the factual content of this book:
Cathy Cale, Frances Cowen, Anthony Chu, Jane Davies, Jane Deal, Inderjeet Dokal, Alison Hayes, Joss Hollway, David Hunt, Caroline King, Nigel Klein, Pippa Kyle, Phil Lee, Keith Lindsey, Eugenio Mercurio, Rodney Meredith, Francesco Muntoni, Neil Murry, Mark Powis, Irene Roberts, Graham Roberts, Ed Schulenberg, Tony Siramanna, Collin Wallace, Paul Winyard, Patricia Woo

chapter 1

Introduction

Paediatric medicine is concerned with identifying and managing conditions that disturb the health of children. This involves not only the treatment of established disease but also the promotion of health and prevention of disease. There is increasing awareness that many diseases that were apparently limited to the adult population have their roots in childhood and fetal life. Birth weight and weight at 1 year have been correlated with death from ischaemic heart disease and respiratory morbidity in adult life. Although health can be defined as the absence of disease, the World Health Organization's definition also recognizes the emotional needs and welfare of the child. It is well recognized that emotionally deprived children may have failure to thrive associated with reduced levels of growth hormone (*see* Chapter 4).

The paediatrician's daily work load can range from the problems of babies born in the second trimester of pregnancy to the emotional difficulties of adolescents in the second decade of life. The paediatrician must be confident in the management of the preterm and newborn infant, be able to persuade and charm the uncooperative toddler and also be able to relate to teenagers with changing emotional and physical characteristics.

Perhaps the most important difference between paediatrics and other branches of medicine is the continuing growth and development that defines childhood. No paediatric consultation is complete without an assessment of height and weight (length, head circumference and weight in infants) which need to be interpreted on appropriate centile charts. The developmental progress of a child is best determined from parental observations and by watching the child's behaviour during play. The developmental progress of older children is largely manifest through education, and information on school progress is invaluable. For example, the sudden onset of unruly behaviour may suggest hyperthyroidism whilst clumsiness noted during games and poor handwriting may point to an undiagnosed congenital hemiplegia.

Communication skills are of vital importance in all branches of medicine and more so in childhood. Small children are limited in their vocabulary (**Fig. 1.1**) and may be unable to explain somatic sensations such as pain. The word 'headache' may be learnt from parents and used to indicate discomfort in any part of the body. For many families English is not the first language and the services of an interpreter may be required. It is not unusual, but it is unsatisfactory for an older sibling to provide this service for his or her parents.

A great problem in paediatrics is lack of cooperation during examination or treatment. Although the teaching in adult medicine is to expose the patient properly before examination, this approach rarely works in young children who are best examined as opportunities present. For example, it is better to slip a stethoscope inside the vest of a sleeping baby (**Fig. 1.2**) and examine the mouth when the baby is spontaneously crying. Similarly, a judgement must be made about the usefulness of information gleaned by examination in relation to the distress caused. For example, there are very few circumstances when digital examination of the rectum is required.

Paediatric Glasgow Coma Scale

4–15 years		<4 years		
Response	**Score**	**Response**		**Score**
Eyes		**Eyes**		
Open spontaneously	4	Open spontaneously		4
Verbal command	3	React to speech		3
Pain	2	React to pain		2
No response	1	No response		1
Best motor response		**Best motor response**		
Verbal command:		Spontaneous or obeys verbal command		6
Obeys	6			
Painful stimulus:		*Painful stimulus:*		
Localizes pain	5	Localizes pain		5
Flexion with pain	4	Withdraws in response to pain		4
Flexion abnormal	3	Abnormal flexion to pain (decorticate posture)		3
Extension	2	Abnormal extension to pain (decerebrate posture)		2
No response	1	No response		1
Best verbal response		**Best verbal response**		
Orientated and converses	5	Smiles, orientated to sounds, follows objects, interacts		5
		Crying	*Interacts*	
Disorientated and converses	4	Consolable	Inappropriate	4
Inappropriate words	3	Inconsistently consolable	Moaning	3
Incomprehensible sounds	2	Inconsolable	Irritable	2
No response	1	No response	No response	1

Fig. 1.1 *The Glasgow Coma Scale (GCS) is an international scale for the assessment of neurological state. The total, or the score for each section, is recorded.*

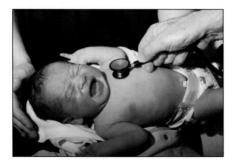

Fig. 1.2 *Auscultation is very difficult when a child is crying.*

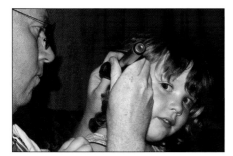

Fig. 1.3 *The examiner rests the hand holding the auroscope on the child's cheek to prevent injury if there is sudden movement.*

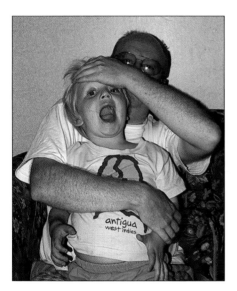

Fig. 1.4 *The throat can be quickly examined if the head and arms are controlled momentarily by the parent.*

A calm, confident, but kind approach usually reassures frightened children and allows the paediatrician to perform an examination and most simple procedures (**Fig. 1.3**). Uncooperative infants can be wrapped in blankets or held firmly by parents (**Fig. 1.4**); older children may tolerate procedures such as lumbar puncture or chest drain insertion with local infiltration of lignocaine but younger children will need sedation or general anaesthesia. Children and babies are smaller than adults and apparently straightforward procedures can be very difficult. Venous cannulation of shocked children can be impossible and if access cannot be established quickly an intraosseous needle must be inserted.

In summary, modern paediatricians must be able to distinguish the normal characteristics of babies, children and young adults from the often subtle features of disease. They must have a high degree of practical ability and communication skills that are essential in dealing with parents and children. Most of these skills can only be learnt at the bedside, but this book aims to serve as a guide to the conditions commonly encountered in general paediatrics.

chapter 2

Epidemiology

THE HEALTH PROFILE

Epidemiology is the study of the distribution and determinants of disease in human populations. By constructing a health profile of the population it is possible to direct resources towards improving the well-being of the population and, in particular, children. A population health profile will include data on:
- the age distribution of the population
- the birth rate, which will indicate how the age spectrum will change in coming years
- the rates of economic disadvantage and overcrowding
- the uptake of immunization and health clinic attendance
- the proportion of minority groups with specific problems.

Definitions of mortality statistics (**Fig. 2.1**) have been derived to allow standardization when collecting data. Although mortality statistics are widely used as indices of child health, they do not necessarily reflect the actual health problems of children. Morbidity is a better indicator of population child health but such data are difficult to collect. An important change in a specific mortality definition is that the stillbirth rate has been extended back from 28 to 24 weeks to reflect survival at these low gestational ages.

Other important roles for epidemiological study are in determining the true natural history and evolution of disease, as well as defining normal variation for the population. This task is impossible for hospital-based research as the patients presenting usually have more severe illnesses and as such tend to have a poorer prognosis. Monitoring the health of a local population can have unexpected benefits in identifying the causes of disease and risk factors as well as the impact of interventions.

SOURCES OF DATA

Epidemiological data are obtained from many sources:
- **A national census** takes place every 10 years in the United Kingdom, and in many other countries, and provides a description of the population.
- **Data relating to health** in the UK are held by the Office of Population Censuses and Surveys (OPCS).
- **Death certification** can produce misleading mortality statistics as there are commonly errors in reporting.
- **Morbidity data,** for example consultations to general practitioners, can be flawed as many patients will not present to medical services to be catalogued but will be treated at home by relatives following advice from pharmacists.
- **Registers** of congenital malformations, cancer and communicable disease exist and are useful as they are generally well supported.

- Direct **epidemiological** studies are carried out to answer specific questions relating to particular populations. Initially they may be purely descriptive, indicating an association between risk factor and disease, but a true link can be demonstrated by a controlled trial.

Key definitions in epidemiology	
Incidence	The number of new cases of a condition occurring in a defined population in a specific time period. A measure of acute or self-limiting episodes
Prevalence	The number of cases of a condition in a population at one moment in time. A measure of chronic conditions
Stillbirth rate	The number of infants born after the 24th week of gestation who do not breathe or show signs of life per 1000 total births
Perinatal mortality	The number of stillbirths and deaths during the first week per 1000 total births
Neonatal mortality rate	The number of deaths in the first 28 days of life per 1000 live births
Post-neonatal mortality rate	The number of deaths after the first 28 days until the end of the first year of life per 1000 live births
Infant mortality rate	The number of deaths in the first year of life per 1000 live births
Age-specific mortality rate	Number of deaths in an age group per 1000 population in the group
Congenital	Present at birth. With no regard to genetic or environmental aetiology
Impairment	Describes a pathological process such as spina bifida, i.e. what is wrong with the patient
Disability	The consequence of an impairment, such as difficulty walking, i.e. what the patient cannot do
Handicap	A disability of body or mind that interferes with the ability to lead a normal life and education, i.e. how it adversely affects the person's life

Fig. 2.1 *Common epidemiological definitions.*

MORTALITY RATES IN CHILDHOOD

Modern obstetric management and better maternal health are probably the reasons why the rate of stillbirths per 1000 total births and the perinatal mortality remain low. Although infant mortality rates continue to decline, over 70% of all deaths in childhood occur in the first year of life (**Fig. 2.2**). The main causes of death in the perinatal period are complications of low birth weight and congenital malformations; post-neonatal deaths are dominated by late deaths from congenital malformations, sudden infant death syndrome

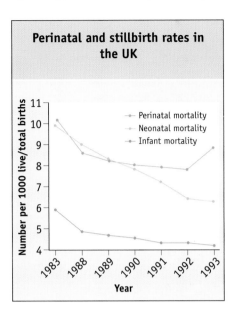

Perinatal and stillbirth rates in the UK

Number per 1000 live/total births

- Perinatal mortality
- Neonatal mortality
- Infant mortality

Year

Fig. 2.2 *Perinatal and stillbirth rates are low in the UK although infant mortality continues to fall. (Source: Office of National Statistics.)*

and low birth weight neonatal survivors. The apparent increase in deaths from congenital malformations has occurred as a result of falling mortality from acquired diseases in the first year of life (**Fig. 2.3a**). There has been a great reduction in the childhood diseases such as whooping cough, diphtheria and polio as a result of immunization, and deaths from pneumonia are uncommon since the development of antibiotics. Deaths from genetic and congenital disease are also less common; this is probably due to antenatal detection and genetic counselling.

In the preschool years, accidents and poisonings are probably the most preventable causes of death. Cancer becomes more common and late deaths from congenital malformations still occur (**Fig. 2.3b**). In older children, from 5 to 14 years, accidents and cancer are the leading causes of death. Half of these accidental deaths are road traffic accidents (**Fig. 2.3c**).

MORBIDITY RATES

When mortality rates are high they can be used to direct provision of health and social services. However, in most industrialized countries mortality rates are low and morbidity is a more important indicator of child health. Morbidity data are, however, harder to collect with accuracy. Hospital admission practice has changed and notification of infectious diseases is probably not complete. Consultations to general practitioners can provide useful data.

DEMOGRAPHY

The social conditions and demographic profile within a population are reflected in the pattern of health in its children. The World Health Organization publishes data relating to

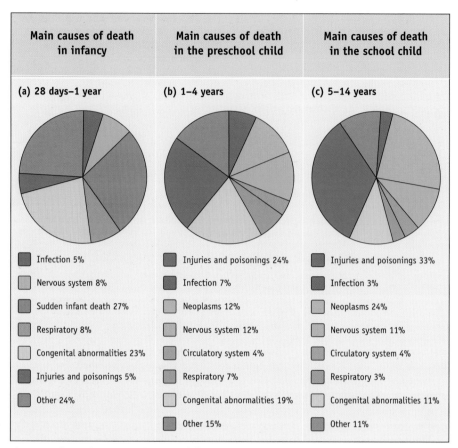

Main causes of death in infancy

(a) 28 days–1 year

- Infection 5%
- Nervous system 8%
- Sudden infant death 27%
- Respiratory 8%
- Congenital abnormalities 23%
- Injuries and poisonings 5%
- Other 24%

Main causes of death in the preschool child

(b) 1–4 years

- Injuries and poisonings 24%
- Infection 7%
- Neoplasms 12%
- Nervous system 12%
- Circulatory system 4%
- Respiratory 7%
- Congenital abnormalities 19%
- Other 15%

Main causes of death in the school child

(c) 5–14 years

- Injuries and poisonings 33%
- Infection 3%
- Neoplasms 24%
- Nervous system 11%
- Circulatory system 4%
- Respiratory 3%
- Congenital abnormalities 11%
- Other 11%

Fig. 2.3 *The main causes of death: (a) in infancy; (b) in the preschool child; (c) in the school child. (From: Platt & Pharoah 1995 Child health statistical review. Arch Dis Child 73(6): 541–548.)*

the world population, age structure and the rate of increase in population size. These data are of particular importance as:

- Inner city dwelling is associated with greater risks of accident in childhood and atherosclerotic disease in adulthood.
- Children from the more advantaged social groups fare better in all measures of health status.
- Falling child mortality rates mean that parents need to conceive fewer children in order to be sure of their survival to adulthood.
- Increasing numbers of children are raised by single parents, who as a group are relatively disadvantaged and whose children are more vulnerable to illness.
- Ethnic minority groups are at risk of different genetic conditions from the rest of the population, such as blood disorders, but may underuse available health resources because of cultural and social differences.

SPECIFIC EPIDEMIOLOGICAL PROBLEMS OF HEALTH CARE PROVISION

SOCIAL CLASS

The Registrar General's social class score rates social class based on the father's occupation. There is a scale from I (indicating professional occupations) to V (describing unskilled manual workers). Differences in mortality and morbidity across these social classes still remain despite having been reported almost 25 years ago (**Fig. 2.4**). The Working Group on Inequalities in Health headed by Sir Douglas Black published its report, known as 'the Black Report' (1980), which demonstrated inequalities of health across the English population. Current data show that these trends continue today.

NEONATAL INTENSIVE CARE OF PRETERM INFANTS

The resources available to a country for provision of health care are finite, and the provision of intensive care for preterm infants is expensive. Advances in technology have allowed survival of infants at 23 weeks' gestation and a birth weight of 500 g (**Fig. 2.5**). Although there are concerns as to the outcome of intensive care, extremely preterm infants do not contribute to the overall impairment and disability rates as there are few infants at these gestations and they have a high mortality. In fact, it is the older gestation infants (greater than 28 weeks) who, although they have a low rate of disability, comprise a relatively large population and produce a large group of children with special needs.

CONGENITAL ABNORMALITIES

The fall in the incidence of neural tube defects seems to have occurred for reasons other than antenatal screening (**Fig. 2.6**) and may be related to folic acid levels in the maternal diet. In contrast, the incidence of Down syndrome remains high despite antenatal serological screening. Refinements to serological testing and use of high resolution ultrasound scanning may change this.

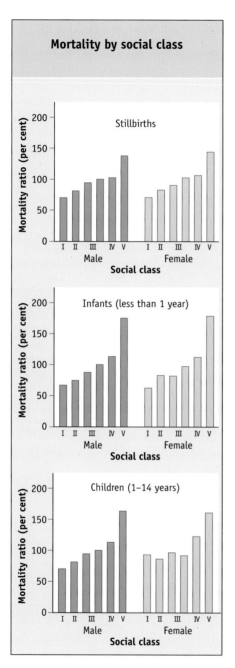

Fig. 2.4 *Mortality by social class. (From: Occupational Mortality 1970–72. HMSO 1978, p. 196.)*

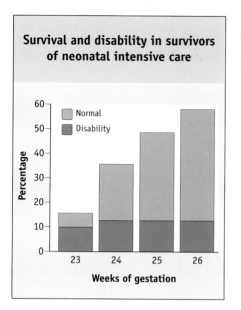

Fig. 2.5 *Survival and disability in survivors of neonatal intensive care. (From: Rennie 1996 Arch Dis Child 74: 214–218.)*

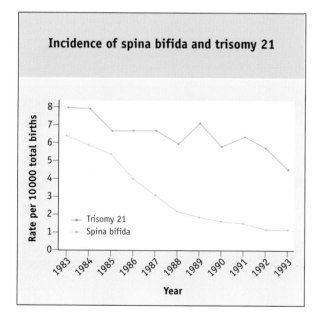

Fig. 2.6 *Spina bifida and other neural tube defects are now rare. Antenatal screening has not had a great impact on the incidence of trisomy 21. (Source: Office of Population Censuses and Statistics.)*

chapter 3

Development

One of the great pleasures of paediatrics is to observe children's development.

As with height and weight, it is important to determine whether development is progressing within the wide range of normality. This can be done by consulting charts that indicate centiles for the times at which certain percentages of children acquire particular skills (**Fig. 3.1**). Thus, walking occurs in 25% of children at 11 months of age, 50% of children at 12 months of age, and 90% of children at 15 months of age. Some, but not all, children lying outside the centiles will have an abnormality, such as cerebral palsy. Although there is a wide range of ages at which skills are acquired, the progression of skills remains orderly, for example sitting precedes walking which occurs before running.

Routine screening of children's development is a relatively inefficient process. Parents are often first to suspect that there is something wrong with their child, and their concerns should be taken seriously as they are usually correct.

DEVELOPMENTAL ASSESSMENT

Progression through key developmental milestones can be sought through history taking and by watching a child's behaviour in the examination room. Even when children choose to cooperate their attention span is short and only 15 minutes is usually available for formal testing.

Development is usually divided into four areas:
- gross motor development
- fine motor development and vision
- speech and hearing
- social development.

GROSS MOTOR DEVELOPMENT

Beginning to crawl and walk are obvious milestones for parents; failure of a child to attain these skills helps to identify cerebral palsy early. The cephalic to caudal developmental progression can be followed in the first months of life. By 6 weeks the infant can raise its head from the horizontal by 90° (**Fig. 3.2**) and by 3 months the infant can prop itself on its forearms (**Fig. 3.3**). Sitting with a straight back is an important milestone as truncal coordination progresses (**Fig. 3.4**). The arms become free to manipulate objects and there is a better view of the environment which accelerates developmental progress. Walking using furniture for support demonstrates power and coordination at a stage when balance reflexes are not fully operational (**Fig. 3.5**). Free walking begins with a wide base which becomes narrower with improving skill (**Fig. 3.6**). There is a wide range of normality in these gross motor skills. Some infants are late in sitting and walking because of a familial tendency. Others may be slow to walk because they are relatively shy or propel themselves

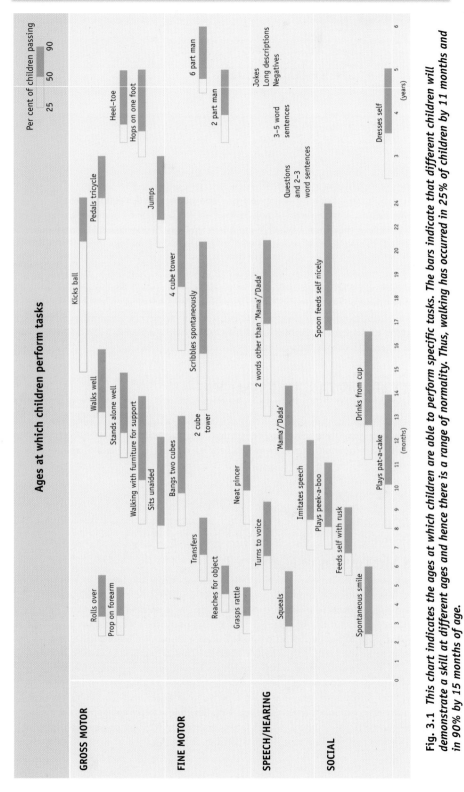

Fig. 3.1 This chart indicates the ages at which children are able to perform specific tasks. The bars indicate that different children will demonstrate a skill at different ages and hence there is a range of normality. Thus, walking has occurred in 25% of children by 11 months and in 90% by 15 months of age.

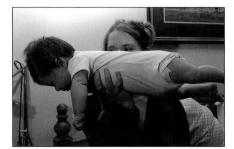

Fig. 3.2 *At 6 weeks a baby can raise its head from the horizontal when placed prone.*

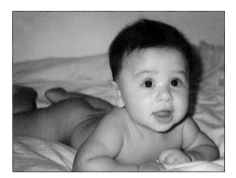

Fig. 3.3 *By 3 months most babies can support themselves on their forearms.*

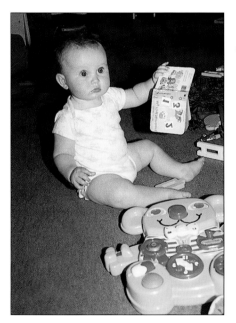

Fig. 3.4 *The ability to sit is important as it allows a better view of the world and frees both hands to manipulate objects.*

by bottom-shuffling. A few will have abnormalities such as cerebral palsy or a neuromuscular disorder. Although boys with Duchenne muscular dystrophy walk late, they often come to medical attention because of late speech development.

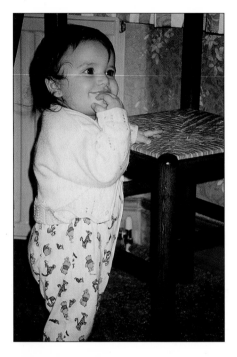

Fig. 3.5 *Infants initially walk holding onto furniture. They have the power and coordination to take steps but lack balance when on their feet. This is known as cruising.*

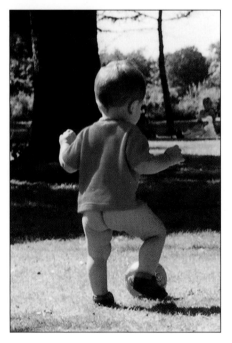

Fig. 3.6 *Walking usually occurs between 9 and 18 months. Initially it is with a wide base for stability.*

FINE MOTOR DEVELOPMENT AND VISION

Visual impairment or a lack of stimulation from the environment can halt developmental progress as good vision is needed for manipulative skills to develop. There is a progression from a whole hand grip to fine finger–thumb apposition (**Fig. 3.7**), and from the isolated use of a hand to coordinated use of both to manipulate objects. Transferring between hands occurs at around 7 months (**Fig. 3.8**) and facilitates the visual rather than oral exploration of objects. Right or left hand dominance is often not established until the second or third year. Strong hand preference before this time might suggest the presence of a hemiplegia.

SPEECH AND HEARING

Hearing is tested routinely at around 8 months by the distraction hearing test (**Fig. 3.9**), as at this age infants are able to turn their heads to sound. The distracter gains the child's attention by non-auditory means and then, hiding any distracting object, stands still. The tester produces high and low pitched noises of about 40 decibels intensity on a level with

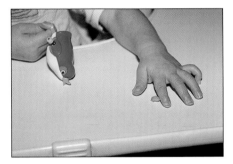

Fig. 3.7 *The neat pincer grip to pick up a small object demonstrates normal neurological function in the hand as well as good visual acuity.*

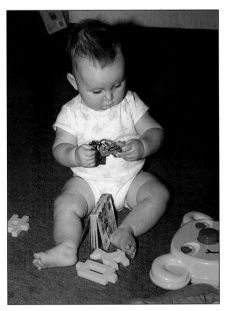

Fig. 3.8 *Transferring between hands usually occurs at about 7 months. However, objects are still placed in the mouth for oral inspection until about 1 year of age.*

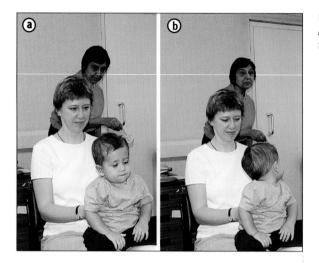

Fig. 3.9(a,b) *Distraction hearing test using a pure tone generator.*

the infant's ears. The distracter then notes whether a response to noise occurred. High risk groups, for example those with family history of deafness, or parents expressing concern that their child does not hear, are evaluated earlier and usually require brain stem auditory evoked responses (BAER). Unfortunately, many children still only come to light with hearing impairment when their speech is noted to be poor at the age of 2 or 3 years. As with gross motor development there are wide variations in the development of speech. Girls tend to speak earlier than boys and some infants have words with meaning at 8 months whilst some normal 3- or 4-year-olds have no words. Twins and triplets often have delayed speech as they use private language to communicate with each other. Autism is associated with a specific abnormality of speech and communication.

Tongue tie is not associated with speech delay.

SOCIAL DEVELOPMENT

The first feature of a child's interaction with other children and adults is a reactive smile which occurs at around 6–8 weeks. By 3 months infants have a general interest in their surroundings and at the age of 4 months most children will look to see where a toy has fallen and anticipate the production of a bottle or breast, showing that they have an understanding of their surroundings. The use of a comb or drinking from a cup shows that the child understands what the object is even though the verbal skills to name it have not yet been acquired (**Fig. 3.10**). Towards the end of the first year infants show casting— deliberately throwing objects to the ground; there is understanding of simple phrases. Self feeding and 2 or 3 word sentences are generally established by 18 months.

Over the next years there is increasing awareness of other children. At 2 years of age they will only play alongside each other but by 3 they can cooperate together. By the age of 5 most children are independent in the daily living skills of feeding, toileting, washing and dressing.

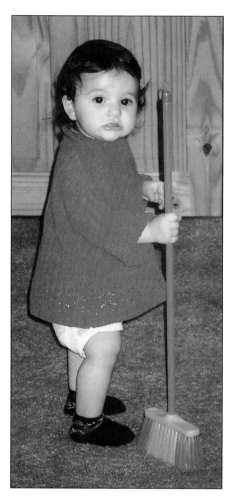

Fig. 3.10 *The appropriate use of this brush indicates an understanding of what it is, although the child cannot yet name it.*

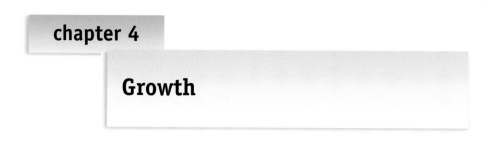

chapter 4

Growth

PATTERNS OF GROWTH IN CHILDHOOD

Growth is one of the characteristics of childhood. It can be thought of as occurring in three phases with differing control mechanisms (**Fig. 4.1**). The most rapid phase is fetal and early infant growth, which is driven mainly by the availability of nutrients; the second phase of growth begins at around 7 months of age when growth hormone is the principal control; finally, the rapid spurt associated with puberty is due to sex hormones augmenting growth hormone effects.

CENTILE CHARTS

Growth centile charts are available for all developed and some developing countries. When evaluating growth it is of critical importance to measure the child's height and weight accurately and then compare against appropriate normal values for the population (**Fig. 4.2**). The 3rd and 97th centiles are each approximately two standard deviations from the median and show the normal height range for most of the population. Growth outside

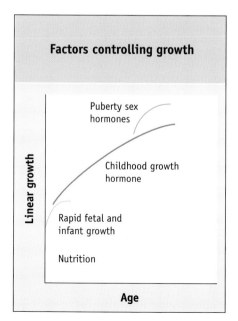

Factors controlling growth

Puberty sex hormones

Childhood growth hormone

Rapid fetal and infant growth

Nutrition

Linear growth

Age

Fig. 4.1 *The infant, childhood, pubertal model emphasizes that different factors control growth at different times in childhood.*

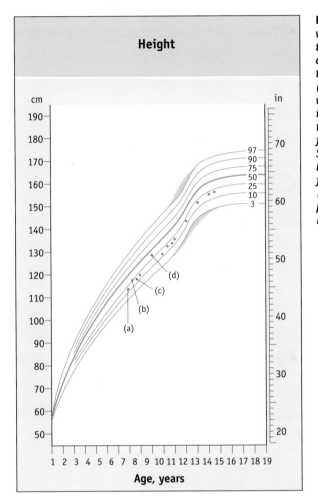

Fig. 4.2 *There is a natural variation in growth during the year: more growth occurs in the spring (a–b) than in the winter months (b–c). Care must be taken when plotting points as an incorrect point (d) can lead to worry and investigation for some years to follow. Standard Buckler–Tanner longitudinal growth chart for British girls. (Reproduced with permission from Castlemead Publications.)*

these centiles may be abnormal, and certainly any child whose growth is crossing centile lines should be suspected of abnormality. It is important to realize that 3% of the normal population also grow on or below the 3rd centile. The same is true for children on or above the 97th centile. In order to identify children with growth failure a lower centile (0.4th) has been suggested as a useful threshold for investigation and treatment.

The growth potential for children with genetic disorders such as achondroplasia and Turner syndrome is often less than for a normal child. Comparing a growth chart for Turner syndrome (**Fig. 4.3**) and a normal female chart it can be seen that a child with Turner syndrome is not only smaller but has a different growth pattern to a normal girl. Special charts for these groups are available.

GROWTH VELOCITY

Velocity charts are derived from careful measurements of children; they show how rapid growth is in infancy and during puberty, and also how slow growth is just before the

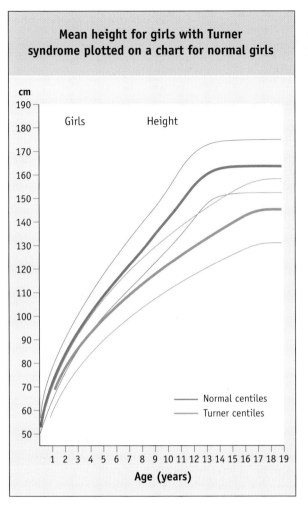

Mean height for girls with Turner syndrome plotted on a chart for normal girls

cm

Girls   Height

Normal centiles
Turner centiles

Age (years)

Fig. 4.3 *Mean height for girls with Turner syndrome plotted on a chart for normal girls.*

pubertal growth spurt. In girls, the pubertal growth spurt occurs approximately two years before that in boys (**Fig. 4.4**). At least 6 months is usually required to establish an accurate velocity in childhood where growth is relatively slow, but in infancy problems can be identified over a matter of weeks due to the rapid growth rate. As puberty varies in its time of onset, an assessment of pubertal status is mandatory before drawing any conclusions about growth.

MEASUREMENT OF GROWTH

Supine length is usually measured up until 2 years of age (**Fig. 4.5**) and standing height thereafter. There is a blip on the centile charts which demonstrates the effect of gravity in the upright position. Careful attention to technique is required to produce accurate and reproducible results. Height also requires to be measured carefully (**Fig. 4.6**), especially in early childhood when the rate of increase in height is very slow. A weight should be put

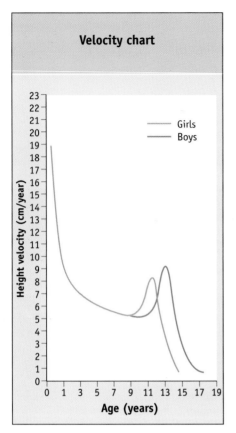

Fig. 4.4 *Velocity charts are derived from normal height charts.*

on the headboard and the child asked to stand straight while an assistant holds the heels in place. Gentle elevation is applied to the head at the mastoid processes to stretch the spine.

Head circumference is measured in a horizontal plane from the occiput to the forehead (**Fig. 4.7**). It should be measured at birth and during health screening in infancy, but graduates of neonatal intensive care units should have head circumference monitored as they are a high risk group for abnormal head growth. Head circumference should be measured in any child who appears to have a large or small head. It is important to plot other family members as a familial large head is common.

VARIATIONS FROM NORMAL

THE SHORT CHILD

Children with familial and constitutional growth delay can be easily identified (**Fig. 4.8a**). In general, those suffering from familial short stature will have always been short and followed a centile line. Therefore they will have a normal growth velocity (although this may lie on the 25th centile for the population) and will be heading for the final height dictated by their parents' height (**Fig. 4.9**). When their bone age (**Fig. 4.10**) is measured it will lie within two standard deviations of their chronological age. In constitutional growth

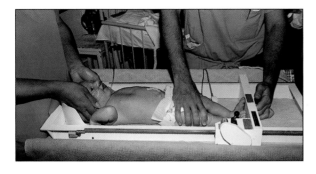

Fig. 4.5 *Measurement of supine length requires two people to hold the head still and also stretch the legs out.*

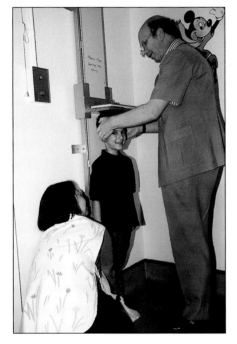

Fig. 4.6 *Height measurement. Height should be measured at every visit to the clinic as, although there may be no concerns about growth initially, many children with chronic illness may have interference with growth potential.*

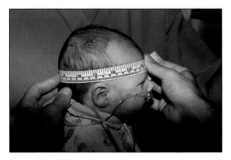

Fig. 4.7 *Head circumference measurement. In babies and infants, head growth should also be carefully measured. Abnormal head growth may indicate disease, for example hydrocephalus.*

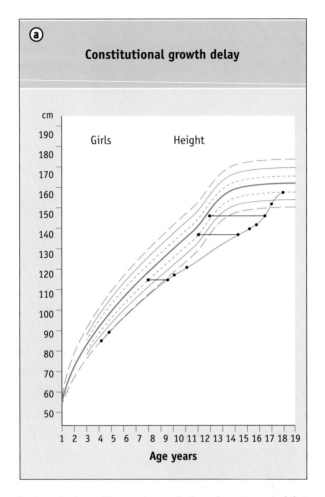

Fig. 4.8(a,b,c,d) *Growth charts illustrating variations from normal. (a) Constitutional growth delay. When other children are enjoying the pubertal growth spurt after about 11 years this girl's skeleton has the growth rate of an 8-year-old; thus she becomes much shorter than her classmates. However, when her skeleton has matured to the point of puberty she also grows rapidly and eventually reaches adult height as predicted by her bone age.*

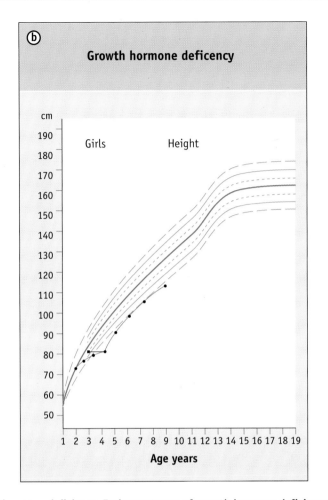

ⓑ

Growth hormone deficency

Girls   Height

cm
190
180
170
160
150
140
130
120
110
100
90
80
70
60
50

1 2 3 4 5 6 7 8 9 10 11 12 13 14 15 16 17 18 19

Age years

(b) Growth hormone deficiency. Early treatment of growth hormone deficiency reduces the amount of height potential that is lost and can never be regained; it also reduces the psychological problems of severe short stature.

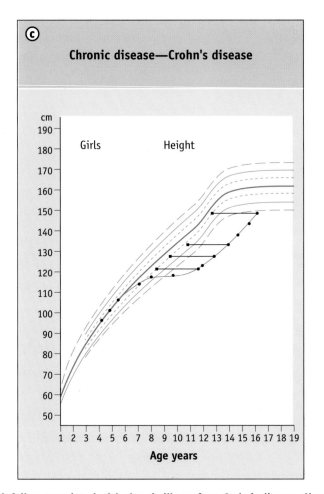

(c) Growth failure associated with chronic illness from Crohn's disease. Chronic inflammation and malnutrition has led to severe growth failure in this child.

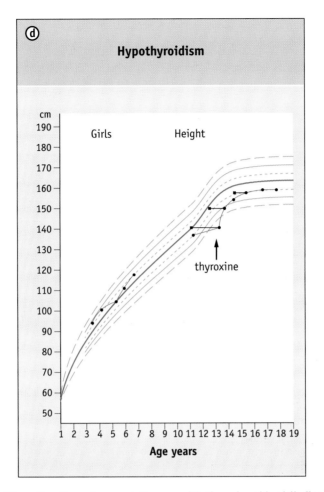

(d) Hypothyroidism. Despite replacement therapy with thyroxine this girl's final height potential has fallen from the 50th centile to the 25th.

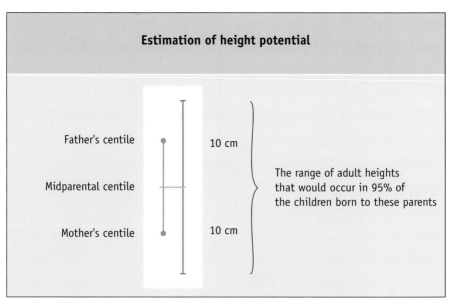

Fig. 4.9 *Estimation of height potential from parental heights. Final adult height should lie within 10 cm of the midparental centile in 95% of cases (see also Fig. 4.2).*

delay, children are short for their chronological age but height is within the normal range for radiologically assessed bone age. Although these children are shorter than their peers in childhood they achieve the normal height predicted by bone age after the pubertal growth spurt.

Those who are growth hormone deficient have an abnormal growth velocity and fall away from the height centiles (**Fig. 4.8b**). They often have central obesity.

Some children are destined to be small. They may have been small at birth for uteroplacental reasons or be part of a normal but short family. They gain height and weight with an appropriate velocity. It is important to gauge the genetic growth potential of a child by plotting the parents' centiles (*see* Fig. 4.9).

Genetic causes for reduced growth are usually apparent by dysmorphic features, such as in achondroplasia. However, short girls with a low growth velocity may have few features to suggest Turner syndrome, and a karyotype (**Fig. 4.11**) should be routinely performed in girls. Similarly, chronic illness associated with growth failure, e.g. renal failure, is usually obvious (**Fig. 4.8c**). However, slowing of growth velocity can be the first indication of hypothyroidism (**Fig. 4.8d**) before other clinical signs develop, and thyroid function tests should be carried out as a routine.

Untreated asthma, like all chronic illness, leads to a reduction in final height. Treatment with corticosteroids can also affect height but produces the pattern of constitutional growth delay with eventual normal height.

UNDERWEIGHT CHILDREN

Failure to gain weight, or failure to thrive, is often the earliest indication of a serious illness; for instance in diabetes mellitus failure to gain weight can precede the usual symptoms of polyuria and polydipsia. However, as with height, there are fluctuations in

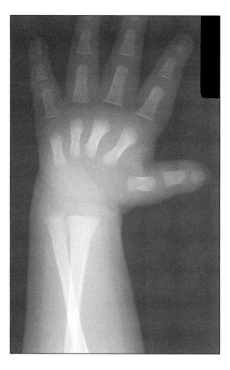

Fig. 4.10 *Severe delay in carpal ossification indicating grossly retarded bone age in a 3-year-old child.*

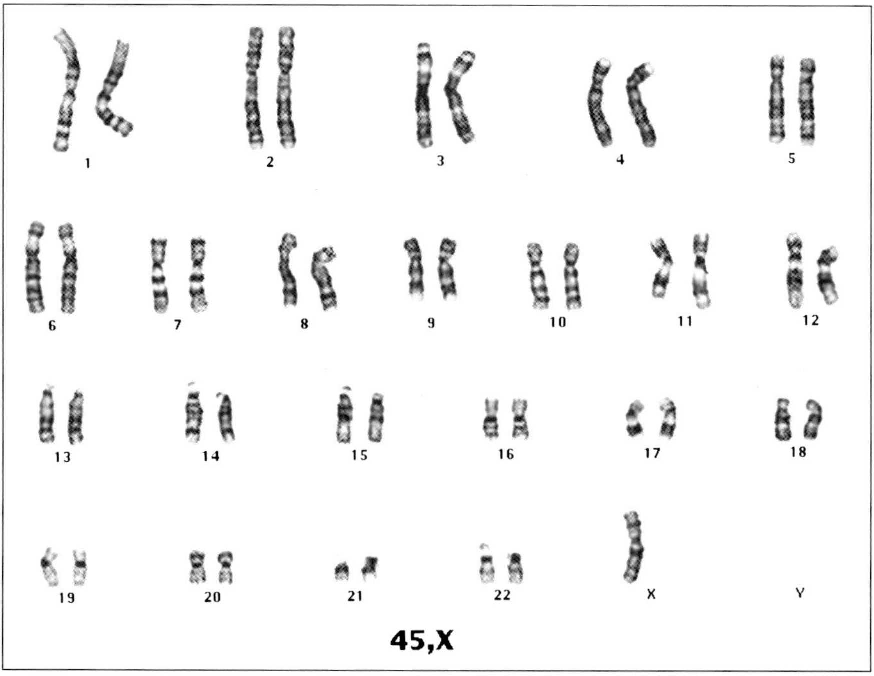

45,X

Fig. 4.11 *Karyotype of Turner syndrome.*

growth rate throughout the year and it is important not to over-interpret short periods of apparent slow growth. Failure to thrive is most commonly a consequence of:

- Poor nutritional intake
- A failure to absorb food (malabsorption)
- Losses from the body, such as protein or glucose leaks from the kidneys
- Excessive metabolic demands, for example heart failure or thyrotoxicosis.

OVERWEIGHT CHILDREN

Obesity is the most common form of malnutrition in developed countries. There is often a family history and the children are excessively tall as well as being heavy. Management of obesity in childhood is extremely difficult as the eating patterns of the whole family need to be changed. Motivation is often lacking until the teenage years and the management is usually to prevent further excessive weight gain while increasing height remodels the child's proportions. Severe calorie restriction during childhood is dangerous as it may interfere with growth.

THE TALL CHILD

A tall child usually comes from a tall family. This is often perceived to be a problem for girls as they may experience difficulty in finding partners. In boys it may be a positive attribute but in the extreme can produce similar social difficulties. It is important to consider hormonal excess, for example precocious puberty or thyrotoxicosis, as although there is increased growth initially, there is final stunting of growth due to premature closure of epiphyseal plates in the long bones. Marfan syndrome is usually clinically obvious: children are very tall with an arm span that is greater than their height, and they have hypermobile joints, a high arched palate, and often subluxation of the lens (**Fig. 4.12**). They are at risk of aortic dissection or mitral valve prolapse.

HEAD SIZE

Head size usually runs in families. A disproportionately small head is, however, usually abnormal and associated with neurodevelopmental problems. A large head in a neurodevelopmentally normal child is usually familial (**Fig. 4.13**).

Abnormalities of head shape are sometimes seen; for example, preterm infants often have longitudinally flattened heads due to the effects of gravity (**Fig. 4.14**). Rarely, premature closure of one or all of the skull sutures (craniosynostosis) may cause a distorted head shape and size (**Fig. 4.15**).

PUBERTY

There is a very wide range of normality with regard to the age of onset of puberty but, once started, it progresses in an ordered fashion. There are standard ratings, described by Tanner, for such obvious signs of puberty as breast development in girls, genital development in boys, and growth of pubic hair in both sexes (**Fig. 4.16**). It is important to realize that girls enter puberty, on average, two years before boys and have the accompanying growth spurt earlier in the process when their breast development begins. Menstruation commences two years after the onset of breast development. The earliest sign of puberty in boys is testicular enlargement, which can be measured with an orchidometer (**Fig. 4.17**). Puberty starts when the testes enlarge to 4 ml, and the growth spurt occurs at the end of puberty when the testicular volume is about 12 ml.

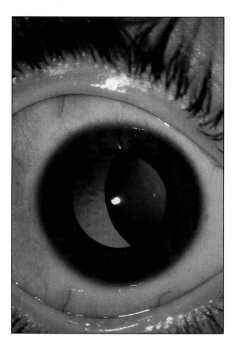

Fig. 4.12 *Dislocated lens in Marfan syndrome. Identification of the cause of tall stature is important as there is a variety of other abnormalities in Marfan syndrome, of which dissecting aortic aneurysm is the most serious.*

Causes of large and small heads

Microcephaly	Macrocephaly
Normal variation (small body and small head) or familial	Normal variation (large body and large head) or familial
Genetic—autosomal recessive microcephaly	Achondroplasia—autosomal dominant
Congenital infection	Expansion of bone, e.g. osteogenesis imperfecta
Perinatal brain injury	
Dysmorphic syndromes	Expansion of marrow, e.g. thalassaemia
Metabolic—infant of mother with uncontrolled phenylketonuria	Hydrocephalus
	Metabolic— mucopolysaccharidosis

Fig. 4.13 *Causes of large and small heads.*

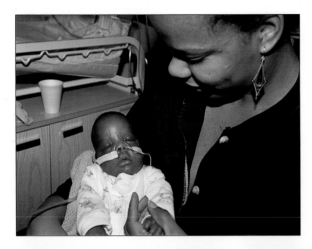

Fig. 4.14 *Scaphocephaly due to prematurity.*

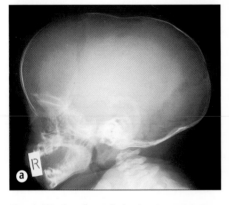

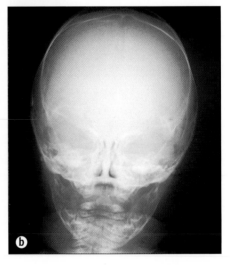

Fig. 4.15 *Scaphocephaly due to premature fusion of the sagittal suture. (a) Lateral skull X-ray; (b) antero-posterior view.*

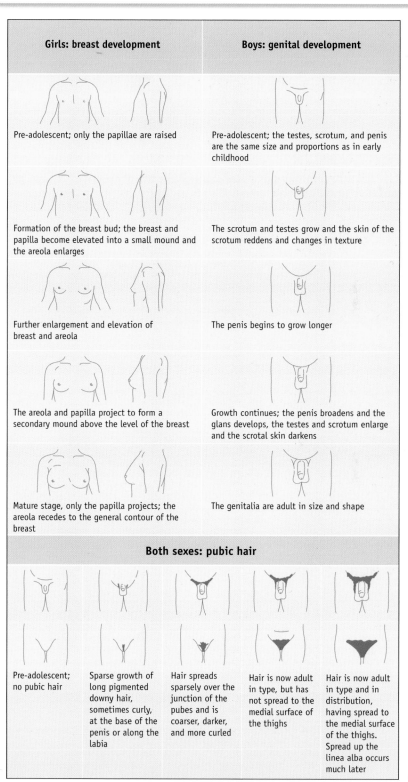

Girls: breast development	Boys: genital development
Pre-adolescent; only the papillae are raised	Pre-adolescent; the testes, scrotum, and penis are the same size and proportions as in early childhood
Formation of the breast bud; the breast and papilla become elevated into a small mound and the areola enlarges	The scrotum and testes grow and the skin of the scrotum reddens and changes in texture
Further enlargement and elevation of breast and areola	The penis begins to grow longer
The areola and papilla project to form a secondary mound above the level of the breast	Growth continues; the penis broadens and the glans develops, the testes and scrotum enlarge and the scrotal skin darkens
Mature stage, only the papilla projects; the areola recedes to the general contour of the breast	The genitalia are adult in size and shape

Both sexes: pubic hair

| Pre-adolescent; no pubic hair | Sparse growth of long pigmented downy hair, sometimes curly, at the base of the penis or along the labia | Hair spreads sparsely over the junction of the pubes and is coarser, darker, and more curled | Hair is now adult in type, but has not spread to the medial surface of the thighs | Hair is now adult in type and in distribution, having spread to the medial surface of the thighs. Spread up the linea alba occurs much later |

Fig. 4.16 *The orderly appearance of secondary sex characteristics.*

35

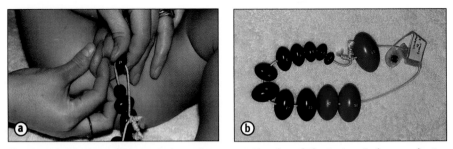

Fig. 4.17 (a,b) *An orchidometer is used to gauge the size of the testes. In boys, puberty has started when the testicular volume is 4 ml.*

chapter 5

Genetics

The instructions to produce an individual are carried as genes (**Fig. 5.1**) on the 23 pairs of chromosomes held within the nucleus. This genotype is expressed and modified by the environment to produce the phenotype—either a structural or a metabolic feature.

Genetic disorders are common in paediatrics.

Many fetuses with chromosomal disorders are lost during the first trimester of pregnancy. Other genetic problems may be manifest at birth, others only later in life, whereas some require an environmental influence or a further genetic mutation before becoming evident. The 2% of children born with a genetic disorder remain known to the health services and have ongoing medical problems.

Genetic disorders are commonly managed by paediatricians but, since each individual disorder is usually quite rare, the skills of a clinical geneticist are essential. As well as making a diagnosis and identifying particular variations of the disorder, further specialized investigations can be performed. Counselling with regard to the risk of recurrence and the possibility of prenatal detection in future pregnancies can be given, as well as information and support.

Genetic definitions	
Genotype	The genetic identity of an individual
Phenotype	The manifestation of the genotype which is often modified by the environment
Gene locus	A position on a chromosome which codes for production of a particular protein, either structural or an enzyme
Alleles	The variants of a particular gene
Homozygous	An individual possessing two identical alleles
Heterozygote	An individual possessing two different alleles
Dominant	An allele that is manifest in the heterozygote
Recessive	An allele that is only manifest in the homozygote state
Mutation	A change in the structure of a gene, often spontaneous and usually deleterious
Syndrome	A recognized pattern of abnormalities that tend to occur together
Sequence	A series of abnormalities that occur as a consequence of an initiating event, e.g. Pierre–Robin sequence

Fig. 5.1 *Some important definitions in genetics.*

Occurrence of genetic disorders

- Half of all spontaneous abortions and 1 in 20 of all stillbirths are due to chromosomal disorders
- One in 40 pregnancies results in a serious congenital abnormality
- 7 per 1000 live births have a chromosomal anomaly
- Two fifths of cases of deafness have a genetic origin
- Half of all cases of blindness have a genetic basis
- Half the cases of mental handicap are due to genetic causes
- Half of all childhood deaths in hospital have a genetic cause
- One third of children admitted to paediatric wards have an inherited disease
- One in three outpatient consultations has a genetic or partially genetic aetiology

THE KARYOTYPE

The 22 pairs of autosomal chromosomes and the single pair of sex chromosomes can be demonstrated by inducing cells (lymphocytes, fibroblasts or fetal cells) to enter mitosis and then arresting cell division in metaphase when the chromosomes condense. A Giemsa stain is used to produce a banding pattern which helps to identify individual chromosomes as well as structural anomalies such as translocations or deletions (**Fig. 5.2**). Very small translocations and duplications can be difficult to identify, even with Giemsa stain. Specific chromosomes can now be identified with fluorescent probes (**Fig. 5.3**).

COMMON CHROMOSOMAL DISORDERS

TRISOMY 21 (DOWN SYNDROME)

Down syndrome is the most common cause of mental retardation. About 94% of trisomy 21 results from non-disjunction of chromosomes during gamete formation (meiosis). Ninety per cent of these cases arise in the ovaries and there is an increasing incidence of non-disjunction with increasing maternal age. Five per cent of cases are due to imbalanced translocations, where a portion of 21 becomes attached to another chromosome and so a gamete can receive the translocated piece of chromosome 21 as well as a normal chromosome 21. A further 1% are due to mosaicism where one cell line in the individual remains normal, while another cell line has an extra chromosome 21. Although the risk of trisomy 21 increases significantly over the maternal age of 35 (**Fig. 5.4**), most babies with Down syndrome are born to younger mothers who produce the majority of births in the population.

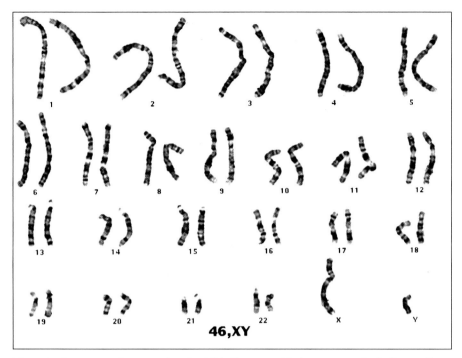

Fig. 5.2 *Karyotype of a normal male child. There are 46 chromosomes including an X and a Y.*

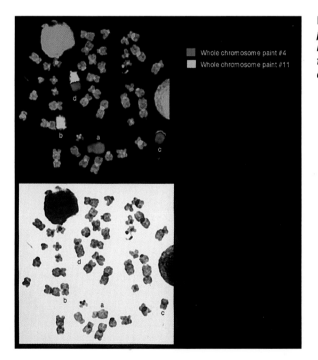

Fig. 5.3 *Chromosome painting. In this case there has been a rearrangement involving chromosomes 11 and 14.*

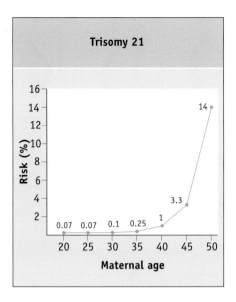

Trisomy 21

Risk (%)

16
14   14
12
10
8
6
4   3.3
2   1
  0.07 0.07 0.1 0.25

20   25   30   35   40   45   50

Maternal age

Fig. 5.4 *Increasing maternal age is the major risk factor for trisomy 21.*

Serum screening is offered to many women and is based on their age and whether there is a decreased serum level of alpha-fetoprotein. This can be refined further if human chorionic gonadotrophin and oestriol levels are also measured. If the estimated risk is felt to be high, amniocentesis and karyotyping can then be performed. Ultrasound provides an alternative to serum testing. Between 9 and 12 weeks'gestation increased thickness of tissue at the back of the fetal neck can suggest chromosomal abnormality. High resolution ultrasound scanning performed at 18 weeks can pick out soft markers such as hypoplasia of the fifth finger or increased sandal gap between the toes, which can also help with antenatal detection.

Clinical features

The facial appearance of trisomy 21 is often noticed by midwives immediately following birth (Fig. 5.5). Not all features of trisomy 21 are present in all individuals.

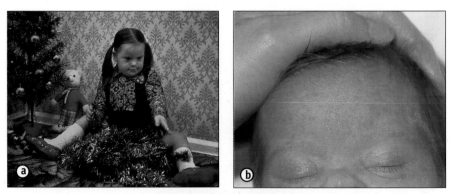

Fig. 5.5 *(a) Appearance of trisomy 21; (b) the eyes in trisomy 21.*

Features of trisomy 21

- Marked hypotonia and often feeding difficulties at birth
- Typical face with central crowding of features, especially when crying
- Palpebral fissures slope upward (outer higher than inner canthus)
- Brushfield's spots (speckling of the iris)
- Brachycephaly (flat back to head), simple ears and short neck
- Small mouth and protruding but normal sized tongue
- Short broad hands with curved little finger (clinodactyly)
- Single palmar creases
- Single flexion crease on little finger and altered dermatoglyphics
- Intellectual impairment, IQ averaging 50
- Congenital heart disease in up to 60% of children
- Duodenal and other intestinal atresias are common
- Increased incidence of leukaemia
- Pre-senile dementia and shortened life expectancy

The hypotonia, feeding problems and facial features are very common, but single palmar creases may be missing in up to 50% of cases (Fig. 5.6). The help of an experienced senior clinician is vital in making the diagnosis. The parents should be counselled before taking blood for karyotyping (Fig. 5.7) and will need careful support over the next few days while they wait for the results. When the diagnosis is confirmed the family need information about the future, an opportunity to ask questions, and time to deal with their emotions. As there is a high risk of serious cardiac malformations it is usual to refer all babies with Down syndrome to a paediatric cardiologist. Long-term support and follow-up is provided by the community paediatricians.

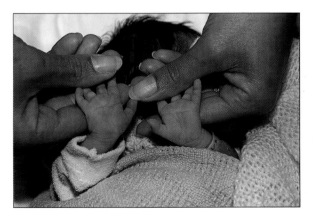

Fig. 5.6 *Single palmar creases are seen in trisomy 21 but are also found unilaterally in 5% and bilaterally in 2% of normal infants.*

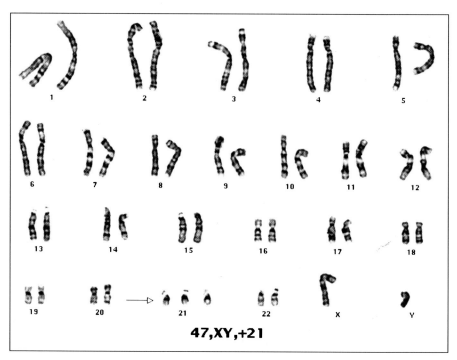

Fig. 5.7 *Karyotype in trisomy 21.*

TURNER SYNDROME (45,XO)

Monosomy X occurs in about 1 in 2500 female live births, but 95% of all XO fetuses abort spontaneously in the first trimester. Non-disjunction at meiosis is the most common cause but translocations of the X chromosome with a loss of material, deletions of the long arm of X, and mosaicism are other causes. At birth, lymphoedema on the dorsum of the feet (**Fig. 5.8**) may be the only sign of Turner syndrome, and the diagnosis is often missed

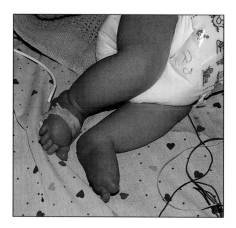

Fig. 5.8 *Lymphoedema on the dorsum of the feet in Turner syndrome.*

until short stature at school age is noted or until a relatively short girl fails to enter puberty. A webbed neck, widely spaced nipples, shield-shaped chest, wide carrying angle and hyper-convex nails are classic but variable dysmorphic features. Coarctation of the aorta is also sometimes seen.

TRISOMY 13 AND 18

Trisomy 18 (Edwards syndrome) and trisomy 13 (Patau syndrome), caused by non-disjunction, occur at a frequency of 1 in 5000–10 000 live births. Infants are growth retarded and have brain, heart and renal abnormalities. The characteristic rocker bottom shaped feet and, in Edwards syndrome, overlapping fingers (**Fig. 5.9**), together with severe dysmorphic features usually allow a clinical diagnosis before karyotypic confirmation. Death usually occurs within the first weeks of life; few children live beyond their first birthday.

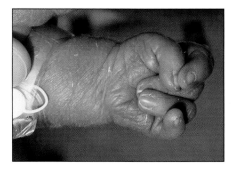

Fig. 5.9 *Overlapping little fingers in Edwards syndrome.*

FRAGILE X SYNDROME

Fragile X syndrome is the second commonest cause of mental retardation and affects 1 in 1000 males. The boys are mentally retarded with macrocephaly and some exhibit autistic features. They have large ears, prominent jaws, long faces and, after puberty, usually have macro-orchidism. Some carrier females have mild retardation. It is possible for a male who is carrying the gene to be unaffected—a so-called 'normal transmitting male'. He will always pass on the abnormal gene to all his daughters who, although unaffected, will be obligate carriers and risk having affected children. Karyotype determination with a folate deficient medium reveals breakages of the X chromosome in 5–25% of metaphase spreads. The molecular defect is due to a highly repeated CGG DNA sequence. Normal individuals have a variable number of these repeats, carriers have more, and affected individuals have an unusually large number of repeats; the number of repeats increases with each generation, particularly during female meiotic division.

DOMINANT INHERITANCE

Dominant disorders are seen when an abnormal allele is expressed in preference to its normal counterpart. Disorders expressing a dominant inheritance tend to affect structural genes, and severe ones are often the result of new mutations (**Fig. 5.10**). An individual with an autosomal dominant disorder has a 50% chance of passing on the abnormal gene to his or her children (**Fig. 5.11**). The spontaneous mutation rate must be considered when counselling parents who have an affected child but are themselves unaffected; in achondroplasia, for example, 80% of cases are due to new mutations.

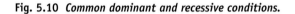

Autosomal dominant and recessive conditions

Dominant	Recessive
Achondroplasia	Cystic fibrosis
Tuberous sclerosis	Spinal muscular atrophy
Neurofibromatosis	Congenital adrenal hyperplasia
Adult type polycystic kidney disease	Phenylketonuria
Bilateral retinoblastoma	Galactosaemia
Accessory digits	
Hereditary spherocytosis	
Myotonic dystrophy	

Fig. 5.10 *Common dominant and recessive conditions.*

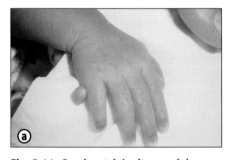

Fig. 5.11 *Dominant inheritance. (a) Accessory digits are commonly seen in paediatric practice and follow a classical autosomal dominant pedigree. If an individual carries the gene for accessory digits an extra digit is always seen; affected individuals have a 1/2 chance of passing the gene on to a child. (b) Mechanism of dominant inheritance.*

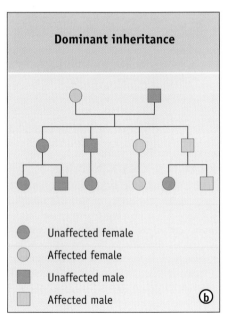

Variable penetrance, that is when some individuals may not exhibit the full phenotype, can also confuse the family pedigree.

RECESSIVE INHERITANCE

In recessive disorders both genes must express the abnormal alleles (**Fig. 5.12**). These diseases are much less common and tend to affect metabolic pathways.

Parents of a child with a recessive disorder each have a copy of the abnormal gene and have a 1 in 4 chance of having another affected child, a 2 in 4 chance of producing a carrier, and a 1 in 4 chance of producing a child without the deleterious gene. A child in

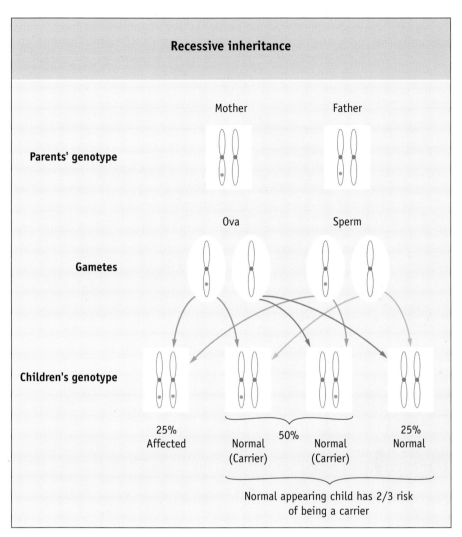

Recessive inheritance

Mother   Father

Parents' genotype

Ova   Sperm

Gametes

Children's genotype

25%
Affected

50%

Normal
(Carrier)

Normal
(Carrier)

25%
Normal

Normal appearing child has 2/3 risk
of being a carrier

Fig. 5.12 *Recessive inheritance.*

such a family who does not suffer from the disease could be entirely normal (1/3 chance) or a be a carrier (2/3 chance).

CONSANGUINITY

If a known carrier (half of whose gametes will be abnormal) wishes to have a child with an unrelated healthy person, the risk depends on the frequency of the abnormal gene within the population. In some communities this may be high, e.g. Tay–Sachs disease in the Ashkenazi Jewish community.

All individuals carry some deleterious alleles that are suppressed by their normal dominant counterparts. If individuals have a common ancestor their children have a higher risk of receiving the same deleterious genes, e.g. first cousins have an eighth of their genes in common and a 3% risk of a child with a recessive disorder. This is an important cause of mortality and morbidity in the western world, but in disadvantaged areas the risk may be relatively small compared to the chances of dying from infectious diseases such as diarrhoea.

SEX LINKAGE

While the Y chromosome determines genetic maleness, the X chromosome carries important genetic information. In the male, a defective gene on the X chromosome must be expressed as there is no alternative. Mary Lyon proposed that, in the female, one of the two X chromosomes, usually the abnormal one, is randomly suppressed; this explains why female carriers of X-linked disorders may occasionally have features of the disorder. However, half of the ova will carry the defective X which will be expressed in a male child or produce a carrier state in a girl (**Fig. 5.13**). For example, Xp21 muscular dystrophy may be manifest in a female carrier by mildly raised creatine phosphokinase levels and large calves but there will be no weakness as half the muscle cells have normal X chromosomes and dystrophin.

MULTIFACTORIAL OR POLYGENIC INHERITANCE

Certain diseases or traits are determined by a collection of genes together with an environmental effect. Some families tend to have more of the genes responsible for a particular trait and so more frequently exhibit the phenotype. Height, congenital heart disease and pyloric stenosis are examples.

DYSMORPHIC SYNDROMES

Many syndromes have a genetic cause (**Fig. 5.14**) and if a cluster of three or more dysmorphic features are found, especially if there is also mental retardation, it is probable that a unifying diagnosis will be found.

Not all individuals with a syndrome will have all the features, and diagnosis can be difficult. Geneticists have therefore produced computer databases and atlases to aid diagnosis. Some conditions do not appear to be genetically determined. For example, the Pierre–Robin sequence (**Fig. 5.15**) is due to hypoplasia of the mandibular area prior to 9 weeks' gestation. This allows the tongue to locate posteriorly and prevents the palatal shelves growing to meet in the midline. After birth, posterior airway obstruction is a problem and is treated by nursing the child prone or with a nasopharyngeal airway. The cleft palate is later closed and the chin eventually catches up in growth.

UNUSUAL CIRCUMSTANCES

GENETIC IMPRINTING
The usual mendelian theory of recessive and dominant alleles holds true for most circumstances. Rarely, the parental source of genetic material is as important as the

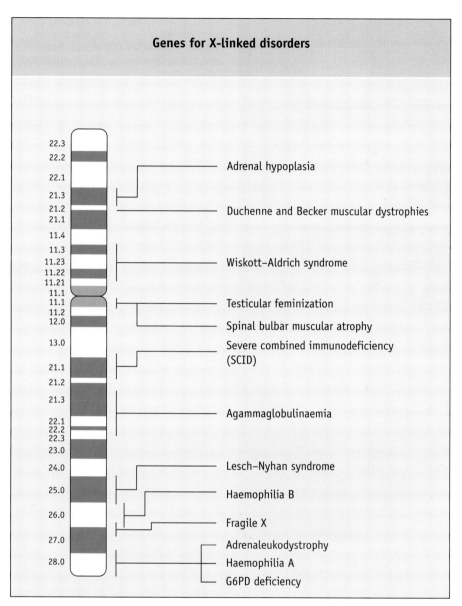

Genes for X-linked disorders

22.3	
22.2	
22.1	Adrenal hypoplasia
21.3	
21.2	Duchenne and Becker muscular dystrophies
21.1	
11.4	
11.3	
11.23	Wiskott–Aldrich syndrome
11.22	
11.21	
11.1	
11.1	Testicular feminization
11.2	
12.0	Spinal bulbar muscular atrophy
13.0	Severe combined immunodeficiency (SCID)
21.1	
21.2	
21.3	
22.1	Agammaglobulinaemia
22.2	
22.3	
23.0	
24.0	Lesch–Nyhan syndrome
25.0	Haemophilia B
26.0	Fragile X
27.0	Adrenaleukodystrophy
28.0	Haemophilia A
	G6PD deficiency

Fig. 5.13 *Diagram of the X chromosome, indicating the position of some of the genes for X-linked disorders.*

presence of the deleterious gene. The best known example is the effect of a deletion on the long arm of chromosome 15. If the deletion is on a chromosome of paternal origin then Prader–Willi syndrome occurs, whereas if it is on the chromosome 15 inherited from the mother, Angelman syndrome (severe mental retardation, absence of speech, and typical gait) results.

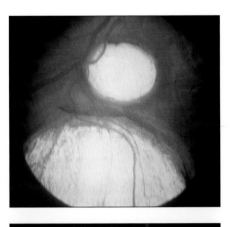

Fig. 5.14 *A coloboma is a defect in the formation of the eye. It is found in the CHARGE association (Coloboma, Heart defect, Atresia choanae, Renal anomalies, Growth, Ears).*

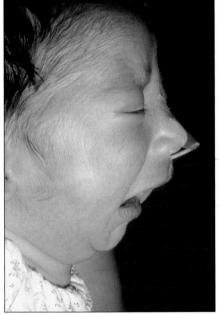

Fig. 5.15 *Mandibular hypoplasia in the Pierre–Robin sequence.*

UNIPARENTAL DISOMY

Uniparental disomy is another rare occurrence where non-disjunction of a parental chromosome occurs during meiosis. The zygote produced initially contains three chromosomes but one of these is rejected. If both chromosomes that originate from one parent remain then uniparental disomy results. This is another mechanism for the Prader–Willi syndrome (**Fig. 5.16**).

GERMLINE MUTATIONS

Germline mutations are new mutations arising during formation of the gametes in the gonads; the somatic cells are unaffected. As some gametes are abnormal there is an increased risk of a genetic disorder in the offspring but this is less than the mendelian risk. For example, a mother who carries the gene for Duchenne muscular dystrophy has a 50%

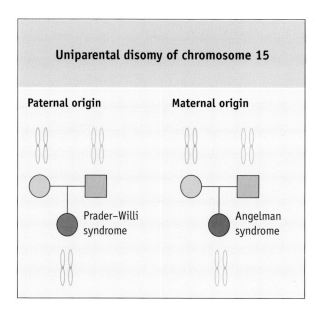

Fig. 5.16 *Mechanism of uniparental disomy. Uniparental disomy results if a child inherits two copies of the same chromosome from one parent, and the corresponding chromosome from the other parent is lost.*

chance of having an affected son. If, however, a mother has a son with Duchenne muscular dystrophy but appears not to be a carrier on DNA analysis, there is still a low risk of recurrence because of possible gonadal mosaicism.

GENETIC COUNSELLING

Genetic disorders are relatively common in medicine but the wide variety means that the individual practitioner can rarely become familiar with them all. The role of the specialist in genetics is to provide a central resource to diagnose genetic disorders and to discuss the condition and its inheritance and therefore risk of recurrence for all members of the affected family. Diagnosis of genetic disorders requires a careful examination of the child and close relatives together with a detailed family history that may encompass three or more generations. Once a diagnosis is made it is possible to determine the future risk of affected children. The options then available to parents can range from carrying on with further pregnancies regardless of risk, in vitro fertilization and embryo diagnosis, antenatal diagnosis and possible termination of affected pregnancy, use of donor sperm or ova, or not to have any more children at all.

ESTIMATING THE RISK FOR FUTURE PREGNANCIES

For healthy parents, the risk of having a child with a genetic abnormality lies in the order of 1 in 50 (2%). If the chances of an affected individual are less than this then the parents are told that they have a low risk. At risks of 1 in 20 (5%) parents are considered at high risk although it must be remembered that the chances of having a normal child are still 95%. For dominant and recessive conditions the risks are higher.

Despite low risk, parents may still wish antenatal diagnosis if possible, as they may not be prepared to accept the low possibility of abnormality.

DIAGNOSIS AND MOLECULAR GENETICS

The progression of a disease gene can be indirectly followed through the members of a family if it lies in close proximity to another recognizable but unique gene combination. Restriction enzymes, which cleave DNA at particular sites, are used to produce fragments, some of which will contain the unique gene sequence. When these fragments are identified, the deleterious gene can also be presumed, with a reasonable degree of accuracy, to be present in the person being tested. Such gene linkage studies are only useful within families known to suffer from an inherited disease and cannot be used for screening in the general population (**Fig. 5.17**). Direct identification of a gene can be performed if an oligonucleotide gene probe is available. Here a short strand of complementary single strand DNA binds specifically to the DNA of the disease gene and is identified on the chromosome by a reporter system, e.g. fluorescence.

The polymerase chain reaction (PCR) is used to make large quantities of DNA from an initial small sample. A series of enzymes activated by cyclical heating and cooling use the initial DNA strand as a template to make millions of identical copies. This allows genetic diagnosis from saliva or a drop of blood—such as that taken and stored after performing the Guthrie test.

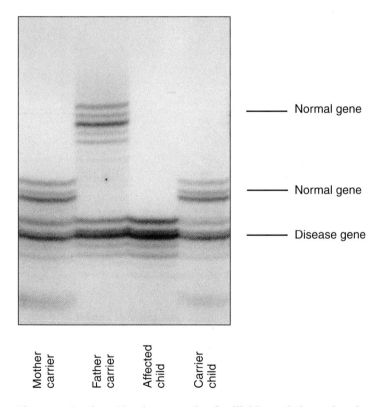

Fig. 5.17 *Southern blot demonstrating familial hypercholesterolaemia.*

chapter 6

Fetal Medicine

The advances in obstetric ultrasound technology and in invasive medical procedures have produced a new specialty concerned with the well-being of the fetus during development.

ULTRASOUND SCANNING AND CONGENITAL ABNORMALITIES

In the United Kingdom, almost every mother will have at least one transabdominal ultrasound scan to confirm pregnancy dates and the number of fetuses.

The expected date of delivery can be predicted using nomograms of crown–rump length (**Fig. 6.1**). Serial measurements of head and abdominal circumference can be obtained during the pregnancy and plotted on nomograms to indicate if fetal growth is progressing well. This is especially important in multiple pregnancy or if the mother has a medical condition such as pre-eclampsia which can lead to fetal growth retardation.

The nuchal fold test is offered at around 12 weeks' gestation. Prominent nuchal tissue at this time is suggestive of chromosomal abnormalities (**Fig. 6.2**). At 18 weeks a scan is done to detect anomalies. Neural tube defects such as spina bifida can be visualized by ultrasound (**Fig. 6.3**). The imaging is sufficiently sensitive and specific for many experts to dispense with maternal serum screening tests.

Genetic abnormalities are often associated with growth failure but other non-specific markers such as nuchal oedema can also alert the examiner. In such cases, and especially if multiple markers are found, it is usual to offer chorionic villus sampling, amniocentesis or fetal blood sampling to obtain a karyotype, although this will not exclude syndromes where chromosomal abnormalities have not yet been identified.

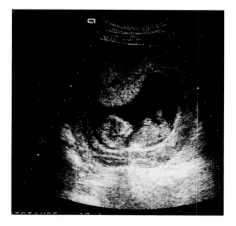

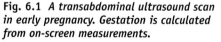

Fig. 6.1 *A transabdominal ultrasound scan in early pregnancy. Gestation is calculated from on-screen measurements.*

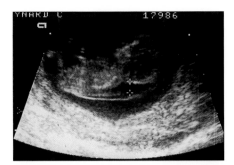

Fig. 6.2 *A prominent nuchal fold at 12–14 weeks' gestation is associated with chromosomal abnormalities in the fetus.*

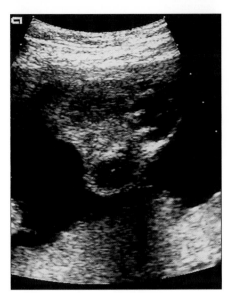

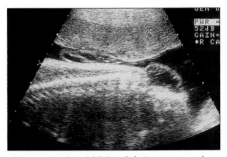

Fig. 6.3 *Spina bifida. (a) Transverse view showing failure of vertebral processes to fuse and exposed spinal cord. (b) Sagittal view showing CSF-filled sac.*

Ultrasound scanning can also detect a variety of disorders requiring surgical intervention in the neonatal period. Duodenal atresia is diagnosed by polyhydramnios and the double bubble sign (gastric and duodenal dilatation) on scanning. Renal anomalies and diaphragmatic hernia are also readily identified. Early diagnosis allows time for discussion and delivery of the mother in a specialized unit with facilities and expertise to stabilize the baby before surgery.

FETAL ECHOCARDIOGRAPHY

The high resolution of ultrasound scanners used in fetal medicine departments allows the routine inspection of the heart and its connections (**Fig. 6.4**). Fetal echocardiography, performed by a paediatric cardiologist, is provided for high risk groups such as those with a family history of congenital heart disease or where a cardiac abnormality is suspected from a previous scan.

Rarely, fetal supraventricular tachycardia produces gross heart failure—hydrops fetalis. This can be detected by ultrasound and the mother can be given drugs, such as digoxin, which will cross the placenta and treat the fetus. Alternatively the fetus can be treated directly.

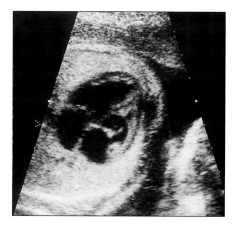

Fig. 6.4 *Fetal echocardiogram showing hypoplastic right heart.*

INVASIVE PROCEDURES

CHORIONIC VILLUS SAMPLING (CVS)

It is possible to biopsy the chorionic villi of the placenta and obtain fetal cells for analysis. Cells can be seen dividing within the specimen and allow a karyotypic result within 24–48 hours. Chorionic villi are a rich source of fetal DNA and therefore many genetic disorders, such as Duchenne muscular dystrophy, thalassaemia and cystic fibrosis, can be diagnosed using molecular techniques. Metabolic biochemical testing can also be directly carried out. If an abnormal result is obtained, termination of pregnancy can be carried out at a much earlier gestation. The risk of fetal loss is 1–2%. This is slightly higher than with amniocentesis, but in experienced hands the increased risk is minimal. CVS is usually performed before 10 weeks when there is no risk of limb reduction defects.

AMNIOCENTESIS

Amniocentesis is the removal of amniotic fluid. This is generally carried out from 15 to 18 weeks' gestation when sufficient liquor volume is present. The ultrasound signals reflect off the amniocentesis needle, showing its position and allowing aspiration of fluid from the amniotic space while avoiding the placenta and fetus (**Fig. 6.5**). Desquamated fibroblasts

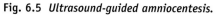

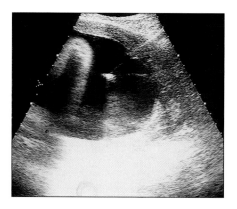

Fig. 6.5 *Ultrasound-guided amniocentesis.*

can be grown for karyotyping and the biochemical composition of the fluid determined. Karyotype and lethicin/sphingomyelin ratio determinations are the main indications for amniocentesis since most genetic disorders can be diagnosed with molecular techniques on chorionic villi. The risk of miscarriage is about 1%.

FETAL BLOOD SAMPLING

Fetal blood sampling can be performed after 18 weeks' gestation and is usually carried out for rapid karyotyping. Blood is obtained at the insertion of the umbilical cord into the placenta, or from the fetal intrahepatic veins. Colour Doppler is used to identify the intrahepatic arteries and a fine needle guided into a vessel (**Fig. 6.6**). Fetal transfusions can also be given in this way. Skin and liver biopsies and aspiration of urine or CSF can also be safely performed by similar techniques.

GENETIC COUNSELLING

Interpretation of ultrasound and other tests usually can only give a probability of normality or abnormality. The need to know if the pregnancy is normal must be balanced against the risks of fetal compromise secondary to an invasive procedure. Invasive procedures should only be undertaken if the information obtained will be relevant to a further intervention. A large part of fetal medicine involves explanations and guidance of parents through such difficult decisions.

MANAGEMENT OF THE HIGH RISK PREGNANCY

During pregnancy, essential hypertension and pre-eclampsia can cause growth retardation or death of the fetus because of impairment of placental function. Regular ultrasonographic assessments of fetal growth and Doppler blood flows give an indication of well-being (**Fig. 6.7**). Normally there is forward umbilical arterial flow throughout the cardiac cycle, both in systole and diastole. Absent end diastolic or reversed diastolic flow is seen in growth retarded fetuses and is a marker for potential compromise. Such infants are also at increased risk of necrotizing enterocolitis. Further redistribution of blood flow is within the fetus may occur to favour the brain over the abdominal organs.

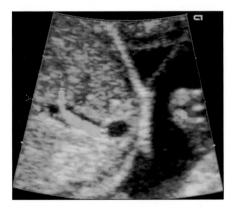

Fig. 6.6 *Fetal blood sampling.*

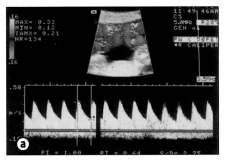

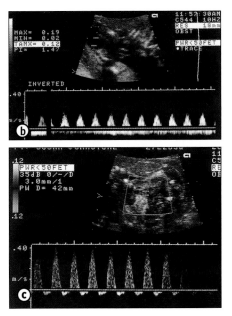

Fig. 6.7 *Doppler wave forms from umbilical arteries showing (a) normal, (b) absent and (c) reversed end diastolic flow.*

DIAGNOSIS AND MONITORING OF MULTIPLE PREGNANCY

Routine ultrasound examination at booking excludes the possibility of undiagnosed multiple birth (**Fig. 6.8**). In particular, high resolution ultrasound is able to distinguish if babies share the same placenta (monochorionicity) and are possibly at risk of feto-fetal transfusion syndrome in which communicating vessels within the placenta and within the two twins allow either a chronic or an acute transfer of blood. The donor becomes anaemic with growth failure while the recipient becomes larger and plethoric. An increased amniotic fluid volume (polyhydramnios) is seen in the recipient and the donor can become 'stuck' to the uterine wall due to oligohydramnios. Reduction of the polyhydramnios by amniocentesis may stabilize the redistribution of blood between the two circulations and delay the onset of premature labour. Following birth the donor is pale and growth retarded and the recipient is plethoric and large (**Fig. 6.9**). It is the recipient who often has most

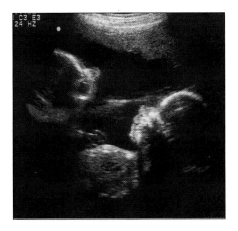

Fig. 6.8 *High resolution ultrasound scanning showing the faces of twin fetuses.*

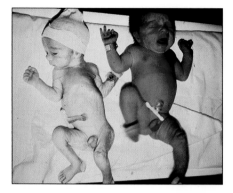

Fig. 6.9 *Feto-fetal transfusion syndrome. The donor is pale and growth retarded but vigorous. His brother is larger and plethoric. (From the Multiple Births Foundation, reproduced with permission.)*

difficulties in the immediate neonatal period with the consequences of polycythaemia (sludging of blood in the microcirculation, hypoglycaemia, and jaundice and often heart failure), while the growth retarded twin is vigorous.

ALLOIMMUNIZATION

Rhesus incompatibility (Rh disease)

Rh disease occurs when a mother with Rh-negative red blood cells generates antibodies against her infant's Rh-positive cells. Severe haemolysis of the baby's cells takes place as the IgG antibodies cross the placenta, causing progressive anaemia as the predominantly extramedullary haemopoietic tissue is unable to produce sufficient red cells. After birth, the continuing haemolysis of cells produces severe jaundice which can cause neurological damage (kernicterus) or death if untreated.

This scenario is now rare as Rh-negative mothers can be given an injection of anti-D to prevent sensitization after miscarriage or childbirth. In fact, the main factor responsible for the reduced incidence of Rh disease was the routine prophylactic administration of anti-D to Rh-negative women after miscarriage or childbirth which began in the late 1960s (Fig. 6.10).

Routine screening for Rh-negative mothers is carried out at booking, and antibody levels are measured in the mother during the pregnancy. If these levels are sufficiently high, serial amniocenteses are carried out to measure the amniotic bilirubin concentration. If these amniotic fluid levels are high, suggesting haemolysis in the fetus, fetal blood sampling can be performed to measure directly the fetal haemoglobin level. Intrauterine transfusions with Rh-negative blood (safe from haemolysis) can then be given to the fetus if there is critical anaemia. Delivery would ideally be planned for around 38 weeks but in some circumstances it can proceed as early as 32 weeks' gestation.

HPA-1 antibodies

Platelets also carry antigens. A minority of mothers have platelets that are HPA-1 negative; if the infant's platelets are HPA-1 positive, antibodies can be generated and cause thrombocytopenia. The first indication of this is often a fatal intracranial haemorrhage. Once the condition has been diagnosed, intrauterine platelet transfusions are required until the baby can be born, usually prematurely.

PLANNING DELIVERY

Decisions in fetal medicine often require a balanced judgement between the hazards of prematurity and neonatal intensive care versus the risks of remaining in a compromised

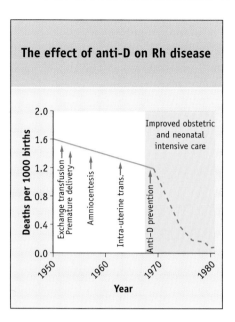

Fig. 6.10 *The effect of anti-D on Rh disease. Although exchange transfusion in the neonatal period was an important milestone in the treatment of Rh disease, the major factor in reducing its incidence was the routine prophylactic administration of anti-D to Rh-negative women after childbirth or miscarriage.*

uterine environment. The pivotal point of the decision will vary with the obstetric and neonatal expertise available at each centre—close liaison is essential. For example, with preterm premature rupture of membranes there is a risk of ascending infection or cord prolapse, but as survival and morbidity of neonatal intensive care fall with each day, it is usually safer for the baby to remain in the uterus until at least 32 weeks.

Tocolysis is the suppression of uterine contractions by drugs such as salbutamol. Delaying an inevitable early delivery is important as corticosteroids, which are given to the mother to enhance surfactant levels in the baby's lungs, take 24–48 hours to be effective.

MULTIFETAL REDUCTION AND SELECTIVE FETOCIDE

As mortality and morbidity increase dramatically in higher order multiple births (four or greater) fetal reduction to two or three embryos may be performed to allow an improved pregnancy outcome.

If there is a major abnormality in one fetus of a multiple pregnancy, parents may decide on selective fetocide in order to protect the lives of the others. The fetal heart of the abnormal twin is injected with potassium chloride under ultrasound control. There is a small risk of inducing labour following the procedure although this is lower the earlier the procedure is performed.

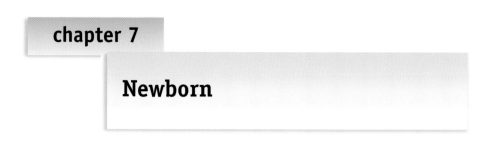

chapter 7

Newborn

Care of the preterm and term infant represents a major part of the general paediatrician's workload. It is important to recognize that the characteristics and diseases of babies are very different to those of children or adults.

RESUSCITATION AT BIRTH

Almost all normal babies adapt to the extrauterine environment without the assistance of midwives and doctors. It is usual for a paediatrician to attend emergency caesarean sections, instrumental deliveries (such as forceps or ventouse), where abnormality is expected, and where there is meconium-stained liquor. Occasionally there will be an urgent call to the delivery room to see an infant that has suffered hypoxic stress or who fails to initiate respiration. Respiratory depression may be due to a drug such as pethidine, which crosses the placenta after about 20 minutes in the mother's circulation. The most important task is to dry the baby well, as heat loss from evaporation can rapidly cause hypothermia and acidosis (Fig. 7.1).

APGAR AND CORD pH

Dr Virginia Apgar, an American anaesthetist, produced a scoring system to aid resuscitation of the newborn. As well as heart rate and respiration, the tone, reflex grimacing and colour were scored to a maximum of 10. The score at 1 minute can be used to assess the need for resuscitation but the heart rate and respiratory effort are the key points (Fig. 7.2). The Apgar score at 5 minutes has been used for prognostic purposes but it is a poor indicator of outcome. The time to first gasp of an apnoeic infant, the pH of the

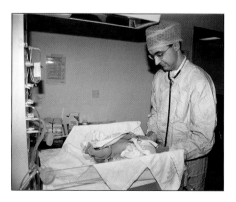

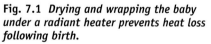

Fig. 7.1 *Drying and wrapping the baby under a radiant heater prevents heat loss following birth.*

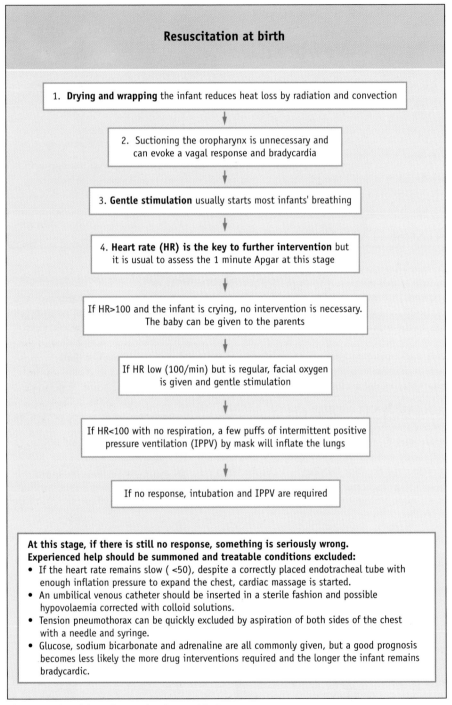

Resuscitation at birth

1. **Drying and wrapping** the infant reduces heat loss by radiation and convection

2. Suctioning the oropharynx is unnecessary and can evoke a vagal response and bradycardia

3. **Gentle stimulation** usually starts most infants' breathing

4. **Heart rate (HR) is the key to further intervention** but it is usual to assess the 1 minute Apgar at this stage

If HR>100 and the infant is crying, no intervention is necessary. The baby can be given to the parents

If HR low (100/min) but is regular, facial oxygen is given and gentle stimulation

If HR<100 with no respiration, a few puffs of intermittent positive pressure ventilation (IPPV) by mask will inflate the lungs

If no response, intubation and IPPV are required

At this stage, if there is still no response, something is seriously wrong.
Experienced help should be summoned and treatable conditions excluded:
- If the heart rate remains slow (<50), despite a correctly placed endotracheal tube with enough inflation pressure to expand the chest, cardiac massage is started.
- An umbilical venous catheter should be inserted in a sterile fashion and possible hypovolaemia corrected with colloid solutions.
- Tension pneumothorax can be quickly excluded by aspiration of both sides of the chest with a needle and syringe.
- Glucose, sodium bicarbonate and adrenaline are all commonly given, but a good prognosis becomes less likely the more drug interventions required and the longer the infant remains bradycardic.

Fig. 7.2 *Algorithm of resuscitation at birth.*

blood leaving the baby in the umbilical arteries and response to resuscitation are better indicators of asphyxia. Bradycardia in a baby is almost always due to hypoxia (**Fig. 7.3**).

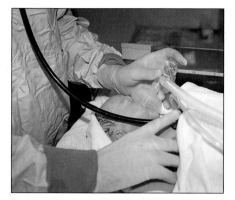

Fig. 7.3 *Bradycardia at birth is due to hypoxia.*

NORMAL EXAMINATION

There are generally three examinations of the newborn infant that take place in hospital.

The first is a brief examination, usually carried out by the midwife, to look for obvious congenital malformations when presenting the baby to the parents following birth.

Over the 24 hours the paediatrician will carry out a full systematic examination of the infant. The baby should be examined in the presence of parents, giving them an opportunity to ask questions. The paediatrician can also enquire about deafness or other conditions that may run in the family. It is prudent to examine the red reflex of the optic fundus when the eyes are open and listen to the heart while the baby is quiet. These are best done before attempting to undress the baby. From then on the examination is usually carried out from the head down, undressing the baby completely. Most obvious abnormalities will have already been spotted by midwives or parents (**Figs 7.4, 7.5** and *see* Chapter 5) but the paediatrician needs to examine for a few specific findings:

- The ocular red reflexes are assessed to ensure that the visual axis is not occluded by cataract or tumour.
- The palate and spine are felt and inspected for defects (**Figs 7.6, 7.7**).
- The hips are examined for instability and the testes and genitalia (**Fig. 7.8**) examined.
- Femoral pulses should be felt to exclude coarctation (*see* Chapter 12), although they often appear normal until closure of the ductus.

Finally, an inspection is made prior to discharge to ensure that no superficial infection, jaundice or feeding problem is present.

INITIATION OF BREAST FEEDING

Breast feeding is the optimal method of infant nutrition (*see* Chapter 10). Breast milk has the correct balance of nutrients, and the fats are easier to absorb than those in formula milks. The potential reduction in the incidence of infections highlights the non-nutritional benefits. It has been suggested that breast feeding reduces the incidence of later eczema.

The earlier and the more frequently the baby is allowed access to the nipple, the more likely breast feeding is to be successful. Suckling triggers the production of prolactin, which

Common minor problems in a neonate

Feature	Significance
Skin lesions	Identification of septic spots is important; haemangiomas and erythema neonatorum are common
Breast enlargement	Due to maternal hormone exposure and can occur in both sexes. Vaginal discharge is also common.
Epstein's pearls	Cysts on palate
Skin tags	Accessory auricles in front of ears can be removed by tying off with cotton
Accessory digits	Inherited in an autosomal dominant fashion and can also be tied off
Sacral dimples	Those over the tip of the coccyx are of no significance. Lumbar pits should be carefully inspected to ensure they are blind ending.
Tongue tie	Almost never interferes with speech
Single palmar creases	Occur unilaterally in 5% and bilaterally in 2% of normal babies. The diagnosis of trisomy 21 is based on a constellation of features.
Two-vessel cord	Is associated with a small increased risk of renal abnormalities

Fig. 7.4 *Common minor problems in a neonate.*

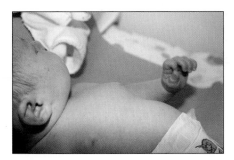

Fig. 7.5 *Neonatal breast enlargement occurs in both sexes due to exposure to maternal hormones before birth.*

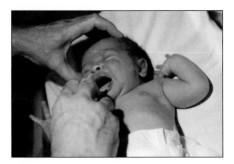

Fig. 7.6 *Inspection of the palate.*

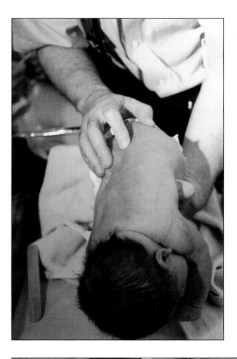

Fig. 7.7 *Inspection and palpation for spina bifida.*

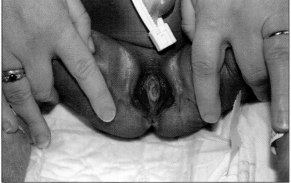

Fig. 7.8 *Vaginal discharge is common in girls, and bleeding may also occur due to withdrawal of maternal oestrogens.*

stimulates milk formation, and oxytocin causes ejection of milk from the breast. There is no correct length of time to allow suckling but babies should be allowed to feed as frequently as they wish. Initially they will take small frequent feeds of colostrum every 1–2 hours, but as milk becomes freely available they will take larger feeds with longer periods in between.

ASPHYXIA–HYPOXIC ISCHAEMIC ENCEPHALOPATHY (HIE)

The fetus copes remarkably well with intermittent hypoxia and variations in placental perfusion. It is only if these factors are present to a severe or prolonged extent that injury develops. Infants born pale and shocked who fail to initiate respiration are said to have 'birth asphyxia' but repeated episodes of asphyxia well before birth may mean that the stresses of birth are poorly tolerated and seen as abnormal fetal behaviour. Rarely, if there is arrest of the fetus in the birth canal or placental abruption, the asphyxia can be directly related to the birth. It is difficult to attribute significance to the cord being around the baby's neck or a knot in the cord as, although noted in asphyxiated infants, these features occur commonly in otherwise healthy babies.

The management of asphyxiated infants is mainly supportive. At birth, normal resuscitative measures are carried out (*see* Fig. 7.2). The baby is transferred to the special care baby unit and stabilized.

- Mechanical ventilation is provided to help control intracranial pressure. Blood gases are checked frequently to keep carbon dioxide levels between 4.0 and 4.5 kPa.
- Myocardial ischaemia is frequently present and may need inotropic support, for example with dopamine.
- Crystalline fluids are restricted in anticipation of the syndrome of inappropriate antidiuretic hormone release (SIADH) or acute renal failure, while the vascular volume is maintained with blood and colloidal solutions as necessary.
- Hypoglycaemia is common and may require the use of strong dextrose solutions to deliver glucose requirements when overall fluid intake is restricted.
- Anaemia, clotting abnormalities and thrombocytopenia may occur and require correction with blood products and parenteral vitamin K.
- Antibiotics are usually given but infection is rarely seen.
- Convulsions are common but are difficult to control with anticonvulsants.
- The progress and degree of organ failure is a guide to overall prognosis. Cranial ultrasound, Doppler measurements of flow in the cerebral arteries, magnetic resonance imaging and spectroscopy (**Fig. 7.9**), and the electroencephalogram (EEG) can also provide prognostic information.

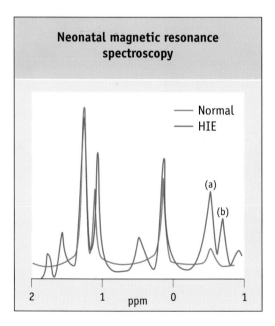

Fig. 7.9 *Magnetic resonance spectroscopy can non-invasively measure the amount of lactate or inorganic phosphate within areas of the brain and indicate increased levels of ischaemic damage. (a) Lactate peak; (b) phosphate peak in HIE.*

BIRTH INJURIES

Birth is a hazardous time, but with modern obstetric practice birth injuries are now uncommon.

NERVE INJURIES

Neck traction during breech extraction or in shoulder dystocia can damage the upper brachial plexus nerve roots, commonly producing an Erb's palsy (**Fig. 7.10**). The hand movements are normal but the arm is held in a 'waiter's tip' position. Spontaneous recovery usually occurs and gentle physiotherapy to avoid contractures can be provided. If recovery does not occur in a few months then surgical exploration is undertaken. Similarly, the facial nerve can be compressed during forceps extraction (**Fig. 7.11**), but this is usually

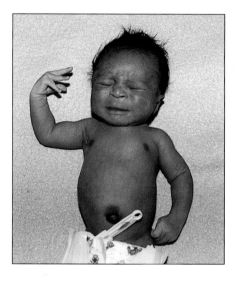

Fig. 7.10 *Left Erb's palsy. The arm is limp, with pronation of the forearm and wrist flexion. The weakness rapidly resolved.*

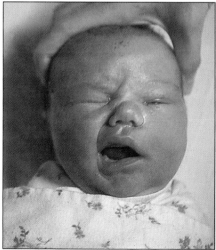

Fig. 7.11 *Facial nerve injury is best seen when the baby is crying.*

65

a temporary phenomenon. Spinal cord bruising or transection is rare but serious. A flaccid paralysis occurs below the area of damage. If the injury occurs above the level of the phrenic nerve roots (C3–5), respiratory failure due to bilateral diaphragmatic and intercostal muscle involvement is seen.

EXTRACRANIAL INJURIES

The presenting part of the scalp can become boggy with a sero-sanguinous fluid due to contact with the cervix; this is termed caput succedaneum (**Fig. 7.12**). A similar oedematous mass on the scalp is produced by the suction cup of a ventouse and is called a chignon. A cephalohaematoma is bleeding under the periosteum of the scalp bones which is limited by the sutures of the skull. In contrast, a subaponeurotic haemorrhage is bleeding into the potential space under the scalp fascia. This is not limited by the sutures and the blood loss can be great enough to produce shock. Any of these bleeds can cause significant jaundice requiring phototherapy but they should never be drained as there is a risk of introducing infection. They all resolve completely with time (**Fig. 7.13**).

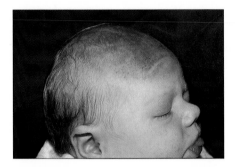

Fig. 7.12 *Caput succedaneum is due to oedema within the presenting part of the scalp and rapidly resolves, often leaving a degree of bruising.*

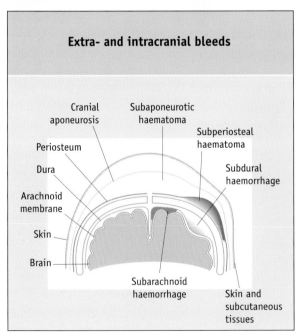

Extra- and intracranial bleeds

Cranial aponeurosis
Subaponeurotic haematoma
Subperiosteal haematoma
Periosteum
Dura
Subdural haemorrhage
Arachnoid membrane
Skin
Brain
Subarachnoid haemorrhage
Skin and subcutaneous tissues

Fig. 7.13 *Diagram of extra- and intracranial bleeds.*

FRACTURES

Fractures can occur during difficult deliveries but are often not noted in the period immediately following birth. A broken clavicle (**Fig. 7.14**) may be noticed only because of an asymmetric Moro reflex or later when a large callus forms over the break. Healing is rapid and complete, although there is often a large amount of callus so that a swelling is palpable at 2 weeks. If fractures of the femur or humerus (**Fig. 7.15**) occur, the limb is splinted against the body for about 10 days.

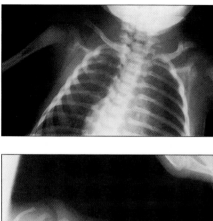

Fig. 7.14 *Fracture of left clavicle.*

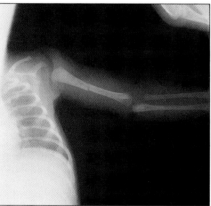

Fig. 7.15 *Fracture of left humerus.*

CONGENITAL INFECTION

Few infections cross the placenta but some, if contracted during the first trimester, may cause abortion or serious defects. Infections acquired later can cause growth retardation, hepato-splenomegaly, thrombocytopenia, a rash, encephalitis and pneumonitis. Infants born with congenital infection often secrete viral particles for long periods and will have IgM antibodies in their blood. Rising antibody titres in the mothers will also confirm a recent infection.

RUBELLA

Infection of the fetus before 22 weeks' gestation incurs a high risk of deafness, and in the first trimester multiple anomalies such as cataracts (**Fig. 7.16**), retinopathy, mental retardation and heart defects are common. Termination of the pregnancy may be considered.

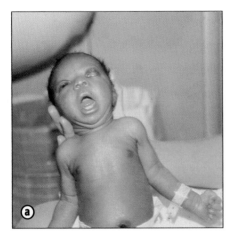

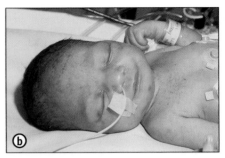

Fig. 7.16 *Congenital rubella infection: (a) congenital cataract; (b) petechial rash.*

Until recently, teenage girls were immunized and pregnant women checked for immunity at the time of booking. All children are now immunized at 15 months and given a preschool booster. This widespread immunization programme aims to raise the level of herd immunity and stop transmission of the infection, particularly to any unprotected women.

CYTOMEGALOVIRUS (CMV)
Up to 5% of pregnant women contract cytomegalovirus; the infection may seem like mild influenza and go unnoticed. The transplacental transmission rate during primary infection is around 50%, but reactivation of previous infection can also affect the fetus. Despite this, 9 out of 10 infants, although infected, will be normal. The remaining 10% may have the general constellation of features associated with intrauterine infection, especially mental retardation and late onset deafness. There is no vaccine.

TOXOPLASMOSIS
Toxoplasmosis gondii, a protozoan parasite of cats (also found in undercooked meat), infects women and crosses the placenta in a similar way to CMV. Although 90% of babies are normal at birth, there is a risk of later chorioretinitis (**Fig. 7.17**) and cerebral effects (**Fig. 7.18**). If a pregnant woman is suspected of contracting toxoplasmosis, spiramycin can

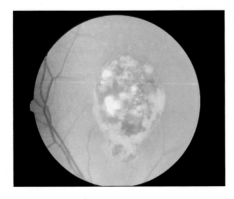

Fig. 7.17 *Congenital toxoplasmosis chorioretinitis.*

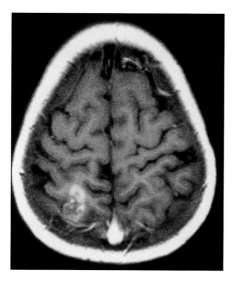

Fig. 7.18 *Cerebral calcification following toxoplasmosis.*

be given to her and then to the baby until 3–6 months of age when the infant can be shown to be free of toxoplasmosis infection by antibody testing.

LISTERIA MONOCYTOGENES

Listeria monocytogenes is a Gram-positive bacterium which is contracted from soft cheeses and undercooked meats. Following a mild flu-like illness, transplacental infection of the fetus can lead to premature labour. There is meconium-stained liquor which, in the absence of a breech presentation, is very unusual in a preterm infant and should be taken as a warning sign. Gentamicin and high dose ampicillin is the treatment of choice. Some babies infected during passage down the birth canal may present some weeks after birth with meningitis.

PARVOVIRUS B19

Parvovirus B19 can produce temporary marrow aplasia in the fetus leading to severe anaemia which may be lethal due to severe heart failure. The appearance of an oedematous baby with pleural effusions and ascites is known as hydrops fetalis.

CHICKENPOX

Herpes varicella zoster can rarely act as a teratogen in early pregnancy. Later acquisition is not a problem provided the infant has had a chance to acquire maternal IgG antibodies. If infection occurs within a few days before or after birth when maternal antibodies are not present, zoster immune globulin and acyclovir can be given to the infant.

HERPES SIMPLEX VIRUS

Genital herpes simplex was regarded as a reason for elective caesarean section to avoid transvaginal infection of the infant. Mothers who have reactivation lesions, either symptomatic or not, should not be deprived of a normal delivery as there is a low risk of infection for the infant; acyclovir can be given if there are any concerns in the first weeks of life.

HEPATITIS B

There is a 90% vertical transmission rate for hepatitis B at any time during pregnancy or thereafter. It is therefore routine to vaccinate all infants born to mothers with hepatitis B at birth and to give further doses throughout the first year. If mother does not carry the anti-Hbe antibody she is regarded as highly infective, and a dose of hepatitis B specific immunoglobulin is also given at birth.

NEONATAL CONJUNCTIVITIS

Sticky eyes are a common problem on postnatal wards (**Fig. 7.19**). Minor discharge with no conjunctival injection suggests a blocked lacrimal duct. There is no need for antibiotics, the eye is kept clean and the child usually grows out of the problem. Passage through the birth canal often results in a minor conjunctivitis. This clears up if the eye is kept clean, but sometimes antibiotic ointment such as 0.5% neomycin is used, after taking swabs. In cases where gonococcal infection is isolated, systemic penicillin should also be given. Conjunctivitis after the first week of life may still be bacterial in origin but chlamydial

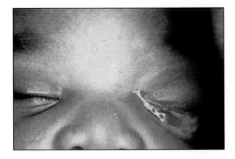

Fig. 7.19 _Neonatal conjunctivitis._

infection becomes much more likely. A special medium is required to culture the organism and, as well as tetracycline eye drops, systemic erythromycin must be given to avoid chlamydial pneumonitis which can follow some months later.

BACTERIAL SEPSIS

Overwhelming infection is often seen in the newborn, particularly in preterm babies. It is important to understand which organisms are likely to be responsible so that antibiotic therapy can be targeted correctly. The baby often presents with general signs of ill health—such as apnoea, increased respiratory rate, vomiting and poor skin perfusion. Blood must be taken for culture and antibiotics should be given intravenously as soon as possible. Intensive care with ventilation and colloid infusions will also be necessary.

In the past, _Staphylococcus aureus_ was a major problem, but in the developing world today Gram-negative organisms such as _E coli_ predominate. However, the commonest organism in meningitis and sepsis in industrialized countries is now the group B streptococcus.

Staphylococcus epidermis was once thought to be non-pathogenic, but is now frequently seen as a systemic infection during neonatal intensive care with invasive procedures such as indwelling venous lines.

Antibiotic therapy with an aminoglycoside or with a cephalosporin, such as cefotaxime, would be appropriate. Ampicillin or amoxycillin should be added to cover the possibility of _Listeria monocytogenes_, which is prevalent on the continent of Europe.

JAUNDICE

More than 50% of all term babies demonstrate jaundice (**Fig. 7.20**). In most babies this is due to a rapid reduction in red cell mass. Bilirubin accumulates as the hepatic enzymes have not matured sufficiently to clear the blood of this pigment. This is physiological jaundice. Bilirubin is normally bound to albumin in the blood. In high concentrations, which are only found during rapid haemolysis, it can cross into the brain and produce brain damage (kernicterus) or deafness. The exact level required to produce damage is not clear but asphyxia, acidosis and prematurity lower the threshold. Generally, serum bilirubin levels are not allowed to exceed 400 µmol/l in term infants without haemolysis and 350 µmol/l in term infants with haemolytic jaundice. Much lower levels are accepted in preterm infants, depending on gestation and other illnesses. Kernicterus is rarely seen since the advent of exchange transfusions and phototherapy. Jaundice in the first 48 hours of life is probably due to rapid haemolysis, for example in rhesus disease or hereditary spherocytosis, and should be carefully investigated (**Fig. 7.21**).

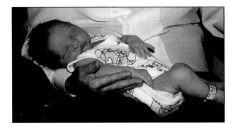

Fig. 7.20 *Jaundice in the newborn may be difficult to detect. It looks like a sun tan.*

Management

Good hydration and an adequate energy intake are important elements in treating jaundice. Phototherapy with light at a wavelength of 450 nm causes a conformational change in the bilirubin molecule which renders the molecule water soluble and allows excretion (**Fig. 7.22**, *see also* **Fig. 7.24**). Babies' eyes are shielded from the light of phototherapy units (**Fig. 7.23**). Overhead radiant light units may cause overheating and a rash in babies. Parents suffer much anxiety over jaundice.

FETAL GROWTH

Growth of the fetus is a good indicator of well-being. Infants that have weights that are disproportionate to their gestational age (if correct) tend to have additional problems:

SMALL FOR GESTATIONAL AGE (SGA) INFANTS

Term infants under 2.5 kg, i.e. the 3rd centile for birth weight, are small for their gestational age and usually have been starved of nutrition in the uterus. There may be apparent sparing of head growth at the expense of the body. As a group, SGA babies are more likely to have asphyxia, require resuscitation, suffer hypoglycaemia and become cold (high surface area and little fat), or have a congenital abnormality or infection.

Hypoxic stress can cause polycythaemia which may require a partial dilutional exchange if the blood is too viscous, and predispose to jaundice (**Fig. 7.24**). Low platelet and white cell counts are also part of this response.

Causes of neonatal jaundice

Non-haemolytic causes

Physiological—slow rate of increase (<40 mmol/l day) peaking during middle of first week of life

Breast-fed babies are more commonly jaundiced than bottle-fed babies

Bruising—cephalohaematoma or intraventricular haemorrhage

Polycythaemia—may be associated with cyanosis, hypoglycaemia or neurological signs from hyperviscosity. If the haematocrit is above 70% a dilutional exchange transfusion is carried out

Delay in passage of meconium—increased entero-hepatic circulation of conjugated bilirubin

Urine infection is often occult

Hypothyroidism—early treatment will prevent cretinism and mental retardation

Galactosaemia. Jaundice in a vomiting, ill baby should suggest this rare condition. Urine contains a reducing substance (Clinitest tablet positive) which is not glucose (glucose test strip negative). A galactose-free diet is required

Haemolytic causes

Hereditary spherocytosis. There is significant jaundice in the first 48 hours of life, family history of the disease (autosomal dominant inheritance), and spherocytes on blood film

Glucose-6-phosphate dehydrogenase deficiency. Should be suspected in non-European male infants (X-linked inheritance)

Haemolytic disease of the newborn. Rh or ABO incompatibility produces spherocytes or haemolytic fragments on the blood film, and the direct Coombs' test is positive

Fig. 7.21 *Causes of neonatal jaundice.*

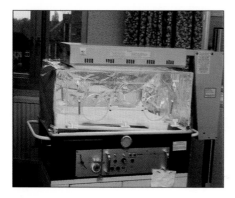

Fig. 7.22 *An incubator is used to control the baby's body temperature when lying fully exposed under a traditional phototherapy unit. Aluminium foil increases the efficiency of the light unit and also shields the room from the bright light.*

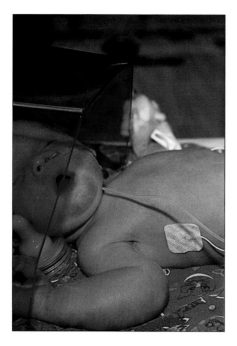

Fig. 7.23 *Plastic shield to avoid dazzling from phototherapy.*

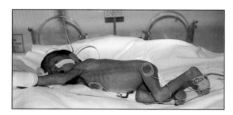

Fig. 7.24 *Small for gestational age baby receiving phototherapy via a fibre-optic phototherapy unit.*

Causes of SGA infants

Maternal
- Poor socio-economic conditions and starvation
- Maternal illness—hypertension
- Smoking, drugs and alcohol abuse

Placental
- Insufficiency
- Multiple pregnancy

Infant
- Congenital infection
- Congenital abnormality

LARGE FOR GESTATIONAL AGE INFANTS

Large for gestational age infants are born to large women or those with diabetes—either known diabetics or those with gestational diabetes. Their large size means that they are at risk of materno-fetal disproportion and birth trauma. Following birth they have a higher incidence of respiratory distress, jaundice and, especially, hypoglycaemia which is a consequence of fetal hyperinsulinism in the face of the maternal hyperglycaemia (**Fig. 7.25**).

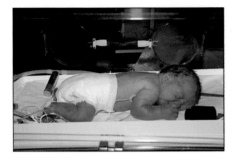

Fig. 7.25 *Large for gestational age infant requiring intravenous dextrose and additional oxygen within an incubator.*

PRETERM INFANTS

Preterm infants (those born before 37 weeks) are not only lacking in size but are developmentally immature and this produces most of the difficulties faced in neonatal intensive care. The main elements in caring for preterm babies are warmth, nutrition and prevention of infection (**Fig. 7.26**).

RESPIRATORY PROBLEMS

Although more common in the preterm infant, respiratory problems occur at all lengths of gestation. In hyaline membrane disease the lungs are of small volume, and on X-ray there

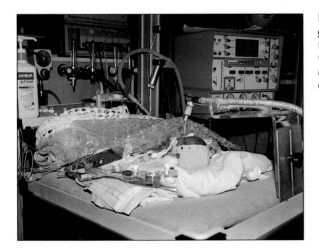

Fig. 7.26 *This 25 week gestation baby is supported with mechanical ventilation. Heat and fluid losses are prevented by covering with bubble-wrap.*

is a ground glass appearance to the lung fields and the presence of air bronchograms (**Fig. 7.27**). Hyaline membrane disease is due to a lack of surfactant which is a protein–lipid mixture that stabilizes the air spaces of the lungs and reduces the work of breathing. Corticosteroids are given to mothers in preterm labour to enhance surfactant production in the fetus prior to delivery, and surfactant can be instilled into the lungs of infants at risk of hyaline membrane disease following birth. Despite these prophylactic measures, babies still require respiratory support which may consist of additional ambient oxygen, nasal continuous positive airways pressure (CPAP) (**Fig. 7.28**) or intubation and ventilatory support (**Fig. 7.26**). A life-threatening complication of ventilatory support is tension pneumothorax (**Fig. 7.29**). The free intrapleural air is removed with a chest drain (**Fig. 7.30**).

Pneumonia with group B streptococcus can also present in this way with a severe illness that can lead to death. It is important to institute early treatment with antibiotics.

APNOEA

The drive to breathe is not firmly established in preterm infants. Pauses in respiration are common and can lead to profound hypoxia. Although it is usually a feature of immaturity, apnoea can also be a symptom of infection, hypoglycaemia or intraventricular

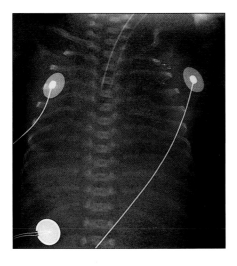

Fig. 7.27 *A typical X-ray of hyaline membrane disease. The lungs are small and there is a ground glass appearance to the lung fields.*

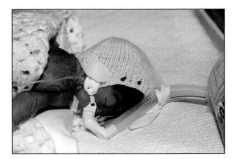

Fig. 7.28 *Nasal CPAP.*

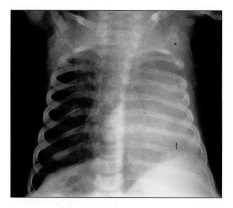

Fig. 7.29 *Tension pneumothorax.*

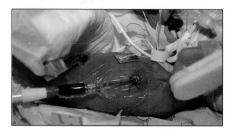

Fig. 7.30 *Chest drain inserted for pneumothorax.*

haemorrhage. Management consists of excluding underlying causes and improving respiratory drive with caffeine or nasal CPAP.

INFECTION

Preterm infants have limited defences against infection. The external barriers of the upper airway and skin are breached by plastic tubes, the skin is thin and fragile, and the immune system is not fully competent. Nosocomial bacteria become pathogens and, as the babies cannot localize infection, septicaemia and collapse quickly occur. The symptoms associated with infection can also be confused with those of other neonatal problems such as a symptomatic arterial duct or apnoea of prematurity. It is therefore usual to take full bacteriological samples (blood cultures, surface swabs, urine, CSF) and start broad spectrum antibiotics before results are available, stopping antibiotics promptly if blood cultures are declared negative at 48 hours. Selection of multiply resistant or unusual pathogens is a problem in intensive care nurseries.

FLUID BALANCE AND NUTRITIONAL DIFFICULTIES

The thin skin and high surface area to volume ratio of preterm infants means that insensible losses can be high and fluid balance is critical. Fluid is initially presented intravenously as dextrose but, as stability allows, total parenteral nutrition can be used. The enteral route is effective in all infants but it must be initially primed with small quantities of milk before its absorptive function and motility are functional. Expressed breast milk, either from the mother or banked, is preferred and can later be supplemented with protein or a specialized preterm formula given to try to achieve rapid growth. Nutritional supplements, especially iron and phosphate, are important as rapid growth will expose any nutritional deficiencies.

NECROTIZING ENTEROCOLITIS

Necrotizing enterocolitis is an inflammatory condition of the bowel heralded by bilious aspirate or abdominal distension. Blood in the stool then follows before the baby collapses as perforation and peritonitis ensue (**Figs 7.31, 7.32**). Treatment is usually with broad spectrum antibiotics and bowel rest for two weeks. If there is evidence of perforation, and the baby is well enough, resections of compromised gut (**Figs 7.33, 7.34**) and/or defunctioning ileostomy can be performed (**Fig. 7.35**). The cause of NEC is not known although a variety of risk factors have been suggested, the major ones being preterm and being fed. Prevention consists of a slow increase in feed volumes and using breast milk which has a protective effect.

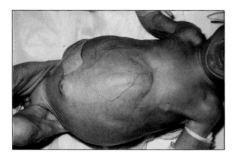

Fig. 7.31 *Discoloured abdomen in perforated necrotizing enterocolitis.*

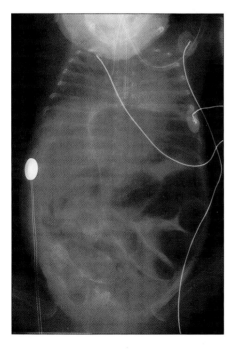

Fig. 7.32 *X-ray showing abdominal free air which outlines the falciform ligament.*

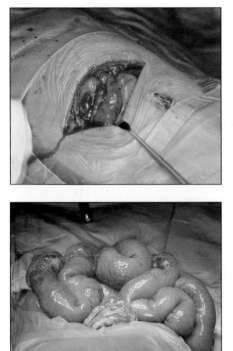

Fig. 7.33 *At operation there is faecal soiling of the peritoneum.*

Fig. 7.34 *Patchy necrosis of the bowel in necrotizing enterocolitis.*

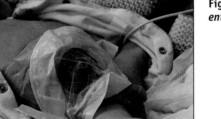

Fig. 7.35 *Ileostomy after necrotizing enterocolitis.*

NEUROLOGICAL PROBLEMS

Intraventricular haemorrhages, due to bleeding from the fragile capillaries on the germinal layer, are common and can lead to parenchymal damage or hydrocephalus.

Periventricular leukomalacia (*see* Chapter 19) is cyst formation within the brain parenchyma following ischaemic lesions caused by episodes of hypotension. Long-term cognitive defects have been noted in survivors of neonatal intensive care.

CARDIOVASCULAR DISORDERS

Initial systemic arterial hypotension is common, especially if maternal hypertension was treated with drugs such as hydralazine or labetalol. Later on, when pulmonary vascular resistance falls and if the ductus arteriosus is still patent, there can be a flow of blood into the lungs producing heart failure. Indomethacin may sometimes act to close a symptomatic patent ductus arteriosus but surgical ligation may be required.

RETINOPATHY OF PREMATURITY

Retinopathy of prematurity describes the formation of abnormal blood vessels in the preterm eye (**Fig. 7.36**). It was prevalent in the 1960s and associated with high oxygen tensions in the blood. Currently, despite careful control of oxygen levels, it still occurs, often in very immature infants, and seems to be associated with the multiple problems of neonatal intensive care. All infants are screened at around 32 weeks' gestation as cryotherapy and laser therapy are effective in controlling the progression of the vascular changes.

JAUNDICE OF PREMATURITY

All preterm infants suffer jaundice which reaches a peak at the end of the first week, in contrast to the third or fourth day in term infants. The management is the same but is often commenced at a lower serum bilirubin level as preterm infants are felt to be more susceptible to kernicterus.

IATROGENIC INJURIES

The provision of neonatal intensive care allows for growth and development but unfortunately the most effective therapies have risks and side-effects; for example, positive pressure ventilation may damage lungs, and extravasation from venous drips and infusions can produce relatively large tissue burns (**Fig. 7.37**).

PARENTS

The stress on parents of having a preterm infant cannot be underestimated. There are deleterious effects on relationships, finances, and other siblings as well as the parent–child relationship. It has been said that sudden infant death syndrome and child abuse are more common in these babies.

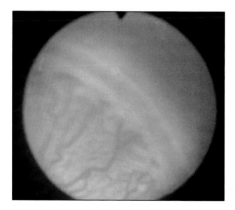

Fig. 7.36 *Retinopathy of prematurity.*

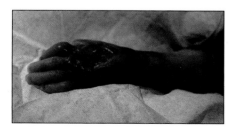

Fig. 7.37 *Soft tissue damage to the hand following an extravasation injury.*

chapter 8

Immunology

The primary organs of the immune system are the thymus, lymph nodes and spleen. The immune system is not confined to a single site within the body but its component cells are distributed throughout all the organs of the body; for example, macrophages are found within the lung and kidney (**Fig. 8.1**) and Kupffer cells in the liver. As well as being able to distinguish between self and foreign material and produce a specific response to remove alien antigens, the immune system retains effective non-specific defence mechanisms.

Defects in any arm of the immune system can produce transient, minor or life-threatening consequences. Deficiencies of the immune system reduce the protection afforded to the body against infections, and dysregulation can produce heightened reactions against the individual's own tissues—hypersensitivity.

MAJOR CELLS OF THE IMMUNE SYSTEM

White blood cells (leukocytes) can be subdivided into different types on the basis of their morphology. The predominant circulating leukocyte is the neutrophil, which is characterized by a multiply lobed nucleus (**Fig. 8.2**). Immature forms, with fewer lobes, are seen in the blood during infection. Approximately 20% of circulating blood cells are lymphocytes, which can be identified by using monoclonal antibodies directed against specific cell surface markers (**Fig. 8.3**). There are smaller numbers of basophils, monocytes and eosinophils.

Many proteins are important in immune responses. These include the components of the complement system and cytokines. These chemical messengers are pivotal in intercellular signalling and mediation of the immune response. Examples are tumour

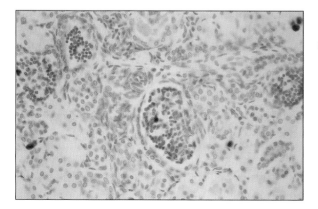

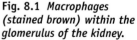

Fig. 8.1 *Macrophages (stained brown) within the glomerulus of the kidney.*

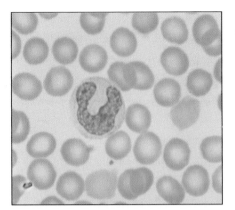

Fig. 8.2 *Mature neutrophil with a multiply lobed nucleus.*

Lymphocytes, their roles and surface markers

Cell	Predominant action	Marker
B cell	Produce antibodies with or without T cell assistance	CD19/20
T cell	Differentiate between self and foreign	CD3
Cytotoxic T cell	Specific direct killing of virally infected and tumour cells	CD8
T helper cell	Involved in regulating cell and antibody mediated immune responses	CD4
Natural killer cell	Direct, non-specific killing of infected cells	CD16/56

Fig. 8.3 *Lymphocyte subtypes.*

necrosis factor (TNF) which can cause tumour lysis and is an important mediator of septic shock, and interleukin 6 (IL6) which is important in the production of acute phase proteins and is also a potent pyrogen.

IMMUNODEFICIENCY

Immune deficiency states are characterized by an increased susceptibility to infection. This may be manifest as frequent infections with common organisms, or infections with organisms that are not usually pathogens for the normal individual. The type of infections and age at presentation are determined by the specific immune defect. Immunodeficiency may be primary (congenital and often genetic) or secondary to drugs and disease states.

NEUTROPHIL DEFECTS

Neutrophils kill organisms by ingestion (phagocytosis) and release of enzymes, oxygen radicals and preformed antimicrobials. Neutrophils are important in fungal and pyogenic bacterial infections such as *Staphylococcus aureus*; dead neutrophils are the main component of pus. The most common cause of neutropenia is chemotherapy for cancers.

Neutrophils, and other blood cell lines, may also be transiently suppressed with viral infections such as parvovirus B19. Primary neutrophil defects are less common. In cyclical neutropenia neutrophil numbers can be documented to fall, accompanied by infections, and then rise over a 3–4 week period. In chronic granulomatous disease (X-linked or autosomal recessive), neutrophil numbers are normal but the cells have a defect in their intracellular 'killing machinery' and although they are able to ingest micro-organisms they are unable to generate a respiratory burst to kill them. In the nitroblue tetrazolium (NBT) reduction test normal neutrophils take up and reduce NBT to form a brown/black deposit, while in chronic granulomatous disease the neutrophils are unable to do this (**Fig. 8.4**).

In the very rare leukocyte adhesion deficiency, neutrophil numbers and intracellular killing mechanisms are normal but the cells are unable to migrate through tissues to the site of infections. These children often present with delayed separation of the umbilical cord and recurrent and very persistent skin infections at sites of minor trauma; pus fails to form at these sites (**Fig. 8.5**).

COMPLEMENT DEFECTS

Activation of the complement cascade causes cell lysis, enhances phagocytosis and improves the efficiency of antibody killing. Defects are rare and produce a variety of clinical pictures:

- An SLE-like disease process with deficiencies of C2, C4 and C1q.
- Increased susceptibility to meningococcal infection with deficiencies of complement components C5–8.
- Hereditary angio-oedema due to C1 esterase inhibitor deficiency. C1 esterase inhibitor is vital in control of the complement cascade. Its deficiency results in an overactive complement system with recurrent angioneurotic oedema. Tracheal obstruction, oedema of the gut mucosa causing abdominal pain and diarrhoea, or areas of circumscribed skin swelling can occur. This absence of erythema and local itching distinguishes it from urticaria. It is inherited in an autosomal dominant manner.

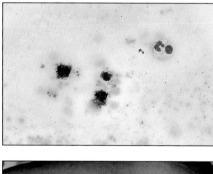

Fig. 8.4 *Neutrophils that are able to generate a respiratory burst can reduce NBT to form a blue-black deposit. The neutrophil on the right is unable to do this.*

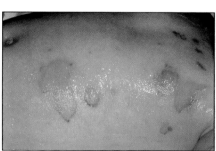

Fig. 8.5 *In leukocyte adhesion deficiency pus fails to form at sites of injury and persistent infection develops.*

HUMORAL IMMUNODEFICIENCY

Several classes of antibody are produced by B cells ($IgG_{1,2,3,4}$, IgA, IgM and IgE).

IgG is passively and actively transported across the placenta to the fetus from the 14th week of gestation, although the majority of the transfer occurs in the third trimester. IgG subclasses 1 and 3 are the first groups of antibody to be produced after birth and reach 50% of the adult values by 6 months of age. Similarly, the fetal production of IgA and IgM is low and increases during the first 18 months of life (**Fig. 8.6**).

Specific defects of a particular antibody class, or a generalized quantitative or qualitative defect of antibody production can occur.

Transient hypogammaglobulinaemia of infancy

Maternal immunoglobulin levels gradually fall after birth, leaving a window from around 3–6 months of age when the infant's immunoglobulin levels are relatively low. Delay in the maturation of immunoglobulin production can occur, allowing frequent minor infections. In particular, production of IgG subclasses 2 and 4 does not mature until after the age of 2, leaving infants vulnerable to infection with organisms with polysaccharide capsules (Hib, pneumococcus, meningococcus).

IgA deficiency

IgA deficiency is found in 1/600 adult blood donors, and most of these people are healthy. The frequency in children is not known. It rarely causes problems unless there is an additional defect in IgG synthesis, usually of IgG subclasses 2 and 4. This produces recurrent ENT and lower respiratory tract infections.

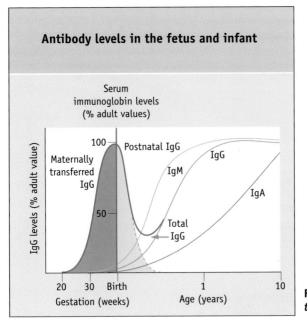

Fig. 8.6 *Antibody levels in the fetus and infant.*

Bruton's disease

X-linked agammaglobulinaemia is the most severe form of humoral immunodeficiency. These boys have no circulating B cells or immunoglobulin because of a failure of B cell development in the bone marrow; they present after maternal immunoglobulin levels have declined. They suffer lower respiratory tract infections and, if untreated, run the risk of developing bronchiectasis.

CELL MEDIATED IMMUNODEFICIENCY

T cells are formed from stem cells in the bone marrow and fetal liver and migrate to and mature in the thymus (**Fig. 8.7**). As part of their normal killing mechanisms, T cells recognize 'self' and will destroy foreign cells or 'self' cells that are displaying foreign antigens.

In cell mediated immunodeficiency there is a defect in T cell numbers or function and, because of the interactions between T and B cells, this always results in a degree of humoral immunodeficiency. Defects in T cell number or function predispose to atypical infections such as *Pneumocystis carinii* pneumonia, tuberculosis, cryptococcal, candidal, and disseminated viral infection (CMV).

Transfusional graft versus host disease

Red cell and platelet transfusions may contain small numbers of active lymphocytes. If the recipient has defective T cell function these cells will not be destroyed by the recipient's T cells. The donor cells instead will recognize the recipient cells as foreign and start to attack them (**Fig. 8.8**). This is usually fatal. Children suspected of having cell-mediated immunodeficiency should receive irradiated blood products as this will kill any lymphocytes.

Di George syndrome

Cell-mediated immunodeficiency is seen in Di George syndrome, which is due to abnormal development of the 3rd and 4th pharyngeal pouches in embryonic life. The thymus is

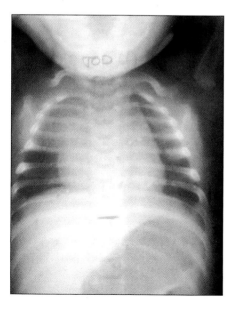

Fig. 8.7 *The thymus gland on neonatal chest X-ray appears as a 'wedge' or 'sail sign'.*

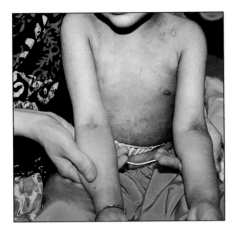

Fig. 8.8 *Graft versus host disease after bone marrow transplantation.*

absent, leading to T cell deficiency and the possibility of graft versus host disease from transfusions. Parathyroid hypoplasia presents as hypocalcaemia; coarctation of the aorta and left ventricular outflow obstruction are common serious cardiac malformations; dysmorphic features (low set ears, hypomandibular and midline facial abnormalities) are also seen. A deletion has been found on the long arm of chromosome 22. Variants of Di George syndrome are now being recognized; patients may present with an immunodeficiency or abnormal facies alone. In recognition of this, the phrase 'Catch 22' is used to describe these clinical syndromes (**Fig. 8.9**).

Chronic mucocutaneous candidiasis

Candidiasis is very common when babies are in nappies (**Fig. 8.10**). However, chronic mucocutaneous candidiasis is due to a specific T cell deficiency. This persistent monilial infection of the skin and nails is often associated with autoimmune hypoparathyroidism and Addison's disease (**Fig. 8.11**).

COMBINED IMMUNODEFICIENCY

Some children have defects in both cell mediated and humoral immunity. At the extreme end of the spectrum are children with severe combined immunodeficiency (SCID). These

Catch 22	
C	Cardiac defects
A	Abnormal facies
T	Thymic hypoplasia
C	Cleft palate
H	Hypocalcaemia
22	22q 11.2 deletion

Fig. 8.9 *Minor variants of Di George syndrome are now being recognized; patients may present with an immunodeficiency or abnormal facies alone. This has been termed 'Catch 22'.*

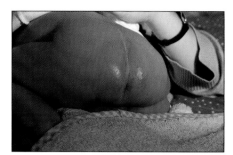

Fig. 8.10 *Normal napkin rash.*

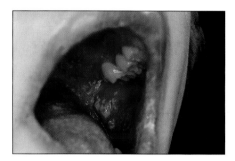

Fig. 8.11 *Oral candidiasis after the neonatal period is suggestive of cell mediated immunodeficiency.*

children lack any humoral or cell mediated immunity. In some variants, lymphocyte numbers are very low (autosomal recessive SCID), whilst in other variants lymphocyte numbers are normal (e.g. X-linked SCID with no T cells but B cells present). These children present early in life, commonly with an atypical infection such as *Pneumocystis carinii* pneumonia, a persistent viral infection such as rotavirus or RSV bronchiolitis, or a disseminated viral infection such as CMV. Unless there is good supportive treatment and bone marrow transplantation, SCID is fatal in early life.

Wiskott–Aldrich syndrome

Wiskott–Aldrich syndrome is an X-linked condition which classically comprises the triad of thrombocytopenia with small platelets, eczema (**Fig. 8.12**) and a progressive humoral and cell mediated immunodeficiency. These children also have an increased susceptibility to lymphomas.

MANAGEMENT OF IMMUNODEFICIENCY

Early diagnosis of immunodeficiency reduces morbidity and mortality. Initial screening tests are simple and universally available, for example T cell counts (**Fig. 8.13**). Functional studies are only performed in specialist centres.

- Live vaccines, e.g. BCG, should not be given to children with cell mediated immunodeficiency as they may cause disseminated disease in this situation. Children with humoral immunodeficiency respond poorly to vaccination, and vaccination responses should be checked 4 weeks after immunization.
- Infections should be treated early with antibiotics.
- Prophylactic antibiotics are often used in children with minor immunodeficiencies, such as a subclass defect, if there is significant morbidity interfering with school. Those with cell mediated immunodeficiency require *Pneumocystis carinii* prophylaxis. Co-trimoxazole is usually given to children.

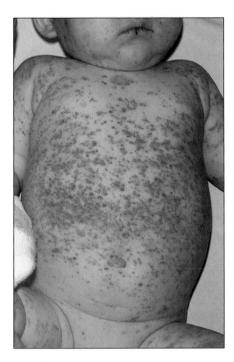

Fig. 8.12 *The rash in Wiskott–Aldrich syndrome is a combination of petechiae and eczema.*

- If there is a significant antibody defect, immunoglobulin replacement therapy can be given; however, it is costly, an intravenous therapy and carries risks of viral infection.
- Bone marrow transplantation is performed in SCID and other serious defects.
- Genetic counselling should be provided as many immunodeficiencies are inherited, often with asymptomatic carriers, and prenatal diagnosis and carrier screening are available for an increasing number of conditions.

HUMAN IMMUNODEFICIENCY VIRUS (HIV)

In HIV infection, lymphocyte numbers decline secondary to viral infection of lymphocytes. This causes a decline in overall lymphocyte numbers with a reversal of the CD4/CD8 ratio. It is increasingly being recognized that there are many differences between the manifestations of disease in the paediatric and adult populations.

The majority of children acquire the infection from their mother in the perinatal period. Others are infected by blood products, e.g. haemophiliacs treated with unscreened factor VIII. Large European studies and data from the USA estimate vertical transmission rates (infected mothers delivering infected children) to be 15%. Higher rates have been reported in the African subcontinent; although some of this is due to reporting bias, higher rates of venereal disease in this population may also contribute.

The mechanism of perinatal infection is not known, and the safest way to deliver an infected mother in the western world is still not clear. The risks of HIV transmission in breast milk must be balanced against the benefits of maternal milk. In particular, in the developing world, the risk to an infant of acquiring a fatal diarrhoeal illness or malnutrition because of bottle feeding may be more than the risk of transmission of HIV.

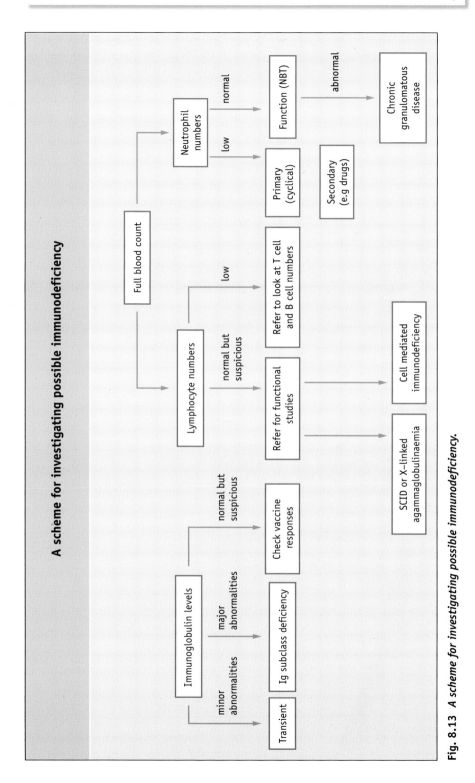

Fig. 8.13 *A scheme for investigating possible immunodeficiency.*

Presentation

Most HIV-infected children present at around 8 months of age, with only 25% presenting after the age of 2 years. Although the commonest presentation is a child born to an HIV mother, a wide spectrum of symptoms can occur which differ from the adult illness.

Diagnosis

Most HIV tests are based on detection of antibody. However, maternal antibody may persist in the infant until 18 months of age, so that antibody testing can not be used in infancy. A variety of alternative techniques are used, including the detection of HIV-specific antigen (p24) and sensitive viral detection techniques using the polymerase chain reaction (PCR). Until a number of negative tests have been obtained and there is clearly no infection, the infant of an HIV-positive mother should be treated as HIV positive and prophylaxis against PCP offered.

Management

As with any immunocompromised child, management is largely symptomatic for specific infections. There are, however, a few specific areas of management:

- A full programme of immunization is advocated except that a killed polio vaccine is used. Pneumococcal vaccine is also given.
- On a worldwide basis, immunization against tuberculosis is still advocated as the risk of dying from TB is greater in the short term than from HIV; in areas of low TB prevalence it is not justified.
- Prophylaxis with co-trimoxazole; Pneumocystis infection, although it occurs at all ages, is particularly dangerous in infants.

Symptoms of HIV infection in children

- Non-specific ill health with hepatosplenomegaly, diarrhoea and failure to thrive
- Lymphoid interstitial pneumonitis—a chronic and progressive infiltration of lymphocytes into the lung
- Progressive neurological disease with developmental regression (**Fig. 8.14**)
- *Pneumocystis carinii* pneumonia (PCP)—a pneumonitis unresponsive to normal antibiotic therapy
- Secondary infectious diseases such as two or more severe bacterial infections within a year, recurrent oral candidiasis, recurrent herpes zoster and simplex dermatitis
- Other illness possibly due to HIV, e.g. hepatitis, cardiac, renal, haematological and skin diseases
- Kaposi's sarcoma is very rare in children

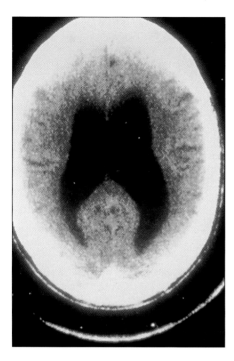

Fig. 8.14 *HIV encephalopathy.*

- Normal childhood infections, e.g. chickenpox, can be life threatening; it is a good idea to avoid infectious contacts and provide specific immunoglobulin if possible.
- Anti-retroviral treatments, such as AZT, may be given.
- Nutritional support.
- Social support for the family, bearing in mind that the parents also are usually infected.

HYPERSENSITIVITY AND ALLERGY

Hypersensitivity is an inappropriately exaggerated immune response, such that the immune process, rather than protecting, damages the body. Allergy is used interchangeably with hypersensitivity and emphasizes the recurrent nature of hypersensitivity.

Gell and Coombs classified the reactions into four types but they usually occur in combination.

TYPE I (IMMEDIATE) HYPERSENSITIVITY

Asthma, hay fever and potentially life-threatening allergies to foodstuffs are caused by immediate hypersensitivity reactions (**Fig. 8.15**). The rapid reaction is due to the activation and degranulation of mast cells. These cells bind IgE on their surfaces which, when linked by antigen, causes release of inflammatory mediators. A delayed component (type IV hypersensitivity) commonly occurs some hours later due to prostaglandin release as part of the inflammatory cascade.

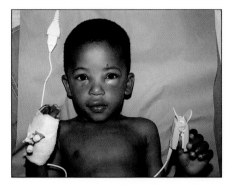

Fig. 8.15 *This boy is allergic to nuts; contact with the oral mucosa has triggered a severe local response with erythema and swelling.*

TYPE II (ANTIBODY MEDIATED) HYPERSENSITIVITY

Antibodies directed to cell surfaces and membranes activate complement and cause lysis. The commonest examples are those of red blood cells: haemolytic disease of the newborn due to Rh or ABO incompatibility is caused by transplacental passage of IgG antibodies that bind to red cells and activate haemolysis by complement (*see* Chapters 7 and 22).

TYPE III (IMMUNE COMPLEX) HYPERSENSITIVITY

Soluble antigen in combination with antibody can form large complexes that circulate in the blood. These complexes are usually mopped up by red cells and removed in the liver but, if there are large quantities, they tend to deposit at sites of filtration or turbulence, e.g. the kidney. Platelet and neutrophil activation can then lead to local endothelial injury. Immune complexes are seen in autoimmune disease or infections where there are large amounts of antigen available.

TYPE IV (DELAYED) HYPERSENSITIVITY

The basis of the type IV hypersensitivity reaction is the response of sensitized CD4+ T helper cells to an antigen, producing a delayed clinical effect 12–24 hours after exposure. The T helper cells release cytokines that attract macrophages, and granuloma formation occurs when the macrophages are unable to engulf and eliminate the antigen. Nickel is a common cause of contact dermatitis (**Fig. 8.16**).

ATOPY

An atopic individual has a tendency to allergy and suffers from asthma, hay fever, eczema or urticaria. There are no really useful tests for allergy but a history of symptoms on

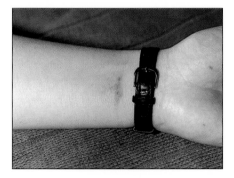

Fig. 8.16 *The patch of eczema on this girl's wrist is caused by nickel from the watch-strap buckle.*

exposure and a reproducible response to the allergen are the key to diagnosis. Unfortunately, delayed onset of symptoms means that the linkage of a precipitant to symptoms can sometimes be difficult. A high level of IgE is usually found in the blood.

Asthma and allergy

Asthma is reversible airways obstruction due to hyper-reactivity of the airways (*see* Chapter 13). The main stimulants are physical conditions (cold, damp or dry air) and viral infections. Allergens such as the faeces of the house dust mite and animal danders can cause immediate symptoms but also a generalized increase in the reactivity of the airways. This often becomes obvious with improvement in symptoms during family holidays and worsening on return home. Not all children have allergies to animals and an objective trial separation should be undertaken before disposing of family pets. Reduction in house dust mite levels is very difficult to achieve. It involves regular damp dusting and vacuuming of bedroom carpets. It is sensible to keep fluffy toys to a minimum in the bedroom and to use a plastic mattress cover.

Hay fever

Seasonal allergic rhinitis is caused by exposure to pollens of grass, flowers and trees. It occurs in the early summer months, often in older children. The recurrent symptoms of sneezing, rhinitis, palatal itching and conjunctivitis (**Fig. 8.17**) when the pollen count is high allow diagnosis without any further investigations. Rarely, a perennial postnasal drip can cause coughing and be mistaken for asthma. Allergic rhinitis is also commonly due to animal danders (**Fig. 8.18**).

The management of hay fever depends on the severity of symptoms. The rapid response to antihistamines such as chlorpheniramine confirms the clinical impression, and if symptoms are mild these agents can be taken as required. More marked symptoms often require regular therapy during the hay fever season. Rhinitis is often not completely

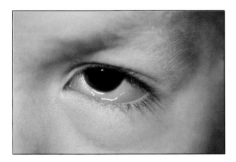

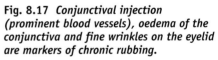

Fig. 8.17 *Conjunctival injection (prominent blood vessels), oedema of the conjunctiva and fine wrinkles on the eyelid are markers of chronic rubbing.*

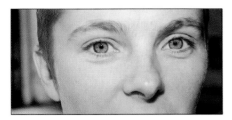

Fig. 8.18 *Repeated rubbing of the itchy nose due to allergic rhinitis has produced a horizontal crease on the nose.*

controlled with antihistamines and a prophylactic topical steroid spray provides good symptomatic relief. Prophylactic sodium cromoglycate eye drops are useful for conjunctivitis but difficult for younger children. A depot steroid injection can be given to provide guaranteed relief for important examinations but this should not be necessary with topical therapy and non-sedating antihistamines.

Allergies and eczema

A particular cause of childhood eczema is dairy product allergy. The onset of eczema on weaning from breast milk onto solids and cow's milk is suggestive, but any child with severe skin problems may respond to a properly organized trial of dietary exclusion. This should be done for a specific time period under a dietitian's supervision as it is easy to allow hidden milk products into the diet or produce a nutritionally inadequate diet.

Cow's milk antigens are also excreted in breast milk and it has been suggested that dietary exclusion of dairy products for a breast feeding mother may help her infant's eczema. It has also been suggested that atopic disease can be prevented by breast feeding and delayed introduction of solids. This remains difficult to prove.

Urticaria

Atopic individuals often suffer weals and erythema caused by a variety of triggers. A hot bath, an allergen or a viral infection may produce a reaction although often no cause can be found (**Fig. 8.19**). Dermatographism is common in urticaria (**Fig. 8.20**). Antihistamines are used for symptomatic relief, and the sufferer usually learns to avoid precipitants.

ANAPHYLAXIS

The term anaphylaxis is reserved for a severe life-threatening allergic reaction. Symptoms start minutes after exposure to the allergen with faintness, fear, itching and feeling unwell. This progresses to circulatory collapse and obstruction to the airway due to oedema. Treatment consists of:

- Adrenaline—given subcutaneously, intramuscularly or intravenously.
- Oxygen is provided, but early intubation or even tracheotomy may be necessary if the airway is compromised.

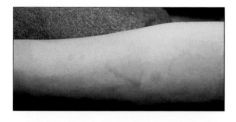

Fig. 8.19 Urticarial rash.

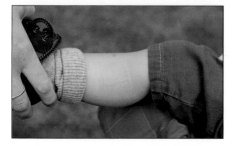

Fig. 8.20 Dermatographism.

- Hypotension is treated with fluids.
- Corticosteroids and antihistamines are given to prevent secondary relapse after the adrenaline has begun to wear off.
- As well as avoiding precipitants, sufferers should wear a medical information bracelet and carry an adrenaline self injector device.

PROVOCATIVE TESTING IN THE DIAGNOSIS OF ALLERGY

The main diagnostic tool is a history of recurrent symptoms with exposure to the allergen. Skin prick testing can be used to confirm hypersensitivity but is not entirely sensitive or specific. Measurement of total IgE or radioallergosorbent (RAST) tests in blood produce similar information but they are expensive and can produce more false positive and negative results than prick testing.

It can be dangerous to test for food allergies because of the risk of systemic anaphylactic reactions. In general, a dilute solution of the food is placed on the skin and then on the lips before being ingested. Progressively stronger concentrations are then used (**Fig. 8.21**). When performing such tests resuscitative measures including hydrocortisone, antihistamines, adrenaline and equipment for intubation must be available.

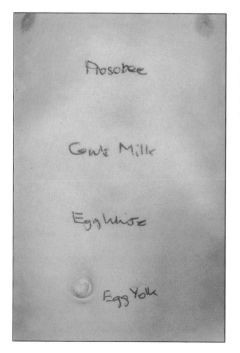

Fig. 8.21 *Food allergen testing. A drop of allergen is placed on the skin and the skin is pricked. Any weal is measured 15 minutes later. A negative control—the dilutant of the test mix—is used to exclude dermatographism, which is wealing due to physical stimulus. Histamine is used as a positive control.*

chapter 9

Infection

Infection occurs when the balance between the host and a potential pathogen is lost. The integrity of the skin, cilia in the respiratory tract, and acid in the stomach are physical barriers to infection. If these are breached, the immune system then fights the infection. Macrophages non-specifically remove foreign material and the T cells and antibodies produced by B cells specifically identify and destroy foreign antigens.

COMMON AND IMPORTANT CHILDHOOD INFECTIONS

Some infections, such as head lice (**Fig. 9.1**) or the childhood exanthems, are a part of normal childhood. They are commonly diagnosed and treated within the family with advice from grandparents, neighbours or local chemists. Inexperienced parents or those without family support often seek medical help. In these circumstances, understanding of the family's perception of illness and a careful explanation of the illness are required.

MEASLES

Measles is rarely seen by hospital doctors these days, largely because of a major reduction in incidence due to vaccination but also because it is easily recognized and managed in the community. It is still a dangerous illness in developing countries.

After a 14 day incubation period, coryzal symptoms (rhinorrhoea, conjunctivitis, a cough and temperature) begin, accompanied by generalized lymphadenopathy. Koplik's spots (**Fig. 9.2a**), white spots on the oral mucosa, occur early and are followed by a blotchy red skin rash that begins on the head and spreads down. The distinctive rash of measles is initially maculopapular and discrete but becomes confluent and may also desquamate (**Fig. 9.2b**). After a few days, recovery begins.

Bronchopneumonia and otitis media are relatively common complications; encephalitis is a rare but serious problem. There is a high mortality from encephalitis and survivors

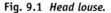

Fig. 9.1 *Head louse.*

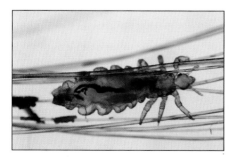

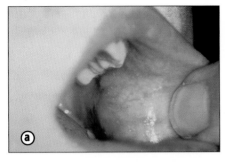

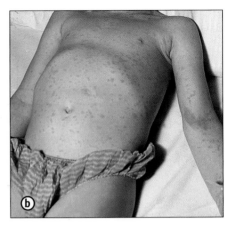

Fig. 9.2 Measles. (a) Koplik's spots are the herald of measles; (b) the distinctive rash of measles is initially maculopapular and discrete but becomes confluent and may also desquamate.

may suffer deafness, convulsions or behavioural disorders. In malnourished children there is a high mortality and morbidity.

Subacute sclerosing panencephalitis occurs up to 10 years after measles and is fatal (*see* Chapter 19).

MUMPS

Mumps has also become much less common following the introduction of the measles, mumps and rubella (MMR) vaccine. This paramyxovirus infection has a 2–3 week incubation period which is often followed by a subclinical illness. As well as the classical picture of bilateral parotid gland enlargement, unilateral gland and submandibular gland involvement are well recognized (**Fig. 9.3**). Pancreatitis and a mild viral meningitis are

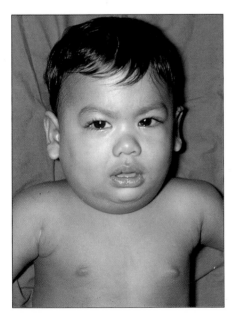

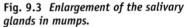

Fig. 9.3 *Enlargement of the salivary glands in mumps.*

common. In post-pubertal boys epididymo-orchitis can occur, but consequent sterility is unusual.

RUBELLA

The importance of rubella relates to its teratogenic effects during pregnancy (*see* Chapter 6). In childhood the infection is mild and often subclinical. There is an incubation period of 2–3 weeks followed by a pink macular rash (**Fig. 9.4**) and lymphadenopathy (especially affecting the occipital nodes).

CHICKENPOX AND SHINGLES

Herpes varicella zoster virus produces chickenpox, and reactivation of the virus produces an infection localized to one or two dermatomes which is called shingles. The incubation period for chickenpox is 14–21 days, following which there is a mild fever and the occurrence of crops of red macules that ripen to papules and vesicles (**Fig. 9.5**) before drying and forming scabs. If left alone, the lesions heal without scarring but children often get pock marks from scratching the itchy lesions. The child is infectious from 2 days before the onset of the rash until up to about a week afterwards, when the rash scabs. Viral particles can be demonstrated in the vesicular fluid. Generally, the younger the child the milder the illness; however, adults, the newborn and immunocompromised patients may have a severe illness with a haemorrhagic rash, pneumonia (**Fig. 9.6**) and even death. A severe illness can occur in those with eczema. Following the rash, children may get an encephalitis which presents mainly as a cerebellar ataxia. The problem almost always resolves with no sequelae.

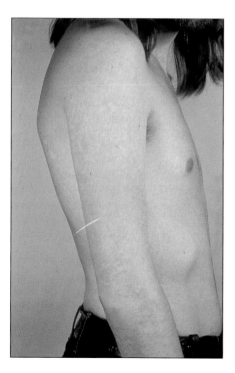

Fig. 9.4 *The typical rash of rubella.*

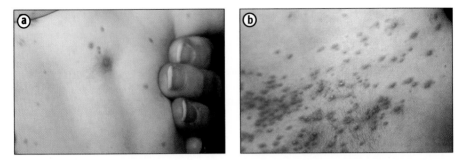

Fig. 9.5(a, b) *The rash of chickenpox. A red macule or papule is first seen; this becomes vesicular before forming a scab. Viral particles can be demonstrated in the vesicular fluid.*

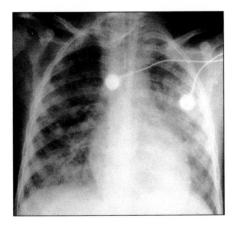

Fig. 9.6 *Varicella pneumonia is a serious complication of chickenpox.*

Immunosuppressed individuals can be given human varicella zoster immunoglobulin and acyclovir. For otherwise previously healthy children, paracetamol for fever and antihistamines such as chlorpheniramine to stop itching are useful. Calamine lotion is not usually used now as it is messy and can allow secondary bacterial infection of spots.

Shingles occurs much less commonly in children than in adults. The word zoster derives from the Greek for girdle and describes the belt-like distribution of shingles (**Fig. 9.7**). It occurs following reactivation of the herpes varicella zoster virus and affects one or two dermatomes (*see* Fig. 9.7). Acyclovir can be useful but the condition is often diagnosed too late for this agent to change its course. In contrast to adults, shingles in children is not associated with post-infection neuralgia. Although there is no association with underlying cancer, shingles is common in children with immunosuppression.

ERYTHEMA INFECTIOSUM (SLAPPED CHEEK DISEASE, FIFTH DISEASE)

Erythema infectiosum was named as being the fifth most important childhood exanthem after measles, rubella, chickenpox and scarlet fever. The cause is parvovirus B19 and it is notable for causing a red rash on the cheeks as if the child had been slapped. There is also a fine red lacy rash on the body (**Fig. 9.8**). There are no other serious features.

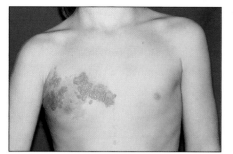

Fig. 9.7 *Shingles affecting a dermatome.*

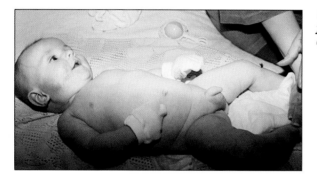

Fig. 9.8 *The red cheeks and fine lacy rash of fifth disease.*

ROSEOLA INFANTUM (EXANTHEM SUBITUM)

Roseola infantum is a viral infection caused by human herpes virus 6 (HHV6). There is a high temperature and malaise which can last for a few days with no other symptoms. The fever then suddenly drops and a macular rash appears which declares the pyrexia to be due to roseola. HHV6 is also implicated in causing many febrile illnesses in small children without the characteristic rash or febrile convulsions.

HAND, FOOT AND MOUTH DISEASE

Hand, foot and mouth disease is common in children and often occurs in epidemics. Vesicles are found on the palms of the hand, soles of the feet, and in the mouth. It is caused by a Coxsackie virus.

INFECTIOUS MONONUCLEOSIS (GLANDULAR FEVER)

Epstein–Barr virus is spread by close contact and affects adolescents in particular but also younger children. Commonly, there is pyrexia, tonsillitis (**Fig. 9.9**), cervical lymphadenopathy, petechial lesions on the soft palate, splenomegaly (**Fig. 9.10**), thrombocytopenia and mild hepatitis. A macular rash can occur and this especially happens if ampicillin is given for the sore throat (**Fig. 9.11**).

Diagnosis is by the Paul–Bunnell or Monospot tests. Contact sports should be avoided if there is splenomegaly as rupture can occur. Postviral fatigue is not a universal finding although lymphadenopathy and splenomegaly can persist for many weeks and raise questions of malignancy.

POLIOMYELITIS

Polio is now uncommon in developed countries but is still an important infection where immunization is not available. Most infections are asymptomatic or have mild symptoms

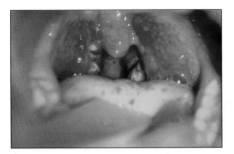

Fig. 9.9 *The typical pharyngitis of glandular fever.*

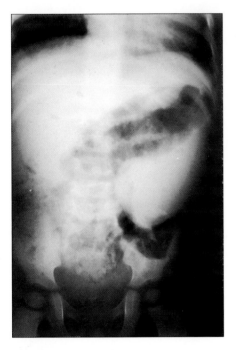

Fig. 9.10 *Splenic enlargement in glandular fever.*

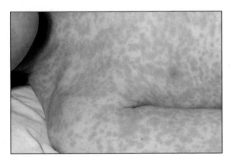

Fig. 9.11 *Drug rash in glandular fever.*

appearing like a mild viral illness. In less than 5% of cases there is central nervous system involvement and meningeal irritation. In a further 1–2% of cases there is paralysis. The anterior horn cells of the spinal cord are mainly involved, causing weakness and respiratory failure, and the bulbar nuclei in the brain stem may also be affected. Recovery from paralysis is variable and may be incomplete.

Oral live attenuated polio vaccine is very effective and safe and has eradicated polio from many countries (**Fig. 9.12**). A killed virus vaccine is also available and should be given to those at risk from live viruses such as children on immunosuppressive therapy and their families.

DIPHTHERIA

Corynebacterium diphtheriae causes a pharyngitis with marked exudate that can obstruct the airway. A neurotoxin produced by the bacteria produces paralysis and myocarditis. The infection is treated with erythromycin to kill the bacteria but antitoxin must also be used to counteract the diphtheria toxin. As with polio, intensive immunization programmes have made this infection extremely rare. However, immunity has now waned in many adults and fresh cases have been reported, especially amongst refugees and in the former eastern block countries.

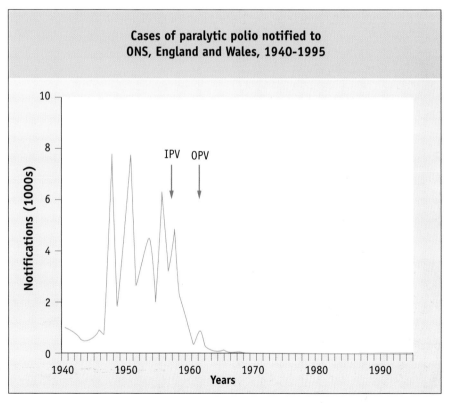

**Cases of paralytic polio notified to
ONS, England and Wales, 1940-1995**

Fig. 9.12 *Reduction in notification of polio following introduction of killed (inactivated polio vaccine—IPV) and then live attenuated vaccines (oral polio vaccine—OPV). Cases of paralytic polio notified to ONS, England and Wales 1940–1995.*

WHOOPING COUGH

Whooping cough is caused by *Bordetella pertussis*. After an incubation period of about one week the catarrhal stage begins; this presents like an upper respiratory tract infection. A cough then develops which becomes more severe and paroxysmal (**Fig. 9.13**) and is terminated by an inspiratory whoop or vomiting. The cough can last for up to 2 months before settling. Babies can become apnoeic and require ventilation, and convulsions may be seen if there is asphyxia from severe spasms. The most common complication is bronchopneumonia.

Before the paroxysmal cough has begun, the organism is identified by taking a pernasal swab and culturing in special media. At this stage there is also a striking lymphocytosis in the blood which provides a strong clue to the diagnosis. Later, serology is useful as the organism is rarely cultured once the paroxysmal cough is established.

Management is supportive with oxygen, suction and nasogastric feeding. Erythromycin is useless once the coughing has started as this is toxin mediated.

The pertussis vaccine is effective and recommended for all children apart from those with a progressive neurological disorder. It is important to note that, although there have been concerns about brain damage as a result of the vaccine, this has never been proven and is rare; the risks of encephalopathy from the illness itself are well documented (**Fig. 9.14**).

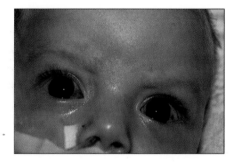

Fig. 9.13 *Conjunctival haemorrhages after prolonged coughing in pertussis.*

SCARLET FEVER

Scarlet fever is due to infection with a group A haemolytic streptococcus (also responsible for tonsillitis, rheumatic fever and glomerulonephritis) that produces an erythrogenic toxin. The initial focus is usually a sore throat or skin infection. A punctate erythematous rash with circumoral sparing is virtually diagnostic. The tongue is initially coated (white strawberry tongue) followed by desquamation to a raw appearance (red strawberry tongue); the skin later peels. Penicillin or, if the child is allergic, erythromycin, produces a rapid recovery.

PERIORBITAL CELLULITIS

Periorbital cellulitis is a serious infection of the soft tissues around the eye. There is local swelling, erythema and tenderness, and the child is also pyrexial (**Fig. 9.15**). The infection usually originates from the ethmoid sinuses in younger children, but in older children it may originate from the ethmoid, maxillary or frontal sinuses, as well as from a dental abscess. In younger children it was commonly caused by *Haemophilus influenzae* but this is rarely the case nowadays since the introduction of the Hib vaccine. Staphylococci and

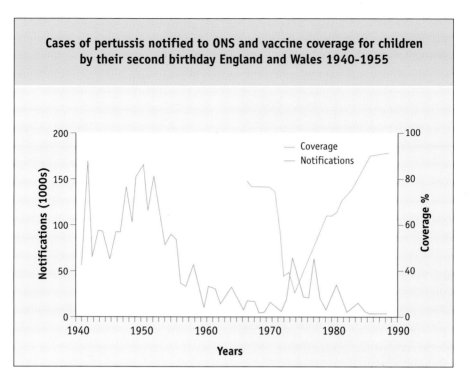

Fig. 9.14 *Resurgence of pertussis and reduction in vaccination due to fears over vaccine safety. Notifications to ONS and vaccine coverage figures for children by their second birthday, England and Wales 1940–1995.*

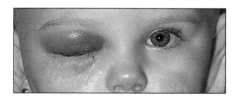

Fig. 9.15 *Orbital cellulitis.*

streptococci are commonly found organisms. Treatment is with broad spectrum intravenous antibiotics, such as cefuroxime, which are also active against staphylococci.

If untreated, the infection can spread to the orbit of the eye with proptosis, painful movements and altered visual acuity. If the infection tracks back towards the brain, cerebral abscess, meningitis or cavernous sinus thrombosis may occur.

BACTERAEMIA AND SEPTICAEMIA

Bacteria often circulate transiently in the blood stream but are rapidly destroyed (bacteraemia). Occasionally they can lodge and multiply, forming local infections such as in bacterial endocarditis after dental extraction. Septicaemia or cerebral abscesses (**Fig. 9.16**) occur in the immunodeficient patient when bacteria multiply in the blood stream. It is toxins produced by the bacteria which often cause shock.

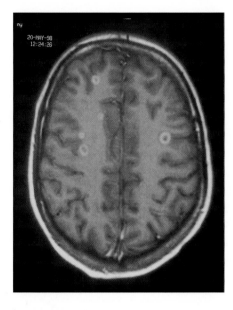

Fig. 9.16 *Multiple cerebral abscesses.*

OSTEOMYELITIS

Osteomyelitis is usually secondary to bacteraemia and involves the metaphyses of long bones. The bacteria responsible are usually staphylococci. The infected limb is painful, and reluctance to walk or use an arm may be an early sign. Erythema and swelling overlying the infection then occur (**Fig. 9.17a**) although bone changes may not occur for 2 weeks (**Fig. 9.17b**). Radionucleotide bone scanning is more sensitive.

MENINGOCOCCAL SEPTICAEMIA

Neisseria meningitidis, as well as causing meningitis, is the most common cause of septicaemia in otherwise healthy children. The bacterium is carried in the nasopharynx in up to 5% of the population. The onset of illness is often with non-specific flu-like symptoms, but on careful examination a rash may be seen. It is initially a petechial red rash that does not blanch on pressure (**Fig. 9.18**). As time passes, more lesions occur and eventually enlarge to form haemorrhagic lesions with a necrotic centre (**Fig. 9.19**). The toxins also produce endotoxic shock characterized by loss of vascular tone, hypotension, oliguria, hypoxic respiratory failure and often disseminated intravascular coagulation. Progression to death can be rapid, and the overall mortality can be 50%.

Management

The key to diagnosing meningococcal infection is a high index of suspicion. The skin of any child who is unwell should be carefully examined for non-blanching lesions. General practitioners should give parenteral penicillin to any child who may have meningococcal infection and rapidly transfer him or her to hospital. Treatment involves a broad spectrum

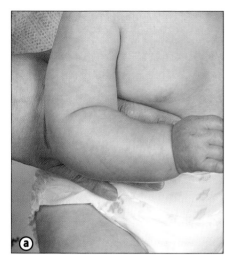

Fig. 9.17 *(a) Osteomyelitis of the distal radius; (b) late X-ray changes.*

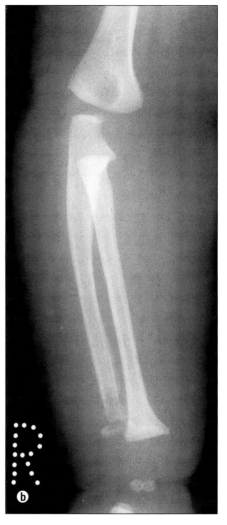

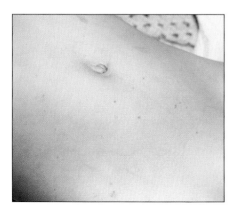

Fig. 9.18 *Petechial rash of meningococcal septicaemia.*

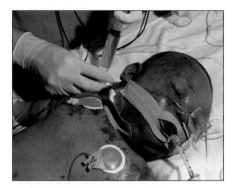

Fig. 9.19 *Massive purpuric rash of meningococcal septicaemia.*

antibiotic such as a third-generation cephalosporin, as there are organisms that are resistant to penicillin, and facilities for full intensive care. The hypotension is treated vigorously: fluid and inotropic support with dopamine should be started early. Blood and other products are often required for disseminated intravascular coagulation. Intubation and ventilation for respiratory failure is usually necessary.

Intravenous antibiotics do not clear the nasopharynx of organisms. Patients and their close contacts must be treated with rifampicin or ciprofloxacin to eliminate nasal carriage.

TUBERCULOSIS

Tuberculosis is once more becoming a problem in the world. It has always been a problem in developing countries but urban populations are now at risk. HIV infection and tuberculosis often co-exist, especially in the African subcontinent and in the drug-using populations of inner cities, and bacterial resistance to isoniazid is increasing.

The pulmonary effects of *Mycobacterium tuberculosis* infection are discussed in Chapter 13. The other primary route of infection is via the gut. In developing countries, tuberculosis commonly produces cervical cold abscesses, but atypical mycobacteria can also infect cervical nodes. It is also possible for the infection to involve the small intestine, causing malabsorption, strictures, tuberculous peritonitis and ascites. Haematogenous seeding to bones, joints, kidneys and meninges may occur. In the young, debilitated or old, miliary TB can occur with pyrexia, weight loss and non-specific ill health. In these groups the skin tests may be negative and sometimes empirical trials of drug therapy are needed.

Diagnosis

The basis of diagnosis is hypersensitivity to tuberculin purified protein derivative (PPD) which is injected intradermally. In those who have met the bacterium and gained immunity there will be a local reaction with erythema and swelling. However, there may be no reaction in the early stages of TB infection, at a time when the immune response is not established, and in malnourished or immunosuppressed persons.

Treatment

Isoniazid has been used widely as the main treatment for tuberculosis infection. Other drugs are added (**Fig. 9.20**) in order to prevent the emergence of resistance and to improve killing efficacy. A common paediatric schedule for treating tuberculosis is 6 months of isoniazid and rifampicin, with pyrazinamide added for the first 2 months. The main reason for treatment failure is non-compliance. Drug resistance is, however, increasingly common, and culture and identification of the bacterium and sensitivities must be carried out. A 3 month course of drugs is given as prophylaxis in children who have been in contact with tuber.

Drugs used in treatment of tuberculosis

Drug	Common side-effect
Isoniazid	Hepatitis
Pyrazinamide	
Ethambutol	Children cannot report the loss of colour vision that commonly occurs
PAS (para-aminosalicylic acid)	
Rifampicin	Turns urine red
Streptomycin	Ototoxic and nephrotoxic

Fig. 9.20 *Drug treatment of tuberculosis.*

KAWASAKI DISEASE

Kawasaki disease is an illness of unknown aetiology suggested by the presence of four out of five principal signs—cervical lymphadenopathy, unremitting fever, conjunctivitis (**Fig. 9.21a**), a characteristic rash (**Fig. 9.21b**) and involvement of mucous membranes—although in some cases three may be sufficient to make a diagnosis. It tends to affect those under 5 years and pathologically it is a vasculitis of small and medium sized vessels.

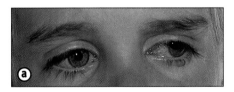

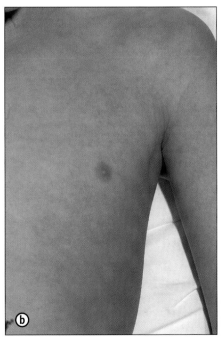

Fig. 9.21 *(a) Conjunctivitis in Kawasaki disease. This boy presented with a high fever and enlarged cervical lymph nodes. His mouth was later noted to be sore. This, with the conjunctivitis, suggested Kawasaki disease. (b) The rash of Kawasaki disease is characteristic but can be overlooked as part of a viral infection or drug reaction.*

Diagnosis and management

In the acute phase there is a neutrophilia, and the erythrocyte sedimentation rate (ESR) and C reactive protein (CRP) are elevated. Other causes of pyrexia are excluded first, but if Kawasaki disease is thought likely, intravenous immunoglobulin is given and produces a rapid recovery. Aspirin specifically controls the pyrexia and is initially given in high dosage. Following resolution of the pyrexia it is continued in low dosage as a transient but marked thrombophilia occurs in the following weeks. In the convalescent phase the digits peel (**Fig. 9.22**) and the platelet count becomes hugely elevated. Echocardiography should be carried out in the convalescent phase as a specific complication is coronary artery aneurysms. It is important to consider Kawasaki disease in febrile children, as the risk of developing aneurysms can be reduced by prompt use of immunoglobulin.

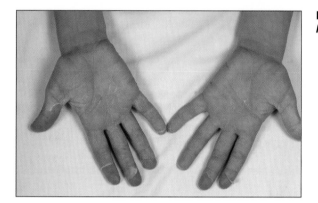

Fig. 9.22 *Peeling digits in Kawasaki disease.*

PRINCIPLES OF INVESTIGATION

Most children who present with a pyrexia will be suffering from a self-limiting viral infection. The task of the paediatrician is to identify this group, explain the benign nature of the infection to the parents and provide advice on making the child more comfortable, e.g. by using an antipyretic such as paracetamol or ibuprofen.

Part of this diagnostic process must involve a consideration of important infections such as meningitis, meningococcal septicaemia, pneumonia, urinary tract infection and Kawasaki disease which require specific investigations such as X-ray or lumbar puncture. The recognition of a sick child is learnt by experience; if in doubt, it is sensible to obtain a second opinion from a more experienced person.

It is also important to recognize that, in the early stages of infection, whether serious or not, the symptoms and signs may be very similar; parents should be warned to return if there are any changes or if they are worried. If they would have difficulty returning or are anxious it may be better to arrange admission of the child and parents to a paediatric ward for observation.

THE SEPTIC SCREEN

In some instances it is not safe to withhold antibiotic therapy until a clear diagnosis can be made. This is particularly the case in babies and infants under a year of age or in older children who present in septic shock. In such cases a septic screen is carried out. The purpose is to examine for all likely sources of infection and then start antibiotic therapy immediately. Nursing observations are made, blood for a full blood count, blood cultures, CRP and glucose are taken, a chest X-ray is performed, and urine is obtained for microscopy and culture. Many would perform a lumbar puncture at this point as well. Broad spectrum antibiotics are given intravenously. If, at 48 hours, blood cultures are demonstrated to be sterile, antibiotics can be stopped and after a further day of observation the child can be allowed home. However, blood cultures may be negative in up to 40% of infections, and if there is a particularly strong suspicion of bacterial infection a full course of antibiotics should be given.

Sometimes meningitis is suspected but the child is too unwell for lumbar puncture to be performed. This procedure can be deferred for a day or so and antibiotic treatment given, but it should always be carried out to check for evidence of meningitis as CSF cell counts and biochemistry remain deranged for up to 72 hours.

INDICES OF INFECTION

The blood count and film are helpful in determining the type of infection. Neutrophilia and a shift to more immature granulocytes indicates bacterial sepsis, whilst lymphocytosis usually points to viral infection. However, in the first three days of life there is a predominant neutrophilia and the normal white cell count can run to 20×10^3. In childhood there is often a mixed picture with neutrophils and lymphocytes in response to infection.

A falling or very high platelet count can be a pointer to infection, and non-specific indicators of inflammatory response such as the C reactive protein (CRP) or erythrocyte sedimentation rate (ESR) are also useful. Individually these are all only moderately sensitive and specific, but together they become very useful.

PYREXIA OF UNKNOWN ORIGIN (PUO)

The term 'pyrexia of unknown origin' is reserved for those fevers that have been present for 14 days and for which no cause has been found, despite investigation. By this time common bacterial infections will have declared themselves and viral infections will have resolved. The investigations required become more invasive and the causative conditions more sinister because, after this time, autoimmune disease and malignancy are more likely.

LYMPHADENOPATHY

Lymphadenopathy is a common finding in childhood and presents the dilemma of deciding how extensively to investigate as, although the majority of cases will have benign rapidly resolving causes, there are also uncommon serious causes, such as cancer.

In general, lymphadenopathy that has been present for a few weeks is likely to be due to infection (**Fig. 9.23**). If it has been present for some months a more serious cause is likely, but if present for longer than this it is unlikely to be due to underlying cancer as malignancy will have declared itself by then. Infants are particularly liable to have infection within the cervical lymph nodes themselves (**Fig. 9.24**).

Most children have a few persistently enlarged cervical nodes due to recurrent viral infections. The absence of nodes in a child who is repeatedly ill may indicate immunodeficiency (*see* Chapter 8).

111

Causes of lymphadenopathy	
Generalized	
Viral	The common exanthems, Epstein–Barr, CMV, toxoplasmosis, HIV
Malignancy	Leukaemia, lymphoma, neuroblastoma
Auto-immune and connective tissue diseases	
Localized (often cervical)	
Tuberculosis	*M. tuberculosis* and atypical organisms such as *M. avium*
Local sepsis	Ear, nose and throat pathologies and dental infection
Malignancy	Hodgkin lymphoma

Fig. 9.23 *Causes of lymphadenopathy.*

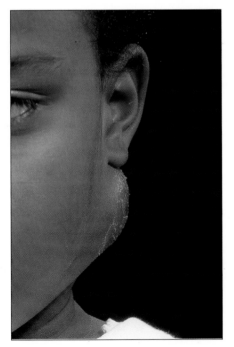

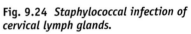

Fig. 9.24 *Staphylococcal infection of cervical lymph glands.*

Management

As well as documenting enlargement of glands around the body, it is also important to examine for hepatosplenomegaly and for evidence of petechiae or bruising which may point to bone marrow infiltration. A full blood count and film, ESR or CRP are helpful as a general screen, and specific serology for common viral illnesses such as EBV or CMV is undertaken. Mediastinal lymph nodes can be seen on a plain chest X-ray. If these investigations are unhelpful it is reasonable to wait a few weeks as in most cases the lymphadenopathy will resolve by itself; some doctors prescribe an antibiotic. Persistent lymphadenopathy requires excision biopsy; needle biopsy or surgical incision and drainage can lead to chronic sinus formation in mycobacterial lymphadenopathy. Excision is often curative (**Fig. 9.25**).

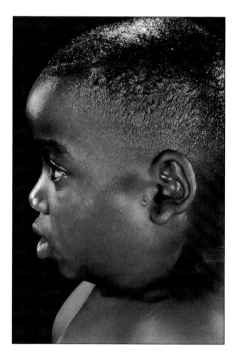

Fig. 9.25 *Tuberculous lymphadenitis.*

chapter 10

Nutrition

NUTRITIONAL REQUIREMENTS AT DIFFERENT AGES

Nutritional requirements, like growth rates, vary with age. Protein requirements in childhood mirror the rate of growth. However, energy requirements remain high between the end of the first year of life and puberty as children are very active during this period of relatively slow growth (**Fig. 10.1**). It is more difficult to indicate how much of each nutrient an individual child should ingest. In 1991, the Department of Health replaced the recommended daily amounts (RDAs) with dietary reference values (DRVs). There are different types of DRV:

- The Reference Nutrient Intake (RNI) for a protein, vitamin or mineral is the amount of the nutrient that is sufficient or more than sufficient to meet the needs of a group of individuals. If the average intake of the group is at the level of the RNI then the risk of a nutritional deficiency is small.
- The Estimated Average Requirement (EAR) relates to the mean requirements of a group for a particular nutrient. Thus, half those in the group will need more than the EAR and about half will actually require less.
- Safe intake is a term used to suggest an appropriate amount of a nutrient if the needs of a group are to be met, but not so large as to cause undesirable effects. It is used for those nutrients for which there is insufficient information to estimate an RNI or EAR.
  Dietitians tend to use RNI when calculating the requirements of an individual child, as the other values relate to the whole population.

Government policy is not usually concerned with the individual, but rather with improving the health of the nation as a whole. Dietary guidelines are produced which relate to the quality of the diet, mainly with regard to adult diseases such as ischaemic heart disease, obesity and large bowel diseases. There are important differences between dietary guidelines and recommended nutritional intake. For example, guidelines advise adults to use semi-skimmed milk, whilst infants and young children need whole fat milk.

BREAST AND BOTTLE FEEDING

Breast milk is considered to have the ideal nutritional composition for babies and young infants. The benefits of breast milk are generally acknowledged (**Fig. 10.2**), but the disadvantaged members of the population, who have most to gain from breast feeding, are less likely to breast feed their children (**Fig. 10.3**).

PROBLEMS WITH BREAST FEEDING

For normal infants there are no nutritional problems with breast milk provided they are weaned onto solids between 4 and 6 months of age. There are specific problems with

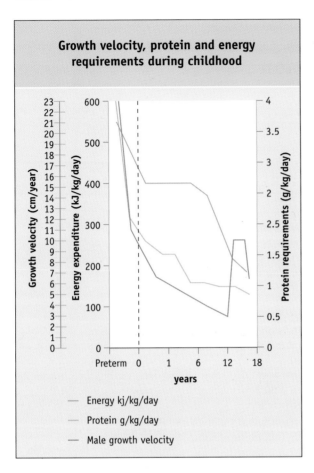

Fig. 10.1 *Comparison of growth velocity to protein intake during childhood. It is clear that protein requirements mirror growth. Energy requirements remain consistently high throughout childhood and reflect the high level of activity in childhood.*

breast feeding which are important for some families. Preterm infants often have increased nutritional requirements (**Fig. 10.4**). These can be met by adding fortifiers to expressed breast milk or using special preterm formulas. The vitamin K content of breast milk is low. It is possible to prevent haemorrhagic disease of the newborn by giving vitamin K to all babies at birth, either as a single intravenous or intramuscular injection, or as a series of oral drops. If oral drops are given at birth to a breast fed baby, 2 further doses are given during the next 6 weeks. Formula milk is fortified with vitamin K and so babies receiving formula do not require further doses of vitamin K.

Mothers with HIV can potentially infect their babies via breast feeding. In many parts of the world, however, the increased risks of death and disease from bottle feeding are greater than the risk of contracting HIV from mother's milk, so breast feeding is recommended (*see* Chapter 8). Similarly, if a mother has open tuberculosis, it is only safe to breast feed if the infant is given isoniazid and immunized with isoniazid-resistant BCG.

Some drugs taken by the mother are present in disproportionately high concentrations in breast milk but the main contraindications to breast feeding usually involve antimetabolites, antithyroid drugs and lithium. The British National Formulary contains information on drugs and breast feeding.

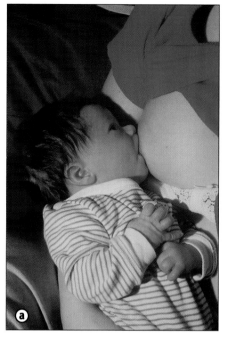

Fig. 10.2 *Breast feeding. (a) Apart from its other benefits, breast feeding is usually a pleasurable and satisfying experience for both the mother and baby. (b) The benefits of breast feeding.*

Benefits of breast feeding

- Presumed optimum nutrient balance of protein, fat, calcium and phosphate
- Improved absorption of fats due to milk lipase
- Low sodium concentration protects against hypernatraemia
- Lactoferrin and secretory IgA protect against infection (gastrointestinal and respiratory), especially important in developing countries
- Reduction in ovulation in breast feeding mothers and reduction in risk of breast cancer
- No need for clean water supply, facilities to sterilize bottles, or finances to buy feed
- Reduction in necrotizing enterocolitis in preterm infants
- Possible reduction in rates of inflammatory bowel disease, diabetes and atopic disease

ⓑ

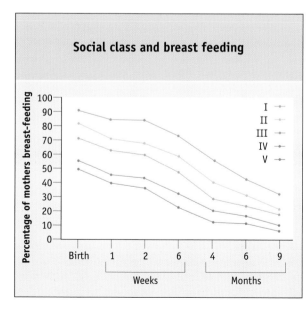

Social class and breast feeding

Percentage of mothers breast-feeding

I
II
III
IV
V

Birth 1 2 6 4 6 9

Weeks   Months

Fig. 10.3 *Social class and breast feeding. More people in social class I breast feed, and for longer, than in social class V. Although breast feeding is convenient and cheap, less than 50% of mothers belonging to social class V are likely to breast feed compared to 90% of those in social class I.*

117

Nutritional requirements of preterm and term infants

Nutrient	Preterm infant (kg/day)	Term infant (kg/day)
Fluid	150–200 ml	150 ml
Energy	130 kcal	100 kcal
Protein	4.0 g	2.0 g
Sodium	2–5 mmol	1.5 mmol
Calcium	4.0 mmol	2.2 mmol
Phosphorus/calcium ratio	2:1	1:1
Iron	45 μmol	5 μmol
Copper	2.5 μmol	1 μmol
Vitamin B_6	45 μg	33 μg
Vitamin K	3 μg	1.6 μg
Suggested total daily intake		
Vitamin A	1000 μg	350 μg
Vitamin D	8.5 μg	20–40 μg
Vitamin C	20 mg	25 mg
Folic acid	65 μg	50 μg

Fig. 10.4 *Nutritional requirements of preterm and term infants.*

FORMULA FEEDS

Many mothers breast feed for a few weeks or not at all, and instead feed their babies on formula feeds. Formula milks are all very similar in composition and are modifications of cow's milk that resemble human breast milk (**Fig. 10.5**). Most formula milks are whey based, containing 60% demineralized cow's milk whey and 40% casein with added fat and other nutrients. Although changing to a formula milk with a higher casein content and iron fortification is often recommended after 4–6 months, there is little reason to do this and babies can remain on the same formula until they graduate to doorstep cow's milk at around the age of 1 year. Additional water may be required by formula fed infants during periods of hot weather; cooled boiled tap water should be provided.

Rarely, a baby will demonstrate an intolerance to cow's milk protein. Cow's milk hydrolysates are used in preference to soya milks in infants less than 6 months of age as up to 30% of infants will also develop soya intolerance. Modern soya based milks are fortified with calcium and are effective feeds; however, as the long-term effects on neural development are not known and they have a high aluminium content, their use is not recommended in the long term.

WEANING

The introduction of solids is carried out between 2 months and 1 year in different households. The current dietary guidelines published by the Department of Health are that the introduction of solids be delayed until 4 months to reduce the incidence of food

Composition of cow's, breast and formula milks

	Cow's milk	Breast milk	Formula
Carbohydrate (g/100 ml)	4.6	7.4	7.2
Fat (g/100 ml)	3.9	4.2	3.6
Protein (g/100 ml)	3.4	1.1	1.5
Calories/100 ml	67	70	65
Sodium (mmol/l)	23	6.4	6.4
Calcium (mg/100 ml)	124	35	44
Phosphate (mg/100 ml)	98	15	33
Vitamin A (µg/100 ml)	38	60	80
Vitamin D (µg/100 ml)	0.02	0.01	1.05
Vitamin E (µg/100 ml)	90	350	950
Folic acid (µg/100 ml)	3.7	5.2	5.3
Iron (mg/100 ml)	0.05	0.08	0.67

Fig. 10.5 *Composition of cow's, breast and formula milks.*

intolerance but not later than 6 months to prevent nutritional deficiencies—especially iron (**Fig. 10.6**). The first foods at weaning are usually baby rice or rusk mixed in a little milk but after a few months infants can manage mashed foods.

PRESCHOOL CHILDREN

By the age of 1 year children should be eating the same type of food as the rest of the family, with modifications to the texture where necessary, and drinking doorstep cow's milk.

Children with food fads and those who are picky eaters are common problems. Although they appear not to eat at all they do manage to take sufficient nutrition to continue growing along their centile. The behavioural aspect is more important than the nutritional component.

OLDER CHILDREN

The child of school age enjoys a wide range of foods and the dietary aim should be to provide the suggested healthy low saturated fat and high fibre diet. Sweets and carbonated drinks that can contribute to caries should be limited. Puberty is an important time as rapid growth will expose any nutritional deficiencies.

VEGETARIANISM

Many families do not eat meat for reasons of religion or lifestyle. Children usually have no problems with such diets if they can assimilate the correct proteins from a varied diet. This is not difficult if eggs and cheese are eaten. Families that are vegan for cultural reasons usually eat ethnic recipes that provide a nutritional balance.

Guidelines on weaning

	0–4 months	4–6 months	6–9 months	9–12 months	12+ months
MILK/DAIRY					
Breast milk/formula milk	———————————————————————→				
Full cow's milk					——→
Yoghurt/custard		————————————————————→			
Hard cheese			grated/cubed ————→		
STARCHY FOODS					
Potato/turnip/parsnip		pureed	mashed	chopped	→
Wholemeal bread/chappatti				————————→	
Breakfast cereals (unsweetened)			———————————→		
Rice		pureed		grains	→
VEGETABLES and FRUIT (fresh, frozen or tinned)					
Carrot/yam/beans		pureed		chopped	→
Peas/baked beans		pureed		whole	→
Cabbage/sprouts/cauliflower		pureed	mashed	chopped	→
Tomato/cucumber/lettuce		pureed	chopped		→
Apple/pear/plum		pureed	finger food		→
Banana/melon		pureed	finger food		→
Tinned pineapple/apricots, etc.			———————————→		
Orange			———————————→		
MEAT and ALTERNATIVES					
Lean meats/liver/chicken, etc.		pureed	minced	chopped	→
Pulses		pureed		grains	→
Fish/fish fingers			pureed	chopped	→
Eggs					

Fig. 10.6 *Guidelines on weaning.*

MALNUTRITION

Throughout the underdeveloped world malnutrition is directly responsible for much morbidity and mortality. The World Health Organization has categorized deficiencies of protein and energy into marasmus, kwashiorkor, and unspecified, i.e. that which does not fit the first two categories. Malnutrition is also seen in developed countries because of uneducated or neglectful parents and commonly in children with chronic illness such as congenital heart disease, cystic fibrosis and gastrointestinal disorders where poor appetite and high energy demands are common problems. Obesity is common in otherwise healthy children.

OBESITY

Obese adults are at greater risk of atherosclerotic heart disease, hypertension, diabetes and early death. Obesity begins in childhood and it is a difficult problem as the habits of the family as a whole need to be addressed (*see* Chapter 21).

MARASMUS

Marasmus is due to insufficient quantities of all nutrients. It occurs throughout the world, often because of a failure of lactation in the mother, or following a prolonged, and often gastrointestinal, illness in the child. Children with marasmus are vigorous and usually hungry but there is a reduction in the rate of linear growth and loss of muscle and subcutaneous fat (**Fig. 10.7**). Biochemical abnormalities are uncommon and will return to normal if adequate nutrition is restored. However, in marasmic children there can be a high mortality from infectious diseases, especially measles.

KWASHIORKOR

Kwashiorkor occurs in developing countries at the time of weaning from breast feeding. The arrival of another infant, financial, or cultural pressures to stop breast feeding mean that the child loses a nutritionally balanced foodstuff and is forced to eat the family food which is usually limited in protein content but high in carbohydrate. Exposure to bacteria in food produces bacterial contamination of the small bowel and gastroenteritis. Appetite is diminished, infants lose their muscle mass but retain subcutaneous fat, and they become oedematous and anaemic with sparse friable hair (*see* Fig. 10.7). Pneumonia, gastrointestinal infection and childhood viral infections such as measles have a high mortality and morbidity in this susceptible group.

MANAGEMENT OF MALNUTRITION

The best way to treat obesity is firstly to identify the problem: this is done by plotting serial measurements of a child's weight and height and those of the parents on centile charts. Advice on changing the diet of the family and increased activity are important measures during childhood (*see* Chapter 21).

Treatment of marasmus, kwashiorkor and unspecified malnutrition is difficult: up to 60% of children may die. Frequent feeding, often via a nasogastric tube, is needed. Protein is usually supplied as semi-skimmed milk; sugar and vegetable oils provide energy. Electrolyte disturbances are corrected and infections treated with antibiotics. These children are at risk of hypothermia.

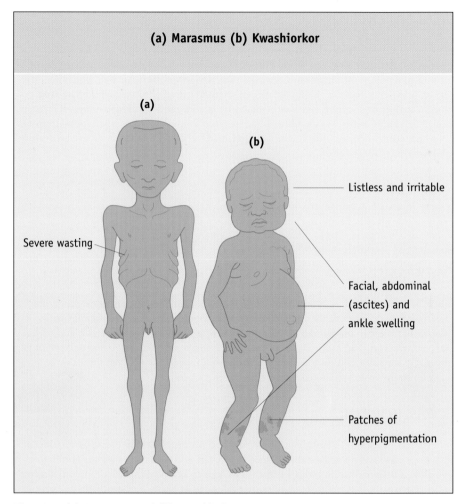

Fig. 10.7 *(a) Marasmus and (b) Kwashiorkor.*

VITAMIN AND MICRONUTRIENT DEFICIENCIES

Vitamin deficiency states are uncommon in developed countries as there is a greater availability of fresh fruit and vegetables, and processed foods are also supplemented with vitamins and minerals. However, lack of the fat soluble vitamins (A, D, E and K) can occur in diseases associated with fat malabsorption, e.g. cystic fibrosis or hepatic disease; such children routinely receive supplements.

Vitamin A deficiency is common in developing countries and causes night blindness, xerophthalmia and corneal scarring. Impairment of the gut mucosa and immunity develop. Studies have demonstrated reductions in infant mortality when susceptible populations receive vitamin A supplements.

Rickets results from inadequate intake or defective metabolism of vitamin D. Vitamin D can be produced in the skin on exposure to sunlight but dark-skinned children living in northern latitudes may not have sufficient exposure and dietary intake may also be insufficient. Rarely, vitamin D deficiency may be secondary to a malabsorption state or an inherited defect of vitamin D biosynthesis. Preterm infants who have difficulty establishing enteral feeds often suffer from rickets due to insufficient phosphate intake. These children are often miserable with failure to thrive. There is ineffective mineralization of bones with bowing of the long bones and softening of the skull. Biochemically, there is a marked elevation in the level of serum alkaline phosphatase and reduction in the calcium and phosphate levels. The bony epiphyses are cupped and frayed on X-rays (**Fig. 10.8**).

Management consists of ensuring sufficient vitamin D, either in the diet or as supplementation.

Zinc deficiency produces a characteristic peeling of the skin to produce raw areas around the mouth and buttocks (**Fig. 10.9**).

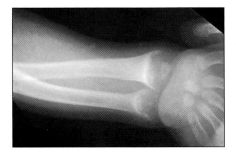

Fig. 10.8 *This child with rickets shows the classical X-ray appearances of cupping and fraying at the ends of the long bones.*

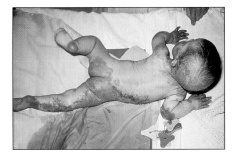

Fig. 10.9 *Zinc deficiency acrodermatitis enteropathica.*

NUTRITIONAL PROGRAMMING

It has always been recognized that small stature can result from growth retardation during fetal life, and that the average height of a population can be limited by nutrition. Recent work has suggested that potential markers of early nutrition such as small size at birth are linked to an increased risk of dying from ischaemic heart disease in later life or the development of risk factors such as diabetes, hypertension and obesity. This concept is known as nutritional programming.

chapter 11

Gastroenterology

Most parents will seek advice at some time about their children's bowels; diarrhoea and vomiting and tummy-ache are common reasons for consultation.

The presentation and management of primarily medical disorders are dealt with in this chapter; surgical problems are discussed in Chapter 24.

VOMITING

Vomiting is the forceful ejection of the stomach contents whereas regurgitation is the effortless return of food. In practice, the distinction between regurgitation and vomiting can be difficult (**Fig. 11.1**). Vomiting is a common symptom in childhood and is usually due to viral gastroenteritis. However, it can be a symptom of a variety of disease states involving the gastrointestinal and other organ systems. This is particularly the case in small babies.

GASTROENTERITIS

Gastroenteritis is a leading cause of death throughout the developing world, and winter epidemics in the UK are responsible for many emergency paediatric consultations.

The initial symptoms are usually vomiting, malaise and pyrexia. Diarrhoea often occurs later and colicky abdominal pain may be prominent enough to suggest a surgical problem. A common pathogen is rotavirus (**Fig. 11.2**). Blood and slime may indicate a bacterial aetiology such as *Campylobacter*, *Shigella* or *Salmonella* spp. Although the diagnosis may appear obvious, it is wise to consider other uncommon but important conditions. In particular, bacterial infection such as urinary tract infection in infants, haemolytic uraemic syndrome and intussusception must be identified as they require specific treatment.

Management of acute infective gastroenteritis

The main problem in gastroenteritis is the prevention and treatment of dehydration. The assessment of dehydration can be performed using clinical signs (**Fig. 11.3**), but the most useful indicator is comparison of the current weight to a recent weight.

The viral infection itself resolves in 7–10 days without specific therapy but the diarrhoea may persist. Stool culture is not usually warranted unless there are unusual features; even if bacteria are cultured from stool, antibiotics are not usually prescribed unless the child is very unwell, as unaided recovery is the rule. If there is no evidence of hypovolaemic shock then oral rehydration is an effective treatment in most instances. Rehydration fluids are formulated to contain electrolytes to replace gastrointestinal losses as well as glucose which allows more rapid absorption of sodium and water from the gut.

Causes of vomiting and regurgitation

(a) Babies and infants

- Possetting. The normal regurgitation of small amounts of milk.
- Wind. It is traditional practice to make a baby belch during a feed to make room for more milk. Breast fed babies tend to suffer less from wind than their bottle fed counterparts. Some babies swallow a lot of air and bring up small quantities of milk in a forceful manner.
- Gastro-oesophageal reflux. The production of relatively large amounts of milk during a feed, soon after or on laying down, should suggest gastro-oesophageal reflux. In practice, the return of milk can be forceful and appear as vomiting.
- Infection. Most infections associated with vomiting will be clinically apparent by a temperature or focal signs, but in the early stages of meningitis lethargy or irritability may be the only other signs and in urinary tract infection there may be no other clues.
- Surgical problems. The presence of bile in the vomit should always suggest a surgical emergency or an obstruction of the bowel distal to the ampulla of Vater. However, the absence of bile in vomit does not necessarily exclude intestinal obstruction. It should also be remembered that vomiting may not occur in low intestinal obstruction until the bowel has become distended with feed.
- Metabolic disorders. Although occurring rarely, congenital adrenal hyperplasia, galactosaemia and other inborn errors of metabolism may declare themselves by vomiting.

(b) Older children

- Gastroenteritis. Vomiting is usually an early symptom in gastroenteritis.
- Surgical problems. Vomiting is an important symptom in the acute abdomen indicating blockage of a smooth muscle lined system or irritation of the peritoneum. Sometimes, however, vomiting may be absent.
- Metabolic problems. The presentation of diabetic ketoacidosis in particular can be dominated by vomiting and abdominal pain. Accidental and non-accidental ingestion of medications or naturally occurring plant toxins can also cause vomiting.
- Behavioural problems. Toddlers with food fads may vomit food if forced to eat.
- Raised intracranial pressure. Typically, children wake with a headache and vomiting and the symptoms subside through the day as intracranial pressure is reduced in the upright position.

Fig. 11.1 *Causes of vomiting in (a) babies and (b) older children.*

Solutions based on rice water are used in developing countries. Small frequent aliquots of the fluid, e.g. a teaspoon every 5 minutes, will trickle through the stomach without accumulating and causing vomiting. The taste of the fluid can be a problem in well, vigorous children, but in more severely dehydrated children there are no problems with cooperation. If a mother is breast feeding it is important to continue this despite the illness as there is a danger of milk production ceasing.

Uncommonly there will be severe dehydration (more than 10%), with hypovolaemic shock; in these circumstances intravenous treatment is mandatory. Initial resuscitation is given as normal saline or albumin to restore effective circulation. The dehydration involving the tissues of the body must be treated more slowly over 24–48 hours. The

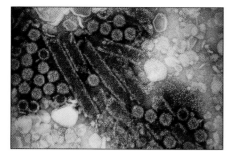

Fig. 11.2 *Rotavirus particles.*

Clinical features of dehydration

5–10% dehydrated	10–15% dehydrated
Thirst and oliguria	Apathy and anuria
Sunken fontanelle, reduced skin turgor and sunken eyes	Features as 5% but with progressive hypovolaemic shock (mottling and cool peripheries)
Elevated creatinine and urea	Acidaemia
Oral rehydration fluids	Intravenous restoration of circulating volume with colloid or normal saline, then correction of body fluid deficit over 24 hours

(a)

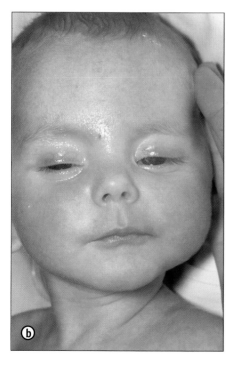

Fig. 11.3 *Dehydration: (a) clinical features; (b) physical appearance.*

(b)

amount of fluid is the sum of the amount of fluid missing (fluid deficit) and the daily requirements of fluid (maintenance), including ongoing losses as diarrhoea.

Usually the body deficit of water and sodium is about the same, producing isonatraemic dehydration. Hyponatraemic dehydration, where more sodium than water is lost, may occur; and when the baby is given an overconcentrated oral fluid this leads to hypernatraemic dehydration.

After 24 hours of clear fluids without further vomiting, small quantities of normal diet can be carefully introduced. Regrading with different strengths of milk is unnecessary. Diarrhoea often persists after the virus has been cleared and is due to disruption of the gut lining and the brush border enzymes. More rarely there is torrential watery diarrhoea on restarting normal diet; this is caused by a temporary lactose intolerance. This post-infectious enteritis usually resolves with a further 24 hours of clear fluids if necessary. Infants sometimes go on to suffer multiple dietary intolerances requiring temporary exclusion of dairy products, gluten and sugars.

GASTRO-OESOPHAGEAL REFLUX

The cardia of the stomach acts as a functional valve keeping food within the stomach. This valve is often lax in babies, and effortless regurgitation of milk into the oesophagus can be provoked by laying down or winding. Possetting, the occasional regurgitation of small amounts of milk, is considered normal but probably reflects incompetence of the cardiac sphincter. Some infants reflux acid in the presence of a competent cardiac sphincter; their problems are not related to posture.

The symptoms of gastro-oesophageal reflux can be severe with vomiting during feeds or often on laying down. Lack of calorie intake can lead to failure to thrive; irritation of the oesophagus by acid can produce oesophagitis. This can be suspected from reluctance to feed, or the presence of faecal occult blood, or be seen on endoscopy (**Fig. 11.4**). Some infants have serious choking, coughing spells or recurrent aspiration of liquids. Up to 50% of preterm infants have reflux and some may have apnoeic spells as a result.

Investigations are often not needed, and a clinical diagnosis and therapeutic trial is usually sufficient. A pH study can be used to confirm the diagnosis in those who do not respond to simple treatment with prokinetic agents and Gaviscon. A pH probe is placed in the mid oesophagus and its position checked radiologically. The pH is recorded over 24

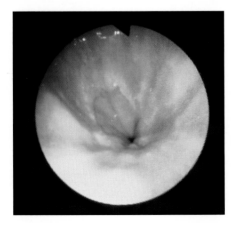

Fig. 11.4 *Endoscopy appearances of reflux oesophagitis.*

hours and the time of feeds noted. Episodes of acid reflux can be identified by examination of the data. Antacids must be stopped before the study (**Fig. 11.5**). Investigations such as barium meal may sometimes be needed to exclude pyloric stenosis and also to exclude malrotation by showing the normal position of the duodenum.

Treatment

Treatment for reflux is staged; most infants tend to outgrow symptoms by 8–12 months as they wean onto solids, assume a more upright posture and the cardia becomes tighter. In severe gastro-oesophageal reflux where drug therapy is ineffective, surgery should be performed (**Fig. 11.6**).

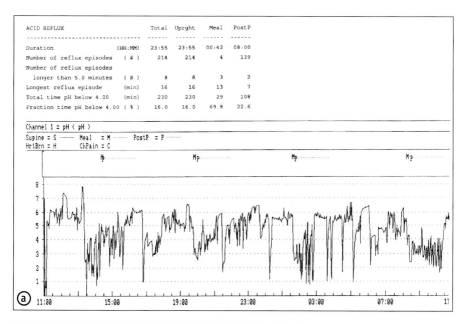

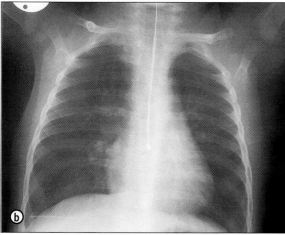

Fig. 11.5 *Investigation of gastro-oesophageal reflux. (a) Data from pH study showing frequent acid reflux; (b) pH probe in mid oesophagus.*

A stepwise management plan for gastro-oesophageal reflux

Minimal symptoms—heavy possetting ⟶ Reassurance to parents

Marked vomiting, no failure to thrive ⟶ Carobel feed thickener or Gaviscon

Vomiting despite the above or failure to thrive ⟶ Metoclopramide or domperidone and
H$_2$ antagonists

Failure of medical therapy ⟶ Investigations

Diagnosis clear—maximal therapy ⟶ Addition of domperidone

Failure of maximal medical treatment ⟶ Surgery

Fig. 11.6 *A stepwise management plan for gastro-oesophageal reflux. Associated oesophagitis should be treated with H$_2$ antagonists such as cimetidine and ranitidine.*

HAEMATEMESIS AND MELAENA

The vomiting or passage of fresh or altered blood causes great concern to parents. In most cases of haematemesis or melaena there is a simple explanation such as swallowed blood during birth (**Fig. 11.7**) or cracked nipple during breast feeding (**Fig. 11.8**). It is sensible to check a clotting profile and blood count to exclude thrombocytopenia or clotting disorders, but if there is no haemodynamic compromise no further action is usually needed. Investigations are undertaken if there are repeated episodes of bleeding or severe anaemia.

Fig. 11.7 *Swallowed blood during birth.*

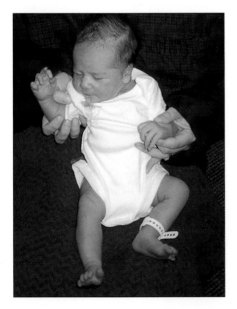

Causes of gastrointestinal bleeding	
Ingested blood	Maternal (cracked nipple or swallowed at birth) or non GI (epistaxis)
Bleeding diathesis	Haemorrhagic disease of the newborn, haemophilia or thrombocytopenia
Vascular causes	Henoch–Schönlein purpura, haemangiomas and telangiectasia
Local causes	Reflux oesophagitis, Mallory–Weiss tears with vomiting, ulcers and gastritis, e.g. stress, peptic, NSAIDs
Surgical causes	Intussusception (a late sign), Meckel's diverticulum
Colitis	• Inflammatory, e.g. allergic and ulcerative colitis, Crohn's disease • Infective, e.g. *Salmonella, Campylobacter, Shigella* and *E. coli*
Anal fissure	• Secondary to constipation • Sexual abuse

Fig. 11.8 *Causes of gastrointestinal bleeding.*

RECURRENT ABDOMINAL PAIN

Ten to twenty per cent of older children and adolescents complain about episodes of colicky mid-abdominal pain which may be severe enough to interrupt schooling and other normal activities. In between the episodes the children appear normal but some of these children also suffer from recurrent headaches and/or episodes of recurrent vomiting. In 95% of cases no underlying cause is found and the child usually outgrows his or her symptoms. It is important in taking the history to ensure that underlying conditions are not overlooked, but exhaustive investigations are seldom helpful. For example, chronic constipation may be found, or epigastric pain radiating to the back, especially at night, might be an indication of peptic ulcer disease. Rarely, episodes of small bowel obstruction may occur due to malrotation, or a Meckel diverticulum may be present. Food intolerance in atopic individuals, abdominal migraine in those with a strong family history, renal calculi, infection or obstruction to the kidney may be causes of recurrent pain.

Most children will grow out of their symptoms, but some may eventually be recognized as having irritable bowel syndrome in adulthood. Although there is little hard evidence to confirm that their personalities are different from those of other children, or that they have problems dealing with stress in their lives, they do benefit from family psychotherapy.

INFANTILE COLIC

Infantile colic is a common self-limiting condition that affects up to 20% of infants from a few weeks to a few months of age. Typically, in the evening there is inconsolable crying, drawing up of the knees and flatus suggesting abdominal pain. This is very worrying to parents and a range of remedies from gripe water to peppermint water are usually tried with varying success. Oesophagitis from GOR or constipation may rarely present in this way.

CONSTIPATION

Constipation can be defined as pain, difficulty or delay in defecation. If the stool is passed easily the frequency is unimportant. Babies fed on formula milk often pass firm stools, and vigorous abdominal contractions are commonly seen.

Preschool children often become constipated during a febrile illness when mild dehydration produces a hard stool. Psychological stress or forceful potty training may also be responsible and there may also be a tear at the anal margin. Pain, experienced in passing the large hard motion, begins a cycle of stool retention and painful passage of further large, hard motions. With chronic constipation the capacity of the rectum increases (mega-rectum) and the call to defecate weakens. Liquefaction of retained faeces leads to overflow soiling which is socially disastrous. By this stage psychological difficulties are universally experienced by both children and parents.

Management of constipation

It is unusual to find any underlying cause such as hypercalcaemia or undiagnosed neuromuscular problems. Occasionally Hirschsprung's disease affecting a short segment of the gut will be present and this causes delay in the passage of meconium after birth. A midstream urine (MSU) should be checked as there is often a coincidental urinary tract infection. An abdominal film is useful in some cases as it demonstrates to the family the degree of the problem (**Fig. 11.9**). There are three main elements to therapy:

1. **The removal of retained faeces.** This is done by softening stools with lactulose or sodium docusate; this may take weeks and soiling may worsen during this time. The gastrocolic reflex can then be amplified by use of senna or sodium picosulphate which clears the atonic rectum and colon, prevents re-accumulation and stimulates a daily bowel action. Occasionally enemas or evacuation under anaesthetic are required.
2. **Maintenance of a regular bowel habit.** A regimen of sufficient faecal softener to produce a soft but not liquid motion, together with a stimulant to amplify the gastrocolic reflex is provided. It may be necessary to provide a booster dose of sodium picosulphate once

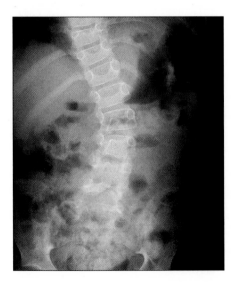

Fig. 11.9 Constipation.

a week or if there is no motion for a couple of days. If an anal fissure is present it is useful to use a smear of lignocaine gel on the anus to prevent pain on defecation. A regular time to defecate, e.g. after breakfast, with a firm foot rest is important. Once there is a regular bowel habit, children's appetites and energy improve and it is easier to introduce roughage and fluid into the diet. Whilst many may dislike fresh vegetables, most children will eat foods such as baked beans and pasta which are good sources of fibre.

3. **Emotional support for the family.** This is as important as the medical therapy. There is often a puritanical zeal for defecation which must be exchanged for positive and relaxed encouragement by the parents. This may need support from the community paediatric nurse or even child psychologist.

Treatment should be continued for at least a year in most established cases. If medical treatment is failing, an anal dilatation under general anaesthetic may help to establish a regular bowel action. At the time, rectal biopsies may be taken to exclude Hirschsprung's disease.

HIRSCHSPRUNG'S DISEASE

Congenital absence of the myenteric and submucosal ganglions from the large bowel produces a narrow non-motile segment. The normal proximal bowel becomes distended with faeces. Only the rectosigmoid is usually involved but sometimes the colon or the entire bowel may be affected. Abdominal distension and vomiting in a neonate who has not passed meconium is the commonest presentation but occasionally an older child with constipation will be found to have an aganglionic segment on rectal suction biopsies (**Fig. 11.10**). The management is surgical, often with a colostomy while the proximal bowel regains tone. The normally innervated bowel is then anastomosed to the anus.

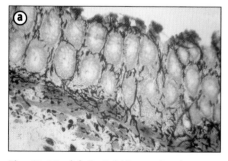
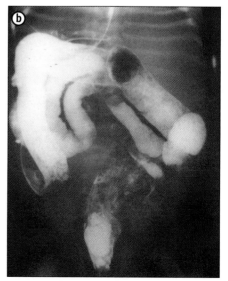

Fig. 11.10 *(a) Rectal biopsy showing absence of the myenteric and submucosal plexuses and proliferation of the proximal nerve fibres in Hirschsprung's disease; (b) X-ray appearance of Hirschsprung's disease.*

CHRONIC DIARRHOEA

TODDLER DIARRHOEA

Many infants who present with chronic diarrhoea are growing normally. The parents complain that after almost all meals there is an urgent defecation with recognizable vegetable matter. This seems to be an exaggerated gastrocolic reflex and improves with time.

No specific therapy is required; parents learn which foods exacerbate the situation and tend to restrict oral intake to meal times. A high fat, low fibre diet can be used to control symptoms.

FAILURE TO THRIVE AND MALABSORPTION

Failure to thrive is an expression used to describe a situation in which a child's growth fails to meet the expected growth rate for a child of that age. It is demonstrated on growth charts by a falling away from a weight centile; linear growth and head growth are initially spared. A thorough history, examination and simple investigations, for example stool culture for *Giardia lamblia* (**Fig. 11.11**), will usually suggest the cause.

- Inadequate nutrient intake is the commonest cause of failure to thrive. This may be due to inadequate availability of food, feeding mismanagement or neglect, or anorexia due to chronic illness or anorexia nervosa.
- Failure to absorb food is associated with gastrointestinal symptoms. There may be vomiting of food, as in gastro-oesophageal reflux, or, if there is malabsorption, offensive smelling diarrhoea that is difficult to flush down the toilet (**Fig. 11.12**).
- Inability to utilize food is the mechanism of failure to thrive in diabetes mellitus. Glucose is available but cannot enter the cells because of insufficient insulin.
- Chronic infection, respiratory and cardiac disease are all associated with increased energy expenditure as well as anorexia.
- Psychosocial problems can affect the child and cause failure to thrive despite adequate availability of food. The mechanism for this is not known.

COELIAC DISEASE

Coeliac disease is a permanent immunological intolerance to the gliadin fraction of gluten, causing atrophy of the villi in the small bowel. The incidence in the United Kingdom has

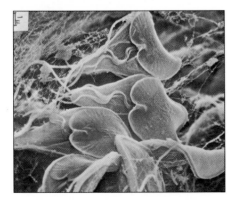

Fig. 11.11 *Giardia lamblia.*

Causes of failure to thrive and diarrhoea

Lactose intolerance	Lactase is present in the small intestine at least for the first few years of life. In Caucasians it continues but for all other races it ceases to be expressed at this time. Diarrhoea can occur in non-Caucasian children due to excessive milk ingestion. The temporary intolerance that occurs in toddlers after gastroenteritis is rarely a problem.
Coeliac disease, food allergy and cow's milk protein intolerance	Coeliac disease is a permanent intolerance to gluten. There are a variety of temporary intolerances and allergies which may produce failure to thrive with solid stools, diarrhoea, vomiting, acute colitis or even anaphylactoid reactions.
Giardia lamblia infection	_Giardia lamblia_ is endemic in all parts of the world and is often circulated by the oro-faecal route. It may be asymptomatic, cause episodes of explosive diarrhoea or cause chronic diarrhoea and failure to thrive. Examination of fresh stool may reveal cysts but examination of duodenal aspirate (the site of infection) is more sensitive. Treatment is with metronidazole. Bacterial overgrowth in the small bowel can also cause problems.
Inflammatory bowel disease	Crohn's disease and ulcerative colitis can present with growth failure and diarrhoea.
Pancreatic insufficiency	Cystic fibrosis commonly presents with malabsorption of fat due to pancreatic insufficiency and a sweat test should be performed in such cases. Shwachman–Diamond syndrome is the rare association of pancreatic failure and neutropenia.
Inborn errors	Sucrase-isomaltase deficiency is a rare inability to break down disaccharides for absorption. There is explosive acidic diarrhoea. Lymphangiectasia and abetalipoproteinaemia (**Fig. 11.13**) are disorders of fat absorption.
Immunodeficiency states	Often due to chronic bacterial, viral or giardial infection.

Fig. 11.12 _Causes of failure to thrive and diarrhoea._

fallen in recent years and this may be related to later introduction of gluten into the diet at the time of weaning.

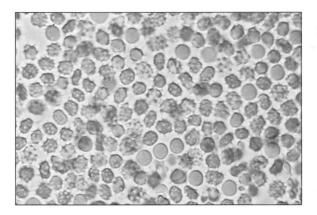

Fig. 11.13 *Acanthocytosis in abetalipoproteinaemia.*

There are a series of presentations:
- The classical presentation of failure to thrive in a miserable and pot-bellied child is rarely seen now (**Fig. 11.14**). There is wasting of the buttocks and bulky malabsorption stools.
- More commonly there is a relatively well child who may have failure to thrive but who often comes to attention because of anaemia due to malabsorption of iron in the affected proximal small intestine.
- Another group are those who have anti-gliadin, anti-endomysial and anti-reticulin antibodies but no clinical disease.

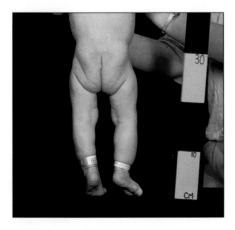

Fig. 11.14 *Wasted buttocks in coeliac disease.*

Management of coeliac disease

Investigation can be initiated by looking for antibodies but this is not specific enough and, since lifelong dietary exclusion of gluten is the management, it is important that the diagnosis be unequivocally confirmed. Temporary food intolerances are common in infants, and a child should also be over the age of 2 before a definite diagnosis is made. The diagnosis is reached by demonstrating typical mucosal atrophy with loss of villi and increased mitotic activity in the hyperplastic crypts while ingesting gluten (**Fig. 11.15a**), reversal of the lesion on stopping (**Fig. 11.15b**), and then recurrence of the atrophy or

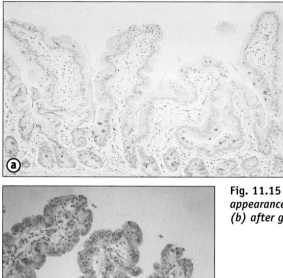

Fig. 11.15 *Jejunal biopsies showing appearances: (a) during gluten ingestion; (b) after gluten exclusion.*

recurrence of typical symptoms on reintroducing gluten. The proximal small bowel mucosa is biopsied by use of a peroral jejunal biopsy capsule. The child is sedated and the capsule positioned radiographically in the jejunum. The capsule is fired by suction and a small piece of mucosa removed. Alternatively, endoscopic guided biopsies may be taken.

Children feel much better and gain weight once on a gluten-free diet. Diet should be continued in adulthood as there is an increased risk of small bowel lymphoma in adults with coeliac disease which probably reverts to normal on a gluten-free diet. Dermatitis herpetiformis and a large joint arthropathy are also rare accompanying features.

ULCERATIVE COLITIS

Ulcerative colitis is a recurrent inflammatory condition of the mucosa; it may be confined to the distal colon and rectum but can also produce a pancolitis. The key symptoms are diarrhoea that may contain blood and mucus, abdominal pain and weight loss. Hypoalbuminaemia can occur due to protein loss from the bowel. The C reactive protein and anaemia reflect the severity of disease. Endoscopy shows characteristic macroscopic changes. The mucosa is friable, and areas of ulceration and regenerating mucosa produce a pseudopolyp appearance. The histological changes of acute and chronic inflammation and crypt abscesses are seen on biopsy (**Fig. 11.16**).

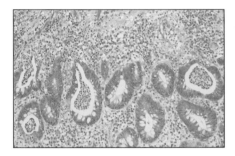

Fig. 11.16 *Histological changes of ulcerative colitis.*

Management of ulcerative colitis

The most worrying presentation is that of a severe fulminating colitis. These children are often very ill and need rehydration, blood and albumin, and total parenteral nutrition. Intravenous corticosteroids and broad spectrum antibiotics are also given. Toxic dilatation of the colon and perforation of the gut are complications that require surgery. For those in remission or with mild disease, topical corticosteroid enemas and sulphasalazine can be used to control the disease.

There is a risk of large bowel adenocarcinoma in adults, and endoscopy is used to monitor for possible neoplastic change at regular intervals. Severe colonic dysplasia is also an indication for colectomy with ileostomy, ileal reservoir or anal pull-through operations.

CROHN'S DISEASE

The presentation of Crohn's disease can be subtle; growth failure, failure to enter puberty or anorexia may be the main features. Diarrhoea and abdominal pain are the more common gastrointestinal symptoms. Peri-anal skin tags or an anal fissure, arthritis, clubbing, erythema nodosum, mouth ulcers and uveitis are other extra-intestinal features.

The disease can affect any part of the gut, from the lips (**Fig. 11.17**) to the anus. A white cell scan is a useful investigation in the diagnosis (**Fig. 11.18**), and the typical lesion seen on biopsy is a non-caseating epithelioid granuloma (**Fig. 11.19**). Although segments of the gut may be disease free, at endoscopy the affected areas show transmural inflammatory changes that can produce a cobblestone appearance (**Fig. 11.20**) and lead to fistula formation, or strictures (**Fig. 11.21**).

Haemoglobin, CRP or ESR, and serum albumin level reflect the severity of the disease.

Management of Crohn's disease

Induction of remission is achieved with a polymeric diet. This is a whole protein liquid feed which excludes other antigenic foodstuffs such as gluten and cow's milk protein, and has been shown to be more effective than steroids in producing remission. It is given for 8 weeks initially and can be used as maintenance therapy as 6 week cycles given every 4 months. Corticosteroids and azathioprine can be used in severe cases. Sulphasalazine is also used as maintenance therapy, especially in Crohn's colitis.

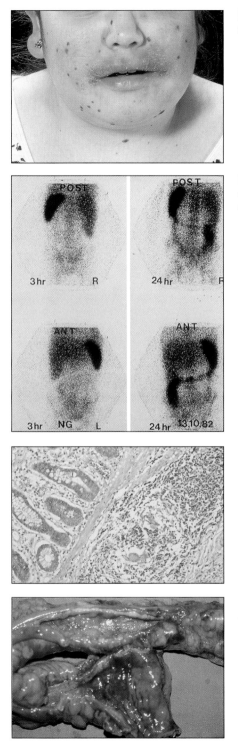

Fig. 11.17 *Crohn's disease involving the lip.*

Fig. 11.18 *Radioactive isotope labelling of white cells which then localize to areas of inflammation in the bowel.*

Fig. 11.19 *Histology of Crohn's disease.*

Fig. 11.20 *Cobblestone appearance of mucosa in Crohn's disease.*

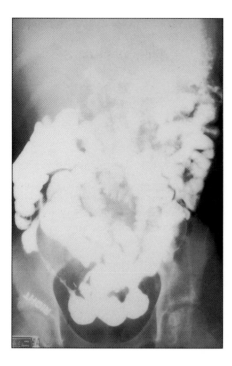

Fig. 11.21 *Barium enema examination showing an ileal stricture in Crohn's disease.*

Dietary measures are important in reversing growth failure; surgery for fistulae, strictures, or resistant disease producing growth failure may be necessary.

LIVER DISEASE

PERSISTENT LATE NEONATAL JAUNDICE

Some babies remain jaundiced after the first 14 days of life. The usual reason for this is breast milk jaundice, which carries no risks for the infant but often generates great anxiety for the family. The bilirubin is unconjugated; provided the baby is clinically well, the only tests to be performed are urine to exclude infection, urinary reducing substances for galactosaemia, and thyroid function tests to exclude hypothyroidism. Phototherapy is not needed, and the jaundice fluctuates but clears over the following weeks.

A persistent conjugated jaundice (more than 17% of the total bilirubin is conjugated) suggests liver disease. It is usually associated with a pale cholestatic stool and dark urine containing urobilinogen; later there may be failure to thrive.

Biliary atresia and neonatal hepatitis are the two main diagnoses to be considered.

Biliary atresia

There is absence or progressive destruction of the intrahepatic bile ducts in biliary atresia. It is the most important diagnosis to be excluded in a jaundiced infant as, if palliative surgery is carried out before 60 days, 80% of babies will achieve satisfactory bile drainage and avoid the need for early liver transplantation. However, the bile duct destruction continues throughout life; cirrhosis with portal hypertension eventually occurs and requires transplantation.

In practice, it is difficult to differentiate biliary atresia from other causes of neonatal hepatitis. Ultrasound, radioisotopic demonstration of impaired biliary excretion and liver biopsy may all be needed to suggest the correct diagnosis. The diagnosis is confirmed at laparotomy when the biliary tree cannot be demonstrated by cholangiography.

The Kasai procedure is a hepatoportoenterostomy—the anastomosis of the jejunum to the severed bile ducts at the porta hepatis.

Neonatal hepatitis syndrome

The collection of disorders representing neonatal hepatitis syndrome all have a similar clinical presentation, either as in biliary atresia or with growth retardation and hepatomegaly at birth. There is a non-specific diffuse inflammatory infiltrate on liver biopsy. A rapid search is made for congenital viral infections such as CMV or HBV; inborn errors of metabolism, such as galactosaemia; α_1-antitrypsin deficiency; and cystic fibrosis. Many babies who receive prolonged total parenteral nutrition suffer this form of liver dysfunction, and sometimes a laparotomy may be needed to exclude biliary atresia.

ACUTE LIVER DISEASE

Most acute disorders of the liver are due to viruses (**Fig. 11.22**). Acute liver failure is uncommon but can follow on from hepatitis A infection and require liver transplantation. Drugs, such as paracetamol in excess, cause liver toxicity, but halothane does not tend to cause hepatitis even after repeated exposure and remains an important anaesthetic agent in childhood. Other causes are Reye syndrome, overwhelming infection and metabolic disorders affecting the liver.

The management of acute liver failure is supportive. Hypoglycaemia is corrected with dextrose; clotting abnormalities with vitamin K and fresh frozen plasma; broad spectrum antibiotics are used to treat and prevent infection; gut bleeding is prevented with H_2 blockers; protein feeds are stopped and the bowel is cleared with regular lactulose to treat the hepatic encephalopathy. Cerebral oedema is treated with fluid restriction and mannitol.

REYE SYNDROME

Reye syndrome is a rare condition in which hepatic failure occurs and there is disruption of mitochondrial function. A variety of triggers, such as viruses and inborn errors of metabolism, have been suggested and aspirin has been incriminated in the pathogenesis. It is important to exclude metabolic disorders of fatty acid oxidation as there are specific measures for these illnesses.

The acute hepatic failure is accompanied by a prominent encephalopathy manifest by altered behaviour and consciousness, cerebral oedema and convulsions. Hypoglycaemia and deranged clotting and liver enzymes with elevated blood ammonia levels are seen, and liver biopsy shows fatty infiltration of the liver. Treatment is supportive and the condition is self limiting although there is a high mortality and morbidity.

CHILDHOOD CIRRHOSIS AND PORTAL HYPERTENSION

Cirrhosis is a pathological diagnosis suggesting extensive fibrosis and regenerative nodules (**Fig. 11.23**). It is the endpoint of a variety of liver disorders and is rare in childhood. Viral infections such as chronic hepatitis B, metabolic disorders such as tyrosinaemia, biliary obstruction as in cystic fibrosis, and biliary atresia and neonatal hepatitis are the commonest causes.

The symptoms of cirrhosis depend on whether there is sufficient hepatic function to meet the body's demands:

Clinical features of viral hepatitis

	Hepatitis A virus (HAV)	Hepatitis B virus (HBV)	Hepatitis C virus (HCV)
Transmission	Faeco-oral route	Vertical spread from mother to infant or lateral spread within families. Treatments involving blood products	Treatments involving blood products
Presentation	Frequently asymptomatic; incubation <3 months. Initial anorexia, pyrexia, nausea and vomiting which settle as the jaundice emerges	Incubation period 3–6 months then similar but more pronounced symptoms than HAV	Incubation period between HAV and HBV, frequently asymptomatic
Diagnosis	IgM antibody for HAV	Hepatitis B surface antigen and antibodies to HBV	HCV antibodies and PCR of viral RNA
Complications	Fulminant hepatic failure rarely occurs. Chronic carrier state does not occur	If the delta agent is transmitted, a chronic state occurs with progressive hepatic damage and increased risk of hepatocellular carcinoma. A few patients have acute hepatic failure	Subclinical carrier state is common with disordered transaminases. Risk of hepatocellular carcinoma
Prevention	Vaccination is available and contacts can be given immunoglobulin	Infants are vaccinated against hepatitis B at birth to prevent vertical transmission. Interferon may be of use	No vaccine

Fig. 11.22   Clinical features of viral hepatitis.

- Encephalopathy may occur during acute infection, due to the nitrogen load from gut bleeding, or with deteriorating hepatic function. Subtle changes in behaviour or sleep pattern can be difficult to identify in children.
- Portal hypertension produces varices in the lower oesophagus (**Fig. 11.24**) and haemorrhoids. Acute bleeding is treated with correction of clotting abnormalities, blood transfusion, and endoscopic sclerotherapy.

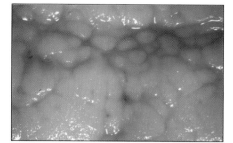

Fig. 11.23 *Cirrhosis.*

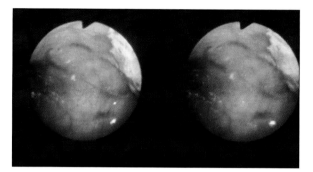

Fig. 11.24 *Oesophageal varices seen at endoscopy.*

- Ascites occurs due to hypoalbuminaemia, sodium retention and renal compromise and the hydrostatic effects of portal hypertension. It is treated with diuretics and sodium and fluid restriction.
- Spontaneous bacterial peritonitis is common.

LIVER TRANSPLANTATION

Liver transplantation is performed for acute or chronic endstage liver failure. As in other transplantation programmes, the child and family require a great deal of evaluation and support. There is difficulty in finding small organs, and a lobe from an adult liver may be transplanted. Deaths tend to occur in the first months from infection (long-term immunosuppression is required), failure of the transplanted liver to function, and thrombosis of the hepatic artery. The 5 year survival is 75%.

chapter 12

Paediatric Cardiology

INTRODUCTION

Cardiac disease is common in children. The disorders are mainly congenital, but in many parts of the world rheumatic fever is becoming more prevalent again. Atherosclerotic heart disease may have its origins in childhood and be due to a combination of inherited and environmental factors. Some diagnoses, such as coarctation, are important as prompt attention can be life saving; others, notably the innocent murmur, simply require an explanation. Echocardiography has revolutionized the diagnosis of heart defects.

INCIDENCE, CAUSES AND RECURRENCE

Congenital heart disease occurs in 8 per 1000 live births; it is the most common congenital abnormality and often accompanies other congenital malformations (**Fig. 12.1**).

Most lesions occur as isolated instances, and polygenic inheritance can be presumed. However, chromosomal errors, autosomal gene defects and teratogens can produce heart lesions (**Fig. 12.2**). Family studies indicate that there is a recurrence risk of about 2% for the next sibling after a child with a heart defect and up to 6% if two children are affected. If the mother has a heart lesion the risk for her offspring can be 5–15%, depending on the lesion. Risks of 50% apply for autosomal dominant conditions, whilst teratogens may not be encountered again and hence the risk for future pregnancies is low.

Frequency of congenital heart lesions	
Lesion	Cardiac defects (%)
Ventricular septal defect (VSD)	33
Atrial septal defect (ASD)	9
Patent ductus arteriosus (PDA)	9
Pulmonary stenosis (PS)	8
Coarctation of the aorta	6
Aortic stenosis (AS)	6
Tetralogy of Fallot	5
Transposition of the great arteries (TGA)	4
Others	20

Fig. 12.1 *Frequency of congenital heart lesions.*

Accurate diagnosis of the heart lesion or syndrome will aid genetic counselling. Karyotyping by chorionic villus sampling or amniocentesis may be indicated.

Aetiology of congenital heart disease

Clinical syndrome	Cause	Associated defect
Down syndrome	Trisomy 21	Atrioventricular septal defect, VSD, PDA
Turner syndrome	Karyotype 45,XO	Coarctation of the aorta, aortic stenosis
Edwards syndrome	Trisomy 18	Septal defects
Noonan syndrome	Autosomal dominant	Pulmonary stenosis, cardiomyopathy
CHARGE (Heart)	Sporadic, genetic	Tetralogy of Fallot, PDA
VATER (VSD)	Sporadic	VSD
Maternal psychosis	Lithium	Ebstein's anomaly (Fig. 12.2b)
Parental epilepsy	Sodium valproate, phenytoin	Coarctation of aorta, aortic stenosis
Congenital infection	Rubella	Septal defects
Marfan syndrome	Autosomal dominant	Prolapsing mitral valve, aortic aneurysm formation
Infant of diabetic mother	Poor glycaemic control	Reversible hypertrophic obstructive cardiomyopathy, increased risk of all lesions

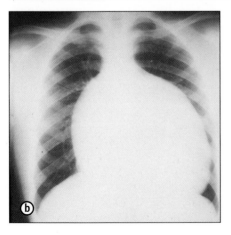

Fig. 12.2 (a) Aetiology of congenital heart disease; (b) X-ray showing appearance of Ebstein's anomaly—ventriculization of the tricuspid valve.

PRESENTATION OF HEART DISEASE

THE FETAL CIRCULATION

Prior to birth, little blood passes to the lungs; instead, the oxygenated placental blood streams through the foramen ovale and the ductus arteriosus to reach the systemic circulation. These channels close following birth, and blood must flow through the pulmonary arteries and the lungs to become oxygenated (**Fig. 12.3**). All blood leaving the heart and passing to the body must pass through the aortic valve and proximal aorta to reach the body, and obstructive lesions such as aortic stenosis and coarctation of the aorta will cause heart failure or shock as the fetal channels close. Similarly, in critical pulmonary stenosis, insufficient blood will pass through the lungs and the systemic blood will remain relatively deoxygenated.

Heart disease in children can present as an asymptomatic murmur, as heart failure, or as cyanosis (which may be episodic).

MURMURS

Murmurs are caused by turbulent blood flow. Although they are often found in the neonatal period, many are not detected until some months later because septal defects can only produce a murmur when pulmonary arterial pressure has fallen sufficiently to produce a pressure gradient across the defect and therefore flow through the hole. The timing of a murmur in the cardiac cycle and its position and radiation across the praecordium often allow identification of the heart lesion. It is always important to listen to the back as the murmurs of pulmonary stenosis, coarctation and patent arterial duct radiate through (**Fig. 12.4**).

Innocent murmurs can occur with structurally normal hearts. Often due to rapid flow through a normal pulmonary valve, e.g. with fever, anaemia or exercise, they can also be generated by vibration of blood in the large veins—a venous hum; others are heard just medial to the apex beat and are caused by turbulent flow over the trabeculae of the ventricles. Innocent murmurs are never associated with symptoms or abnormal signs. They are soft and systolic, and the second heart sound has normal splitting on inspiration. Variation on standing or turning the neck helps to make the diagnosis of a venous hum. If there is any doubt or parents need reassurance an echocardiogram performed by a paediatric cardiologist is essential.

CYANOSIS

Children often have blue extremities, may go blue around the mouth, or have blue lips due to vasomotor changes when cold or unwell. A blue tongue, however, indicates central cyanosis. Central cyanosis is caused by deoxygenated blood entering the systemic circulation (**Fig. 12.5**). If this is due to primary lung disease it can be corrected by giving 100% oxygen (the hyperoxia or nitrogen washout test); however, this is not the case in deoxygenated cyanotic heart disease where blood either bypasses the lungs or enters the systemic circulation. With time, cyanosis leads to polycythaemia which improves oxygen delivery to the tissues but predisposes to a high risk of thrombo-embolism and stroke. If there is a right to left shunt, cerebral abscesses may occur as bacteria are not filtered out in the lungs but can enter the systemic arterial circulation.

Clubbing of the fingers occurs with cyanosis in congenital heart disease. It is also seen in cystic fibrosis, cirrhosis of the liver and infective endocarditis (**Fig. 12.6**). There is initially a spongy feeling to the nail bed, then loss of the nail fold angle, increased curvature of the nail and finally a drumstick appearance to the finger.

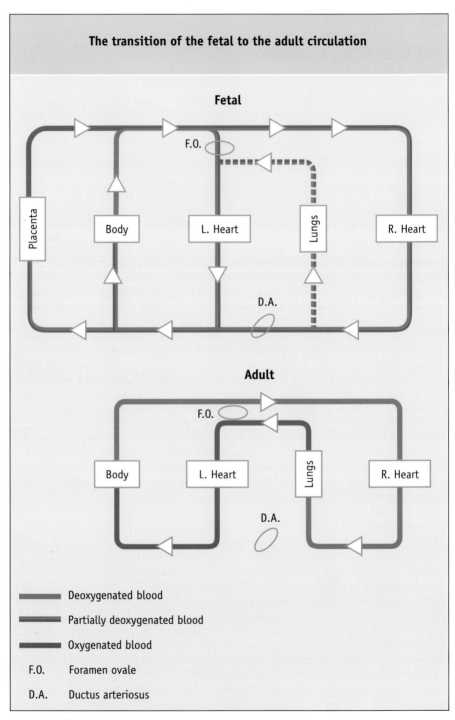

Fig. 12.3 *The transition of the fetal to the adult circulation.*

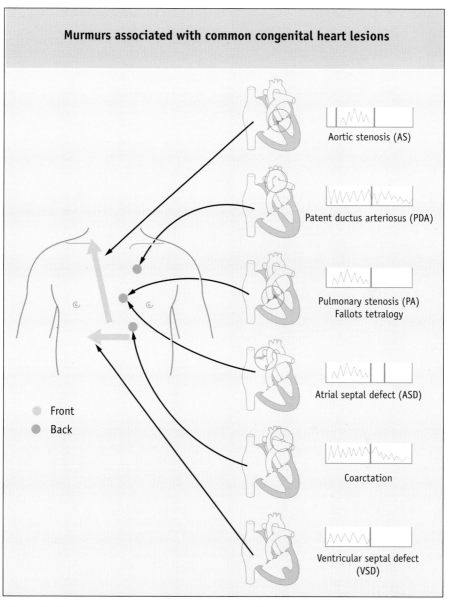

Murmurs associated with common congenital heart lesions

Aortic stenosis (AS)

Patent ductus arteriosus (PDA)

Pulmonary stenosis (PA)
Fallots tetralogy

Atrial septal defect (ASD)

Front
Back

Coarctation

Ventricular septal defect
(VSD)

Fig. 12.4 *Murmurs associated with common congenital heart lesions. The sites at which murmurs are classically heard are indicated on the left, and the intensity of the murmur is shown on the right.*

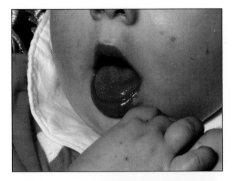

Fig. 12.5 *Children often have blue extremities due to vasomotor changes when cold or unwell. Similarly, they may go blue around the mouth or have blue lips. A blue tongue, however, indicates central cyanosis.*

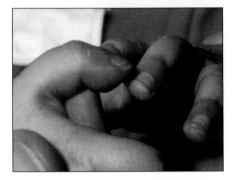

Fig. 12.6 *Clubbing in an infant with complex cyanotic heart disease. Clubbing is also seen in cystic fibrosis, cirrhosis of the liver and infective endocarditis.*

Transposition of the great arteries

In transposition of the great arteries the aorta and pulmonary artery originate from the wrong ventricles so that blood returning from the lungs is sent back into the lungs via the left ventricle and systemic venous blood is passed into the aorta from the right ventricle (**Fig. 12.7**). Persistence of the arterial duct and mixing of blood flows across the foramen ovale or a ventricular septal defect (VSD) provide oxygenated blood for the body. When there is little mixing and/or pulmonary stenosis, the infant will be deeply cyanosed.

During the first weeks of life transposition of the great arteries is the most common cause of cyanotic heart disease. Conversely, if there is a large communication between the two sides of the heart and no restriction to pulmonary blood flow, the cyanosis will be mild but, as the pulmonary resistance falls following birth, increasing amounts of blood will be recirculating through the lungs and heart failure will develop.

There may be no murmurs in transposition of the great arteries unless there is turbulence due to stenosis or a large flow across the pulmonary valve. The diagnosis is usually made when the duct closes and the baby becomes severely cyanosed. It is urgent to make a diagnosis before the baby becomes acidotic and sick. Echocardiography demonstrates the abnormal anatomy. The X-ray classically shows a narrow superior mediastinum and a large heart ('egg on its side'), and the ECG indicates right ventricular hypertrophy.

A prostaglandin infusion will usually reopen the arterial duct and temporarily improve cyanosis, but a balloon atrial septostomy (Rashkind procedure) is usually required and can be carried out in the intensive care unit under ultrasound guidance. During the Rashkind procedure a deflated balloon is passed into the right atrium and across the foramen ovale.

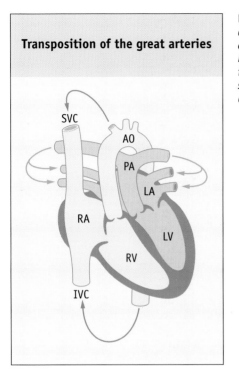

Transposition of the great arteries

SVC
AO
PA
LA
RA
LV
RV
IVC

Fig. 12.7 *In transposition of the great arteries the aorta and pulmonary artery originate from the wrong ventricles so that blood returning from the lungs is sent back into the lungs via the left ventricle and systemic venous blood is passed into the aorta from the right ventricle.*

It is then inflated and withdrawn sharply to produce a large tear in the atrial septum which improves cyanosis (**Fig. 12.8**). The definitive operation is an arterial switch procedure which involves transecting and correctly re-implanting the great vessels; this is carried out when the baby is stable.

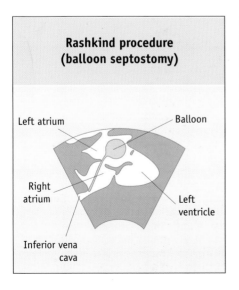

Rashkind procedure (balloon septostomy)

Left atrium
Balloon
Right atrium
Left ventricle
Inferior vena cava

Fig. 12.8 *Rashkind procedure. During the Rashkind procedure a deflated balloon is passed into the right atrium and across the foramen ovale. It is then inflated and withdrawn sharply to produce a large tear in the atrial septum which improves cyanosis.*

Tetralogy of Fallot

After the first year, the tetralogy of Fallot is the commonest cause of cyanotic heart disease. The four elements of the tetralogy are a consequence of anterior deviation of the intraventricular septum. A large VSD is produced, the pulmonary outflow tract (infundibulum) becomes narrowed, and the aorta appears to override the VSD. The right ventricle is exposed to high pressures, and hypertrophies (**Fig. 12.9**).

Although infants with the tetralogy are usually pink at birth, as they grow they may become increasingly cyanosed and clubbed as the pulmonary stenosis becomes more significant and blood flow to the lungs is reduced. Hypercyanotic spells—episodes of sudden severe cyanosis—are pathognomonic of tetralogy of Fallot. The episodes are caused

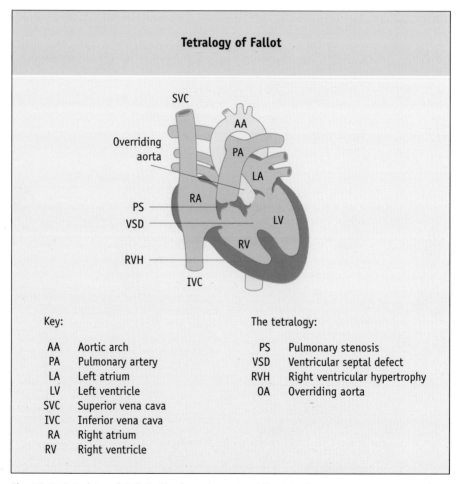

Tetralogy of Fallot

Key:

AA	Aortic arch
PA	Pulmonary artery
LA	Left atrium
LV	Left ventricle
SVC	Superior vena cava
IVC	Inferior vena cava
RA	Right atrium
RV	Right ventricle

The tetralogy:

PS	Pulmonary stenosis
VSD	Ventricular septal defect
RVH	Right ventricular hypertrophy
OA	Overriding aorta

Fig. 12.9 *Tetralogy of Fallot. The four elements of the tetralogy are a consequence of anterior deviation of the intraventricular septum. A large VSD is produced, the pulmonary outflow tract (infundibulum) becomes narrowed and the aorta appears to override the VSD. The right ventricle is exposed to systemic pressures and hypertrophy develops.*

by infundibular spasm and may be life threatening. Older children tire easily during play and are seen squatting as they recover (**Fig. 12.10**). This is because the vasodilatation produced during exercise causes a drop in systemic resistance and blood flows across the VSD away from the lungs and into the systemic circulation. Squatting compresses the inferior vena cava and increases systemic resistance, directing blood through the pulmonary stenosis and into the lungs rather than across the VSD.

Clinical examination also shows the parasternal heave of right ventricular hypertrophy, and an ejection systolic murmur representing flow across the narrowed pulmonary outflow (not the VSD).

The diagnosis is made with echocardiography but occasionally angiograms are required to make a proper assessment of the morphology of the heart (**Fig. 12.11**). The X-ray shows a boot shape to the heart because the hypertrophied right ventricle is prominent. The right ventricular hypertrophy can also be demonstrated on ECG (**Fig. 12.12**).

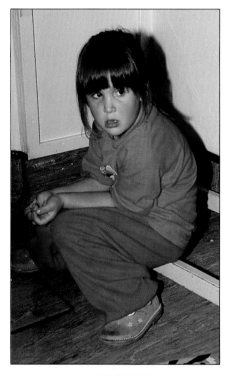

Fig. 12.10 *Squatting increases systemic vascular resistance and improves pulmonary blood flow in tetralogy of Fallot.*

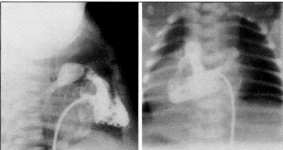

Fig. 12.11 *This angiogram clearly shows the hypertrophied right ventricle and infundibular stenosis in tetralogy of Fallot.*

153

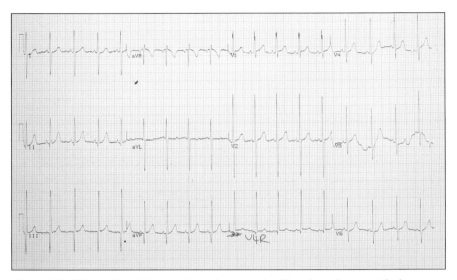

Fig. 12.12 *ECG showing right ventricular hypertrophy. There is an intraventricular conduction defect, a tall R wave in V4R (an extra lead placed over the right ventricle) and an upright T wave in V1.*

Propranolol can be used to prevent or treat spells. However, in symptomatic infants an artificial connection (shunt) between the systemic circulation and the pulmonary arteries can be constructed; this improves pulmonary blood flow and allows growth before further surgery is carried out (**Fig. 12.13**). The definitive repair involves closing the VSD and widening the pulmonary outflow with a pericardial patch if necessary.

Complex cyanotic congenital heart disease

Many rarer forms of congenital heart disease are associated with cyanosis. The severely disordered anatomy can be delineated by echocardiography. Children are usually cyanosed from birth and become clubbed. Treatment is initially to improve pulmonary blood flow during infancy, with a shunt, before an attempt to provide a definitive repair when the child is larger. It is often impossible to produce a biventricular heart as one ventricle may

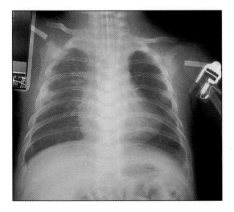

Fig. 12.13 *This infant with tetralogy of Fallot has had a shunt surgically inserted between the right subclavian artery and the right pulmonary artery. The improved blood flow can be seen as increased pulmonary markings in the right lung field.*

be too small to function. In these cases the superior and inferior venae cavae can be connected directly to the pulmonary arteries and the heart used to pump blood to the body (Fontan circulation).

HEART FAILURE

The heart can fail because of an inability to force blood through an obstruction, e.g. aortic stenosis, coarctation or pulmonary stenosis, or because of impaired function, e.g. cardiomyopathy or an arrhythmia. Persistent arterial duct, or atrial and ventricular septal defects all cause symptoms of heart failure when there is a large volume of blood shunting from the left (systemic) to the right (pulmonary) side of the circulation and the heart cannot manage to fulfil the body's requirements as well as recirculate blood through the lungs (**Fig. 12.14**). If the heart fails gradually, the symptoms and signs of heart failure

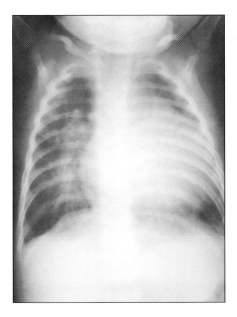

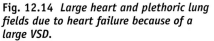
Fig. 12.14 *Large heart and plethoric lung fields due to heart failure because of a large VSD.*

Symptoms of heart failure

- Breathlessness and sweating—especially on feeding
- Failure to thrive
- Recurrent chest infections
- Fluid retention and paradoxical weight gain
- Tachycardia and gallop rhythm
- Hepatomegaly
- Elevated jugular venous pressure

develop. Treatment of heart failure is directed at the underlying cause but supportive measures such as nasogastric feeding of infants and use of diuretics may be needed.

Some shunts may be asymptomatic in childhood, but in later life the chronically increased pulmonary blood flow may lead to the Eisenmenger syndrome. Progressive elevation in pulmonary pressure causes reversed, or right to left, shunting of blood and increasing cyanosis. At this late stage heart–lung transplantation is the only option.

PATENT ARTERIAL DUCT

In fetal life, the arterial duct connects the pulmonary artery and the aorta to allow blood to short-circuit from the lungs to the body. Sometimes the arterial duct does not close after birth, and systemic arterial blood can flow into the lungs when the pulmonary artery pressures fall. In preterm infants this can lead to heart failure or inability to wean from ventilatory support; in other children an asymptomatic murmur is heard during a health check. Classically, there is a continuous murmur of blood flowing across the duct throughout systole and diastole. A loud second heart sound indicates elevated pulmonary artery pressure and a plethoric chest X-ray the large shunt of blood. Echocardiography will identify the open duct.

Pharmacological closure with indomethacin can be effective in preterm infants but ligation at thoracotomy may be necessary. In larger children it is now possible to close a patent duct with an occlusion device held on the end of a catheter and inserted through the femoral vein.

VENTRICULAR SEPTAL DEFECT

A rough systolic murmur suggests a VSD (**Fig. 12.15**); its intensity does not reflect the size of the hole. The activity of the cardiac apex, the loudness of the second sound and

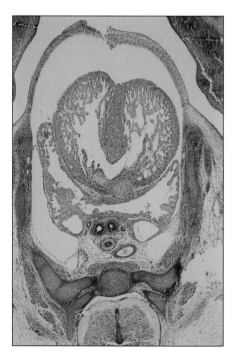

Fig. 12.15 *Ventricular septal defect in a developing mouse.*

symptoms of heart failure describe the magnitude of the shunt. As with a patent arterial duct the effects on the heart are demonstrated by left ventricular hypertrophy on ECG and plethoric lung fields on the X-ray, but echocardiography and colour Doppler imaging will identify the turbulent jet through the lesion.

Many lesions close spontaneously through childhood, but if there is heart failure resistant to treatment with diuretics, surgery with cardiopulmonary bypass is needed. Even if there are no symptoms but a defect is large and thought unlikely to close, surgery is essential to prevent the Eisenmenger syndrome.

ATRIAL SEPTAL DEFECT

Atrial septal defects cause wide fixed splitting of the aortic and pulmonary components of the second heart sound. The preferential flow of blood through the defect into the more distensible right ventricle produces a flow murmur at the pulmonary valve.

The X-ray may be normal or reveal plethoric lung fields and a large heart. There is right axis deviation on the ECG. Children are usually asymptomatic but closure is usually undertaken if the defect is large because of the danger of irreversible pulmonary hypertension in early adult life.

ATRIO-VENTRICULAR SEPTAL DEFECT

Atrio-ventricular septal defect is a more severe lesion and is commonly seen in infants with Down syndrome. As well as an atrial defect there is a large ventricular defect and the two are linked by a single valve rather than the usual tricuspid and mitral valves. The diagnosis is suggested by finding fixed splitting of the second sound, suggesting an atrial defect, together with left ventricular hypertrophy suggesting a ventricular defect. Echocardiography will fully characterize the defect.

AORTIC STENOSIS

In aortic stenosis the valve is often thickened or bicuspid. If it is critically stenosed, the infant will present in the neonatal period with heart failure as the arterial duct closes. In milder disease a murmur may be the only finding, but fatigue, dizziness, or loss of consciousness on exercise can occur. The pulse is of low volume and prolonged, there is a systolic murmur radiating to the neck accompanied by a thrill in the supraclavicular notch, and an opening click is heard to precede the murmur. The ECG (**Fig. 12.16**) is useful to monitor the development of left ventricular hypertrophy. There are large voltage complexes which may be accompanied by ST depression in the leads that lie over the left ventricle (V5 and V6). Echocardiography will demonstrate the abnormal valve and any other accompanying lesions. The pressure gradient across the valve can be measured using the Doppler principle; relief of the stenosis is required if the gradient is greater than 60 mmHg. This can be done during a catheter study when pressures can be measured directly and a balloon used to stretch the valve. Valvuloplasty can also be performed at open surgery. The valve will eventually need replacing in adult life.

COARCTATION OF THE AORTA

Coarctation of the aorta occurs near the origin of the ductus arteriosus just below the subclavian artery and probably arises because of ectopic ductal tissue spilling into the aortic wall. When the duct closes, the aorta is pinched and the severe obstruction produces cardiomegaly and pulmonary oedema. The body distal to the coarctation is deprived of blood, leading to cardiogenic shock with acidosis, oliguria and absent femoral pulses.

A prostaglandin E_2 infusion is used to re-open the arterial duct. Surgical repair of the coarctation is performed once the acidosis and heart failure are stabilized. The area of

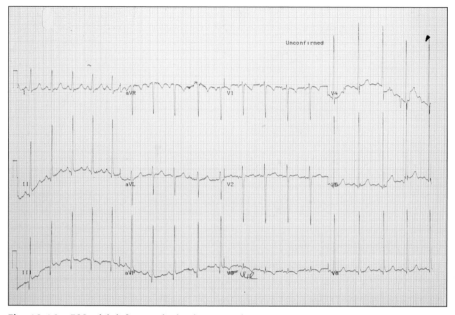

Fig. 12.16   ECG with left ventricular hypertrophy.

narrowing can be excised and an end-to-end anastomosis performed, or the area can be widened using a flap formed from the subclavian artery (**Fig. 12.17**) or a Goretex patch.

Mild coarctation may present later in childhood with weak or absent femoral pulses and hypertension in the upper body. A systolic murmur of the coarctation may be heard on auscultation of the back. Collateral vessels bypassing the area of aortic narrowing may be felt to pulsate over the scapulae and be seen as rib notching on the chest X-ray. Surgery is again required to widen the narrowing and halt the hypertension. Balloon dilatation of aortic coarctation does not seem to be successful as a primary treatment, but may have a role if the surgical repair becomes narrow later in life (**Fig. 12.18**).

PULMONARY STENOSIS

In mild cases of pulmonary stenosis the child will be pink and asymptomatic but have a systolic murmur radiating through to the back. With more severe stenosis there may be limitation of exercise tolerance and right ventricular hypertrophy (*see* Fig. 12.12). If, in conjunction with the pulmonary stenosis, there is also a VSD, this will allow deoxygenated blood from the right ventricle to pass into the systemic circulation and produce cyanosis. The diagnosis is made by echocardiography and the gradient across the valve can be measured by Doppler ultrasound. Treatment by valvuloplasty during cardiac catheterization is usually successful.

EXTRACORPOREAL MEMBRANE OXYGENATION (ECMO)

In many conditions in which the heart or lungs have failed but recovery is expected to occur soon, the body can be supported by an external pump and oxygenation system (**Fig. 12.19**). This technique is a modification of the bypass machines used during open

Surgical repair of coarctation of the aorta

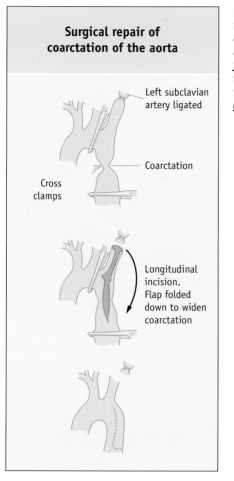

Left subclavian artery ligated

Coarctation

Cross clamps

Longitudinal incision. Flap folded down to widen coarctation

Fig. 12.17 *The subclavian flap repair is the commonest operation performed for coarctation. The subclavian artery is ligated and the proximal stump opened to form a flap which can be folded down to widen the area of narrowing. Collateral vessels provide blood to the left arm which grows and functions normally.*

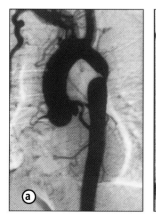

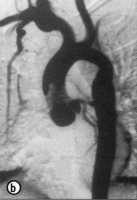

Fig. 12.18 *Angiograms showing appearances (a) before and (b) after balloon dilatation of previously repaired but re-stenosed coarctation. (The left subclavian artery was used in the initial flap repair.)*

159

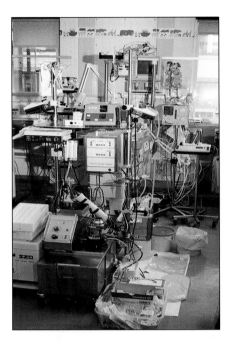

Fig. 12.19 *ECMO machine.*

heart surgery. In order to obtain a sufficient flow of blood through the machine the right atrium and the internal carotid artery are cannulated (**Fig. 12.20**).

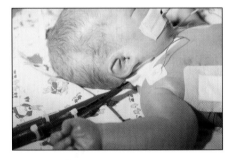

Fig. 12.20 *Large cannulae inserted into the internal carotid artery and right atrium for ECMO.*

ARRHYTHMIAS

PAROXYSMAL SUPRAVENTRICULAR TACHYCARDIA

Paroxysmal supraventricular tachycardia is the only frequently encountered arrhythmia in children. It occurs in normal hearts but particularly in Ebstein's anomaly (*see* Fig. 12.2b) and the Wolff–Parkinson–White syndrome. The abnormal connections in Wolff–Parkinson–White syndrome are suggested by the short PR interval and slurring on the upstroke of the R wave (**Fig. 12.21**). Palpitations may be felt by older children when the supraventricular tachycardia occurs and they may feel faint and become unwell. Babies do not tolerate the tachycardia and rapidly become shocked. Vagal manoeuvres such as the diving reflex are very effective at terminating a paroxysm but if this fails an intravenous bolus of adenosine, which blocks accessory pathways momentarily, is usually effective in stopping the arrhythmia and confirming the diagnosis of supraventricular tachycardia (**Fig. 12.22**). Cardioversion may be required in an ill infant. Flecainide or digoxin is used to prevent recurrence; catheter ablation of the abnormal connections with radio frequency is a permanent solution.

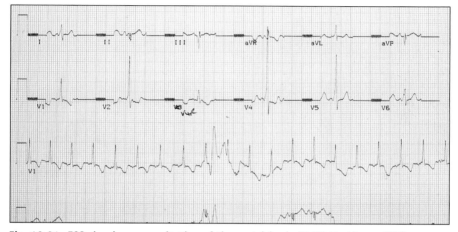

Fig. 12.21 *ECG showing pre-excitation of the ventricles in Wolff–Parkinson–White syndrome.*

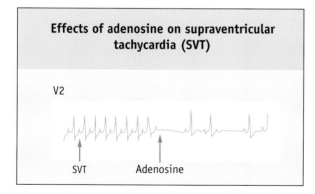

Fig. 12.22 *ECG showing effect of adenosine on supraventricular tachycardia.*

CONGENITAL HEART BLOCK

Infants whose mothers have autoimmune disease and carry anti-Ro antibodies may have complete heart block. There is no relationship between the P waves and the QRS complexes on the ECG (**Fig. 12.23**). The low heart rates that can occur are often well tolerated but pacemakers are usually inserted (**Fig. 12.24**).

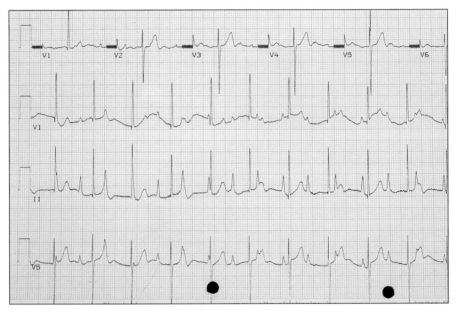

Fig. 12.23 *ECG showing complete heart block.*

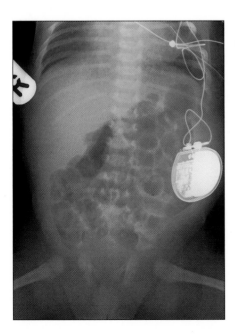

Fig. 12.24 *Pacemaker inserted in neonate for congenital complete heart block.*

BACTERIAL ENDOCARDITIS

In bacterial endocarditis the area of endocardium that is struck by turbulent blood becomes infected, often by *Streptococcus faecalis* released during minor operations or dental work. These bacteria form and harbour in vegetations (**Fig. 12.25**). The child is unwell and the emboli produced from the vegetations may cause splinter haemorrhages seen in the nail beds, necrotic skin lesions and haematuria. The spleen is usually enlarged and there are often changes in the cardiac signs. The white cell count and ESR are raised. Bacterial endocarditis should be considered in any child with a heart lesion and an unexplained pyrexial illness. Serial blood cultures are taken to identify the organisms before a minimum of 6 weeks' intravenous antibiotics are given.

Consideration of antibiotic prophylaxis and good dental hygiene is important for all children with congenital heart disease.

RHEUMATIC FEVER

Rheumatic fever is a systemic illness, thought to be of an autoimmune nature, caused by a preceding group A streptococcal throat infection. After an interval of a few weeks, a migratory polyarthritis, rash and pancarditis occur. A pericardial rub, and murmurs due to regurgitation through inflamed heart valves may be heard. St Vitus' dance is a chorea that is sometimes seen. Treatment is mainly symptomatic with analgesia for the arthritis but as the illness settles the valves may be left scarred with residual mitral or aortic regurgitation and stenosis. Repeated episodes are common and prophylactic penicillin is used to avoid further streptococcal infections.

HYPERTENSION

Hypertension is uncommon in children, and most mild cases are essential in origin. More severe hypertension is often due to primary renal disease such as glomerulonephritis and

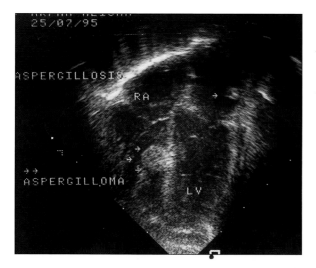

Fig. 12.25 *Large vegetations in a child with fungal endocarditis.*

renal artery stenosis, coarctation of the aorta, or endocrine causes such as phaeochromocytoma or Cushing syndrome. Repeated measurements with the correct size of cuff are essential to identify children with hypertension; normal values for age are found in standard textbooks.

ISCHAEMIC HEART DISEASE

Ischaemic heart disease is the major cause of death in adults. Its origins lie in a genetic predisposition to atheroma compounded by the effects of the modern lifestyle. Although familial hypercholesterolaemia (**Fig. 12.26**) does occur in an autosomal dominant fashion, it is rare. Prevention of heart disease is based on dietary reduction in saturated fats, avoidance of smoking, and regular exercise.

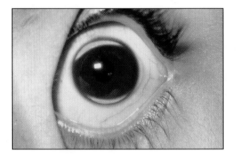

Fig. 12.26 *Arcus senilis in hypercholesterolaemia.*

chapter 13

Respiratory Disorders

Respiratory disorders account for about half of all paediatric consultations. The average young child has up to eight viral upper respiratory tract infections (URTIs) each year and this is especially true if there are older siblings to bring infections home; it is not uncommon to meet a child with a constantly runny nose. Passive exposure to cigarette smoke, gas heaters and cooking, and the inner-city atmosphere are all implicated in this high morbidity.

THE UPPER RESPIRATORY TRACT

THE COMMON COLD (CORYZA)

Rhinorrhoea, cough with clear phlegm, pyrexia, diarrhoea and vomiting, earache or rash in a relatively well child is strongly suggestive of a viral infection, usually with one of the many strains of rhinovirus. Paracetamol for the child and a reassuring explanation for the parents is all that is usually required. If there is evidence of a secondary bacterial bronchitis, with green phlegm, antibiotics can be given.

TONSILLITIS AND PHARYNGITIS

Pharyngitis, or a sore throat, is usually caused by an adenovirus, rhinovirus or group A streptococcal infection. The tonsils are masses of lymphoid tissue that guard the throat and often enlarge in response to a viral pharyngitis. Tonsillitis (**Fig. 13.1**), infection of the tonsils themselves, is much less common and usually due to group A streptococcal infection or Epstein–Barr virus.

In both conditions, the child has a sore throat with difficulty swallowing, is pyrexial and ill. Examination reveals inflammation of the tonsils or pharyngeal wall, often with an exudate. It is not easy to distinguish between viral pathogens and bacteria, and antibiotics such as penicillin are usually given for severe symptoms. Ampicillin and its derivatives are

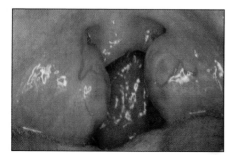

Fig. 13.1 Tonsillitis. Viruses are responsible for two thirds of the cases of tonsillitis seen, but clinically it is difficult to differentiate these from bacterial infections.

avoided as they can cause a diffuse maculopapular rash if the child has glandular fever (*see* Fig. 9.11).

PERITONSILLAR ABSCESS

A peritonsillar abscess, or quinsy, is rare and usually occurs in adolescents. Intravenous penicillin is given and any collection of pus is drained. This is usually an indication for tonsillectomy when the infection has settled.

Recurrent tonsillitis disrupting schooling is also cited as a reason for tonsillectomy. This is controversial as the tonsils (like the adenoids) become smaller after the age of 6 years; also, many apparent episodes of tonsillitis are in fact pharyngitis and will continue after the operation. Upper airway obstruction by large tonsils, leading to obstructive sleep apnoea, is also an indication for operation. Similarly, adenoids are often removed if they obstruct the posterior nasal space and cause snoring or if they block the origin of the Eustachian tube and lead to glue ear.

SINUSITIS

Sinusitis is not a problem in young children as the sinuses are not fully developed. Pain over the eyebrow together with a temperature in the older child should raise concerns of frontal sinusitis. Prompt antibiotic treatment.

ACUTE OTITIS MEDIA

Infection of the middle ear is a common finding in children. The cause can be viral or bacterial but it is not possible to distinguish them clinically. The child may appear irritable and miserable with a pyrexia but no localizing features. The diagnosis may be missed unless the eardrums are inspected for bulging redness with prominent blood vessels. Antibiotics are often given but spontaneous resolution often occurs when pus in the middle ear discharges through the tympanic membrane. Recurrent infections are seen in immunodeficiency states and with glue ear.

GLUE EAR

It has been estimated that up to 90% of children will have at least one episode of glue ear—an accumulation of fluid in the middle ear in the absence of acute infection. It occurs because of eustachian tube dysfunction and loss of ventilation to the middle ear causing a vacuum effect. Thus there is increased production of mucus and poor drainage of secretions. The condition is intimately associated with acute otitis media as infection leads to chronic effusion and effusion predisposes to infection. There is an association with parental smoking. Glue ear is very common in Down syndrome and almost universal in cleft palate.

The effect of glue ear is to muffle sound; low frequencies tend to be affected more than high. Some children will have marked interference with hearing and sometimes speech, leading to difficulties at school, but often the condition goes unrecognized, especially if unilateral. The appearances of the eardrum are variable but classically the drum is dull (**Fig. 13.2**) and there is loss of the light reflex. Pneumatic otoscopy (puffing air at the drum and looking for movement) is a method of diagnosis, as is tympanometry (**Figs 13.3, 13.4**) which is measurement of the resonance of the eardrum and middle ear cavity.

Management of glue ear

As glue ear has a fluctuating course and often resolves by itself, it is sensible to wait some months before intervening. The aim of surgery is to improve hearing; if the glue ear is unilateral or there is minimal hearing loss and no other disturbance of speech or schooling,

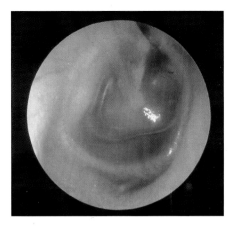

Fig. 13.2 *Glue ear.*

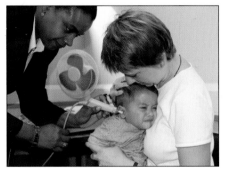

Fig. 13.3 *Tympanometry is a sensitive method of detecting glue ear.*

surgery may not improve matters. For those with chronic effusions causing problems the usual approach is to place a ventilation tube (grommet) in the eardrum (**Fig. 13.5**). This produces improvement while the device is in place but grommets fall out within 6–12 months, often with recurrence of effusion. Large adenoids may exacerbate glue ear, and adenoidectomy may be of use.

STRIDOR

ACUTE STRIDOR

Stridor is an inspiratory whooping noise caused by obstruction to airflow above, or at, the level of the glottis, whilst expiratory wheeze indicates obstruction below the cords in the small airways, as seen in asthma.

The common causes of acute stridor all constitute medical emergencies. Epiglottitis, croup (laryngo-tracheobronchitis) and inhaled foreign body may be distinguished on clinical grounds.

Foreign body — There is usually a history of aspiration when a foreign body lodges in the upper airways. Coughing and spluttering accompanies the onset of stridor which may vary in pitch or intensity as the object moves. It is always important to consider a foreign body, especially in small infants, as urgent removal by bronchoscopy is required. Many foreign bodies are not visible on X-rays but they can act as a ball valve and cause overinflation of

167

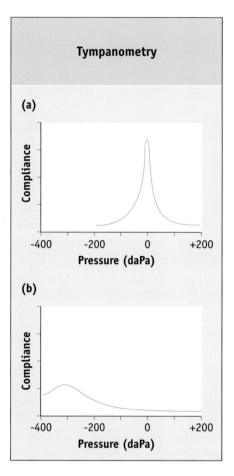

Fig. 13.4 *Tympanometry. The compliance of a normal tympanic membrane is recorded as a bell-shaped curve (a). In glue ear there is a flattening of the curve and the peak is shifted towards negative pressure due to fluid in the middle ear and the partial vacuum (b).*

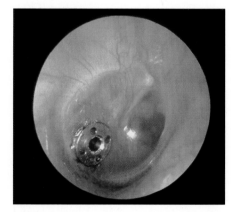

Fig. 13.5 *Grommet in eardrum.*

one lung (**Fig. 13.6**) and persistent abnormalities of perfusion/ventilation even after removal (**Fig. 13.7**).

Croup — Croup begins as a coryzal illness with an increasingly prominent barking cough and progressive stridor. It is often caused by para-influenza b. Stridor is worse at night or when the child is upset. Increasing recession, tachycardia and desaturation indicate worsening airways obstruction. Nebulized budesonide on admission may reduce severity of the symptoms; if airways obstruction is imminent, adrenaline may provide temporary relief while arrangements are made to provide an airway by intubation.

Epiglottitis — Epiglottitis is a pyrexial illness caused by *Haemophilus influenzae* type b. It is now much less common because of the Hib vaccine. The child is toxic with rapidly worsening stridor and drooling and does not cough. Attempts to view the throat can lead to complete obstruction of the airway and should not be attempted. If the diagnosis is

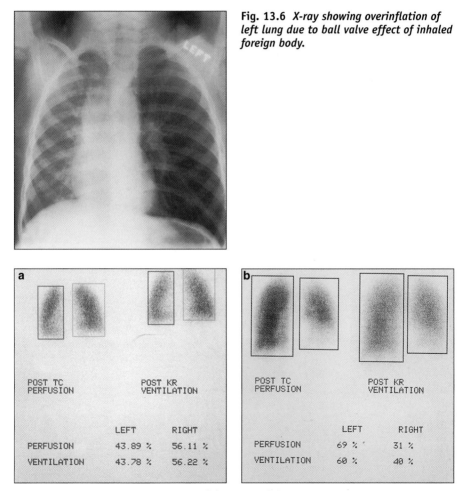

Fig. 13.6 *X-ray showing overinflation of left lung due to ball valve effect of inhaled foreign body.*

Fig. 13.7 *Ventilation–perfusion scan: (a) normal, (b) right basal perfusion–ventilation defect following inhalation of foreign body.*

169

suspected the child should be taken to theatre where the epiglottis can be inspected and intubation performed (**Fig. 13.8**). A swollen and cherry-red epiglottis is diagnostic, and swabs can be taken for bacterial culture; antibiotics such as cefuroxime or ampicillin, that are active against Haemophilus, are used.

CHRONIC STRIDOR

There are a number of possible reasons for a history of stridor from early infancy. Most cases are due to a floppy larynx—laryngomalacia—but a congenital web, vocal cord paralysis, and subglottic stenosis after prolonged intubation (**Fig. 13.9**) are other causes. A vascular ring around the trachea and oesophagus is a rarer cause—both dysphagia and stridor may be present. Although many lesions can be corrected surgically, tracheostomy is often needed (**Fig. 13.10**).

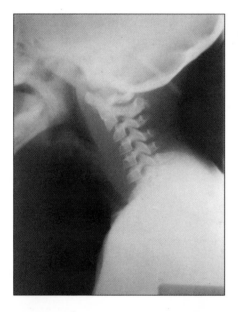

Fig. 13.8 *X-ray showing swelling of the epiglottis which occludes the airway.*

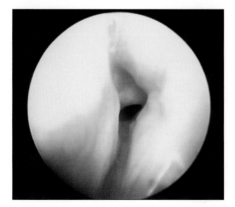

Fig. 13.9 *Subglottic stenosis following prolonged neonatal intubation.*

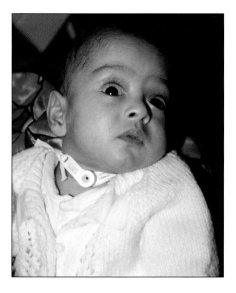

Fig. 13.10 *Tracheostomy.*

THE LOWER RESPIRATORY TRACT

BRONCHIOLITIS

Bronchiolitis is confined to infants under the age of 10 months. The illness is caused mainly by respiratory syncytial virus (RSV) and occurs in winter epidemics. The diagnosis is made on clinical grounds from a coryzal illness which quickly leads to tachypnoea (**Fig. 13.11**), overinflation of the chest, and wheeze. Crackles may be heard on auscultation, and the pneumonitis may produce cyanosis.

X-rays demonstrate overinflation and areas of collapse due to occlusion of smaller airways by oedema and slough (**Fig. 13.12**). RSV can be identified in nasopharyngeal secretions by immunofluorescence. Infants may need oxygen and nasogastric or even intravenous fluids; they usually recover over a few days. Some babies become apnoeic and require ventilation. Ribavirin, a nebulized antiviral agent, is costly and probably adds no real clinical benefit. Nebulized ipatropium bromide or salbutamol is usually ineffective. Antibiotics are not required except for secondary infection.

Fig. 13.11 *Normal respiratory rates.*

Normal ranges for respiratory rates	
Age (years)	Respiratory rate (breaths/min)
<1	25–35
1–5	20–30
5–12	20–25
>12	15–25

171

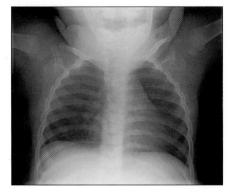

Fig. 13.12 *Bronchiolitis.*

PNEUMONIA

Pneumonia is infection of lung parenchyma; it is either confined to lung segments (lobar pneumonia) or is diffuse and peribronchial (bronchopneumonia). Bacterial pneumonia often follows a viral infection or occurs in association with an underlying predisposing condition such as immunodeficiency, cystic fibrosis, anatomical abnormalities, or aspiration.

In practice, many postviral infections probably go unrecognized as antibiotics are prescribed in the community for cough and a temperature before clinical or radiological signs are established (**Figs 13.13–18**).

The causative bacteria and, therefore, appropriate therapy can be deduced from the child's age and clinical presentation (**Fig. 13.19**). Many children with pneumonia are relatively well and can often be treated with oral antibiotics provided they can tolerate oral intake. However, if there is any doubt it is always safer to give intravenous antibiotics initially.

CLINICAL FEATURES

Infants and young babies with pneumonia may present only with signs of systemic illness and pyrexia. Alternatively, tachypnoea may be the only sign indicating an infection in the chest. It is therefore sensible to take an X-ray of any infant in whom pneumonia may be a possibility. In older children the picture is more typical. There is a cough which may produce purulent sputum and tachypnoea. Grunting, nasal flaring and cyanosis (due to

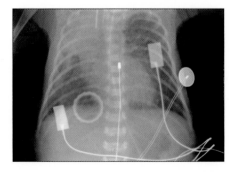

Fig. 13.13 *Right upper lobe consolidation/collapse in a preterm infant.*

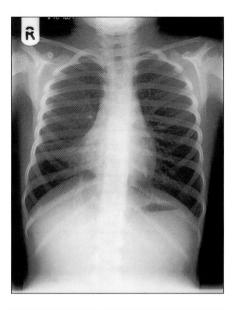

Fig. 13.14 *Right middle lobe consolidation suggested by loss of right heart border.*

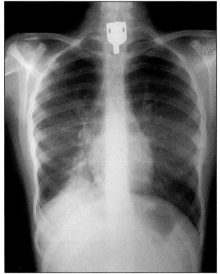

Fig. 13.15 *Right lower lobe consolidation indicated by loss of right hemidiaphragm.*

V/Q mismatch) are all signs of severe disease. It may not be possible to demonstrate the classical physical signs of dullness to percussion, increased vocal fremitus, bronchial breathing and crepitations. Similarly an X-ray may not show opaque lung tissue in the early stages.

PATHOGENS

Streptococcal pneumonia

Streptococcus pneumoniae is the commonest bacterial cause of pneumonia, especially in the younger child. There is an acute illness; the child is pyrexial and looks toxic, often

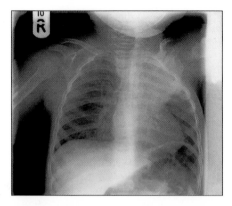

Fig. 13.16 *Left upper lobe consolidation.*

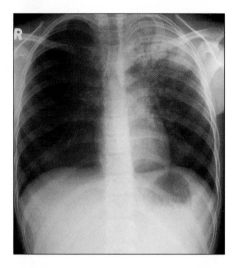

Fig. 13.17 *Left upper lobe collapse/consolidation.*

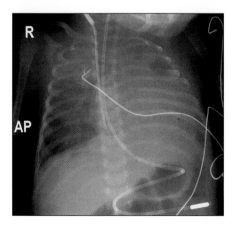

Fig. 13.18 *Left lower lobe collapse/consolidation.*

Antibiotic choices for pneumonia in childhood

Age group/cause	Organisms	Antibiotic
Neonates	Group B streptococcus, coliforms and *Staphylococcus aureus*	Penicillin and an aminoglycoside (gentamicin or amikacin), or a third generation cephalosporin (cefotaxime).
Infants	Pneumococcus, *Haemophilus influenzae, Staphylococcus aureus* (particularly with cystic fibrosis)	Amoxycillin or a cephalosporin. If ill or *Staph. aureus* is likely then flucloxacillin and gentamicin.
Children	Pneumococcus, *Haemophilus influenzae, Mycoplasma pneumoniae*	Amoxycillin or a cephalosporin. If Mycoplasma is likely, consider erythromycin.
Aspiration/foreign body	Secondary infection with *Streptococcus pneumoniae* or *Haemophilus influenzae*	Amoxycillin or cephalosporin. Metronidazole is not necessary as anaerobes are sensitive to usual antibiotics.
Immunosuppressed	Gram positive organisms and Pseudomonas, Klebsiella	Broad spectrum coverage such as piperacillin or ceftazidime, with gentamicin.
	If central venous catheters, coagulase negative staphylococci	Vancomycin if line infection is suspected.
	Fungal infections	Systemic antifungal therapy.
	Pneumocystis carinii pneumonia (PCP)	Co-trimoxazole for PCP.

Fig. 13.19 *Antibiotic choices for pneumonia in childhood.*

having referred shoulder tip or abdominal pain. The radiograph shows lobar consolidation. Classical clinical signs of bronchial breathing, dullness to percussion and coarse crackles are often found. There may be a pleural effusion which can cause stony dullness on percussion, decreased breath sounds and vocal fremitus. Rapid improvement occurs after antibiotics are started. Some children are at increased risk of pneumococcal infection. These include children with nephrotic syndrome and hyposplenism, particularly those with sickle cell disease. Such children are given long-term prophylactic penicillin and pneumococcal vaccination.

Staphylococcal pneumonia
Staphylococcal pneumonia is a rare but potentially devastating pneumonia, usually affecting infants under 1 year of age. The infant is extremely sick. Lobar changes occur, often accompanied by empyema and multiple lung abscesses (Fig. 13.20). Prolonged antibiotic therapy, drainage of the pus and stripping of thickened pleura may be required. Tests for cystic fibrosis must always be done.

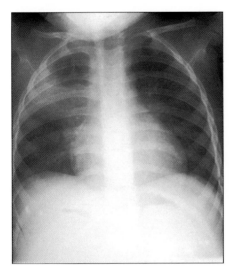

Fig. 13.20 *Cavitating consolidation in staphylococcal pneumonia.*

Viral agents

Viruses are probably the commonest causes of pneumonia in childhood. The usual types are respiratory syncytial virus (RSV), adenovirus (**Fig. 13.21**), influenza and para-influenza. All produce a spectrum of clinical illness, from mild tachypnoea in a child with a head cold to a gravely ill infant with marked cardiorespiratory distress. RSV and adenovirus are especially dangerous in small infants.

The degree of respiratory embarrassment parallels the degree of lung involvement, but apart from crackles there may be no other signs. Patchy diffuse changes or areas of segmental collapse that may be due to mucous plugging can be difficult to differentiate from bacterial infection and it is sensible to give an appropriate antibiotic to cover this eventuality.

The mortality and morbidity from viral infections is low, but adenovirus can cause obliterative bronchiolitis—destruction of the smaller airways.

Mycoplasma

Mycoplasma is a common but often unrecognized pathogen affecting children of school age and young adults. There is a generalized illness with pyrexia and malaise which may overshadow the respiratory signs, but X-rays show dramatic shadows (**Fig. 13.22**). Rising IgM titres to Mycoplasma are diagnostic, and cold agglutinins produce rouleaux on the

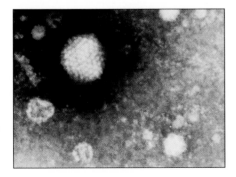

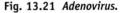

Fig. 13.21 *Adenovirus.*

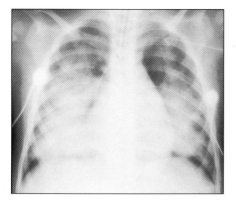

Fig. 13.22 *Mycoplasma pneumoniae.*

blood film. Culture of the organism is difficult. Untreated, the illness is self limiting but erythromycin is usually given and may shorten the duration.

UNUSUAL CIRCUMSTANCES

If pneumonia is recurrent, slow to clear, or recurs in the same areas it is as well to think of an underlying cause, e.g. foreign body, congenital abnormality (**Fig. 13.23**), aspiration, cystic fibrosis, immunodeficiency, HIV or tuberculosis. Abnormalities in cilial structure and movement are associated with recurrent chest infections (**Fig. 13.24**) and many of these children also have dextrocardia.

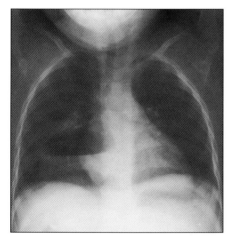

Fig. 13.23 *Bronchogenic cyst causing recurrent infection.*

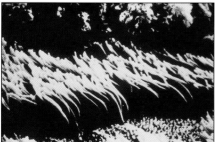

Fig. 13.24 *Cilia taken from the nose can be examined for their beating.*

TUBERCULOSIS

Tuberculosis is returning as a major worldwide problem. Primary infection can occur anywhere in the body, including the lungs, cervical glands and gastrointestinal tract. When it occurs in the lungs there may be a minor peripheral lesion but massive hilar lymphadenopathy (**Fig. 13.25**). This leads to lobar collapse. Systemic spread of the bacteria is responsible for miliary tuberculosis, which has a characteristic X-ray appearance (**Fig. 13.26**). Caseating pulmonary tuberculosis is seen in adults after secondary infection or reactivation of dormant bacteria.

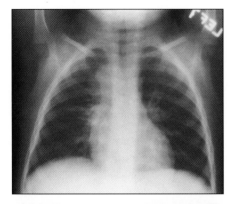

Fig. 13.25 *Massive hilar lymphadenopathy due to tuberculosis.*

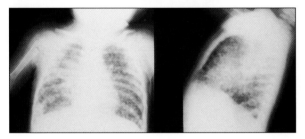

Fig. 13.26 *Miliary tuberculosis.*

CYSTIC FIBROSIS

Cystic fibrosis is the most common severe inherited disease of the white population, occurring in 1 in 2000 births. It is due to expression of a defective gene complex on chromosome 7 which is inherited in a recessive fashion and leads to an abnormal chloride channel on cell membranes. Thick inspissated secretions are produced and lead to the different features of the disease.

Pulmonary features

Abnormally thick mucus predisposes to a vicious cycle of stasis, recurrent bacterial and viral infection, damage to the airways, bronchiectatic change and further accumulation of secretions (**Figs 13.27, 13.28**). The possibility of cystic fibrosis should be entertained after an unusually severe chest infection, or if there are recurrent bacterial infections or persistent chest symptoms of cough and wheeze. In infancy, the common pathogens encountered are *Staphylococcus aureus* and *Haemophilus influenzae*. Later, colonization with *Pseudomonas aeruginosa* is inevitable (**Fig. 13.29**). *Pseudomonas cepacia* has been associated with rapid deterioration in some patients.

Treatment is primarily preventive with regular physiotherapy (**Fig. 13.30**). Postural drainage and percussion is used in younger children and babies, but forced expiration exercises—huffing—are effective in older children. Chemoprophylaxis with flucloxacillin and with nebulized aminoglycosides may be of value, and acute exacerbations are treated aggressively with intravenous antibiotics.

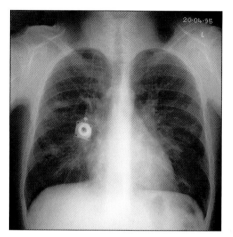

Fig. 13.27 *Chest X-ray in cystic fibrosis. A permanent vascular access device (Portacath—see Fig. 13.28) is also seen.*

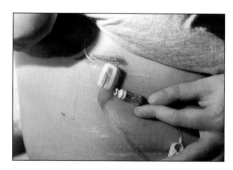

Fig. 13.28 *Portacath immediately after surgical placement.*

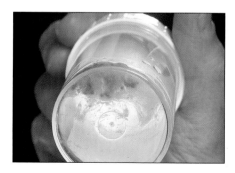

Fig. 13.29 *Sputum plugs in cystic fibrosis.*

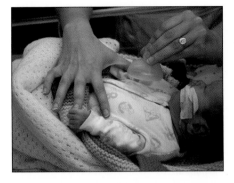

Fig. 13.30 *Physiotherapy in a baby with cystic fibrosis.*

Complications such as haemoptysis, pneumothorax and aspergillosis are not uncommon and eventually cor pulmonale and respiratory failure supervene. Reversible airways obstruction is often seen in cystic fibrosis, and bronchodilators may improve lung function. As damage to the lungs progresses, extended palliation by means of heart–lung transplantation is an option.

Gastrointestinal features

Abnormally thick and sticky meconium may lead to delay in passage of the first stool, or rectal prolapse in the neonate. Obstruction may be seen at birth with meconium ileus. Older children suffer meconium ileus equivalent (MIE) which is a subacute bowel obstruction caused by inspissated faeces in the terminal ileum and caecum (**Fig. 13.31**). MIE can be diagnosed easily by ultrasound (which may also reveal fibrosis of the bowel secondary to enzyme therapy) and is treated by gastrograffin given by mouth or enema with plenty of water.

Failure to thrive, with a greasy stool and voracious appetite, is a common presentation due to pancreatic insufficiency. Treatment consists of taking pancreatic enzyme replacements as capsules with meals and extra vitamin supplementation to avoid deficiency from fat malabsorption. Nutritional support with high energy intake is required for normal

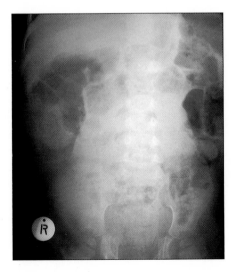

Fig. 13.31 *Meconium ileus equivalent.*

growth; gastrostomy and overnight feeding is sometimes needed. Progressive destruction of the endocrine pancreas leads to diabetes mellitus in some children and usually requires insulin.

Biliary cirrhosis and portal hypertension are often encountered and there is an increased incidence of gallstones in young adults.

Diagnosis

The gold standard is pilocarpine iontophoresis—the sweat test. A weak electrical current aids absorption of pilocarpine into the skin which then produces maximal sweating. One hundred milligrams should be collected; in cystic fibrosis the sweat sodium level is greater than 60 mmol/l. If there is a borderline result administration of fludrocortisone can be used to suppress sweat electrolytes in normal subjects. It should be remembered that babies may not sweat for some weeks after birth.

A useful screening test is the immunoreactive trypsin level. This pancreatic enzyme is present in an increased concentration in the blood of young babies with cystic fibrosis. However there are many false positive results and the diagnosis must be confirmed by a sweat test.

There are over 200 mutations for the cystic fibrosis gene. Gene probes are available for 85% of these and can confirm the diagnosis, especially if there is a family history. Prenatal diagnosis by chorionic villus sampling is possible. Affected males are subfertile, as the sperm have reduced motility, but females have normal fertility. As life expectancy is increasing, genetic counselling is also becoming very important for the sufferers themselves.

ASPIRATION AND GASTRO-OESOPHAGEAL REFLUX

Recurrent aspiration of gastric contents due to gastro-oesophageal reflux or disordered swallowing leads to recurrent chest infections, coughing and wheezing. Patchy shadows are seen at the lung apices in supine infants and basally in those with an upright posture (**Fig. 13.32**). Video fluoroscopy, pH probe monitoring and a search for tracheo-oesophageal fistula with bronchoscopy may be necessary.

ASTHMA

A traditional definition of asthma is recurrent episodes of reversible airways obstruction manifested by wheeze, coughing and dyspnoea. However, in contrast to adults, in childhood 'all that wheezes is not asthma'. Other causes of wheezing, such as an inhaled foreign body, cystic fibrosis, gastro-oesophageal reflux or aspiration, should be considered. Viral infections such as RSV and rhinovirus commonly produce acute wheezing in small infants as part of an acute illness. In the years after bronchiolitis or prolonged neonatal ventilation, children can exhibit bronchial reactivity and wheeze readily with URTIs.

There are two main patterns of symptoms in childhood:

- Infantile asthma, formerly known as 'wheezy bronchitis', in the under 2 year age group; this often occurs without an atopic background during viral URTIs. The airways obstruction is due to inflammation of the airway walls, mucus partially occluding the lumen, and a degree of bronchoconstriction in infants with small airways. There is some response with the inhaled anticholinergic drug, ipratropium bromide, and the beta adrenergic agonist, salbutamol, but oral corticosteroids have little effect. Prophylaxis

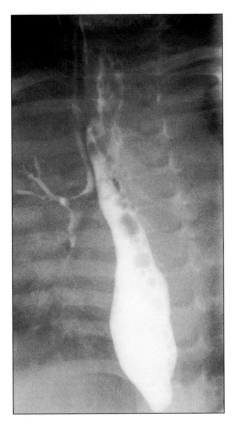

Fig. 13.32 *Aspiration into the pulmonary tree during an upper gastrointestinal contrast study.*

with inhaled sodium cromoglycate or steroids is similarly ineffective, and repeated admissions to hospital are often necessary when the child is acutely ill. The symptoms subside as the child grows out of infancy.

- Other children often have intermittent wheezing from infancy but, in contrast, usually have a family history of atopy and settle into an adult pattern of asthma. Coughing and wheeze can be triggered by viral infections; nocturnal coughing is prominent. Bronchial hyper-reactivity in these children produces symptoms on exercise, when laughing, in cold weather and, in some, on exposure to animal danders. The underlying pathology is a hypersensitivity response via histamine release and degranulation of mast cells.

Diagnosis

In infantile asthma there is usually recurrent prolonged wheezing. It is of great importance to exclude rarer causes of wheezing. The chest X-ray should be relatively normal in infantile asthma. In atopic asthma the diagnosis is made from the history as there may be no symptoms or signs between attacks. It is often useful for the child to keep a diary of symptoms which can be used to chart the response to treatment and correlate viral infections and environmental triggers. In children over the age of 5, peak flow readings can also provide useful information (**Figs 13.33, 13.34**).

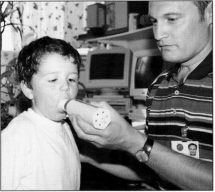

Fig. 13.33 *Peak flow meter.*

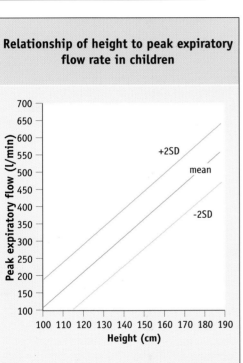

Relationship of height to peak expiratory flow rate in children

Fig. 13.34 *Relationship of height to peak expiratory flow rate in children.*

Management

The aim of therapy is to provide a normal unlimited lifestyle. General advice includes avoidance of cigarette smoking in the home, keeping allergen levels low by stopping pets entering bedrooms, frequent damp dusting, and limiting fluffy toys and carpet in the bedroom to reduce the levels of house dust mite.

For intermittent mild symptoms the first step is an inhaled beta agonist, such as salbutamol or terbutaline, delivered by an appropriate device. A metered dose inhaler and spacer is preferred for small children and should be available for use in a severe attack (**Fig. 13.35**). A dry powder inhaler is preferred by children older than 5 years.

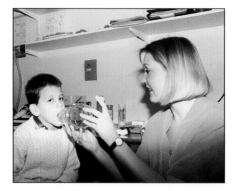

Fig. 13.35 *Metered dose inhaler and spacer.*

If symptoms are frequent, prophylactic therapy is required. Sodium cromoglycate, a mast cell membrane stabilizing drug, is often tried first for those with mild symptoms. It is available as an aerosol for use with a spacer but poor compliance is a common problem as it needs to be taken 3 or 4 times per day.

For children with more severe problems, particularly if symptoms have required hospital admission, inhaled steroids (beclomethasone, budesonide or fluticasone) are required. They are taken twice daily via a spacer and the mouth rinsed afterwards. A relatively high dose is taken first to control symptoms and then reduced to the minimum effective dose. Systemic corticosteroids are sometimes needed. Where possible, these are given on alternate days to reduce adrenal suppression.

Parents often worry about the effects of steroids on growth, but the long-term effects on children of exercise limitation and feeling unwell throughout the whole of childhood must not be ignored. Untreated asthma can lead to growth failure, but inhaled steroids are unlikely to do this except in cases where large doses are required.

The acute attack

Acute attacks tend to occur in the autumn months when children return to school and colds are more common. It is usual for symptoms to increase over a couple of days before cough, wheeze and breathlessness become disabling. Use of bronchodilators via a spacer can be vital at this time as children may not be able to use dry powder inhalers. If symptoms are worsening despite high dose salbutamol every 3–4 hours, the child should be seen by a doctor and a short 1–3 day course of high dose steroids given. This short course of steroids should clear the chest but will not interfere with long-term growth. Some children have attacks that progress rapidly and can be life threatening. These children are often provided with steroids to take immediately and salbutamol in nebulized form. They should have direct access to the hospital ward.

In hospital the basis of treatment is nebulized bronchodilators and steroids, which in severe cases can both be given intravenously. Aminophylline is often effective but reserved for severe attacks when other measures have failed.

The severity of the attack can be judged in many different ways. Pulse oximetry is important as it reveals hypoxia from ventilation–perfusion mismatch in the lungs. A low peak expiratory flow rate (PEFR) will also be recorded if the child is able to use the meter. A chest X-ray is usually not necessary if there is a good response to treatment but is important if there is any suggestion of pneumothorax. Areas of fleeting collapse are common in acute asthma attacks and do not necessarily indicate infection (**Fig. 13.36**). Difficulty in speaking and sitting quietly are important signs as fatigue determines the need

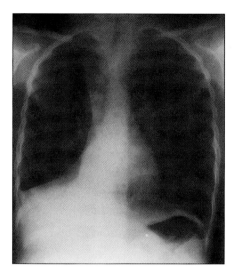

Fig. 13.36 *Chest X-ray of acute asthma attack. There is overinflation, right upper and left lower lobe collapse.*

for ventilatory support. Pulsus paradoxus (pulse pressure lower in inspiration than expiration) indicates severe asthma if the difference is more than 20 mmHg. Arterial blood gases do not contribute to management as the pCO_2 remains relatively normal until clinically obvious exhaustion occurs. Mechanical ventilation is difficult but rarely is needed.

CHRONIC LUNG DISEASE OF PREMATURITY

After neonatal intensive care for respiratory distress syndrome, in very preterm infants, there appears to be iatrogenic damage to the lungs from ventilation. Survivors often have reduced ventilatory capacity and require supplemental oxygen (**Fig. 13.37**). The situation improves as they grow new lung tissue but careful attention to nutrition and care during

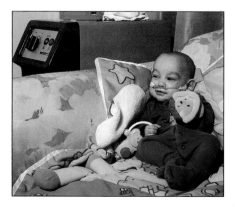

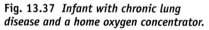

Fig. 13.37 *Infant with chronic lung disease and a home oxygen concentrator.*

185

intercurrent infections is required. This is provided by community neonatal nurse specialists, who make it possible for these babies to be cared for at home.

ABNORMALITIES OF THE CHEST WALL AND DIAPHRAGM

Pectus excavatum is usually an isolated finding, and usually is of no clinical significance apart from the cosmetic aspect (**Fig. 13.38**). In contrast, pectus carinatum is a boat-shaped chest which occurs because of pulling on the lower rib margins by the diaphragm while the chest is still pliable. It is seen in conditions with increased work of breathing such as long-standing untreated childhood asthma or chronic lung disease of prematurity (**Fig. 13.39**).

Diaphragmatic hernia can present in two ways:

1. Ultrasound scanning can diagnose a diaphragmatic hernia before birth, or a clinical diagnosis can be made at the time of birth because of persistent cyanosis. The prognosis in these babies depends on the degree of accompanying lung hypoplasia (**Fig. 13.40**).
2. Alternatively, a hernia may present with vomiting or a chest infection in an older baby or child. The prognosis is better for this group as there is not usually lung hypoplasia (**Fig. 13.41**).

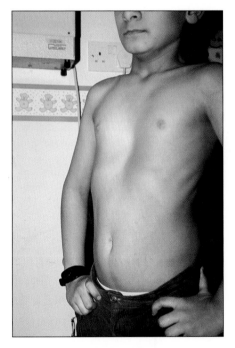

Fig. 13.38 *Pectus excavatum.*

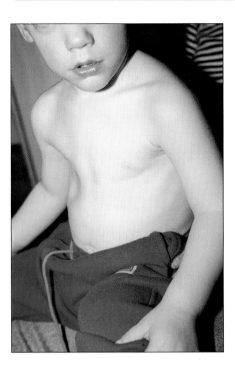

Fig. 13.39 *Pectus carinatum.*

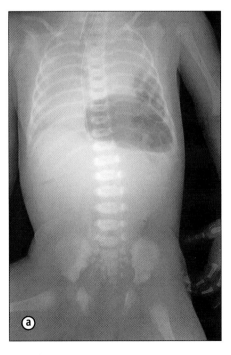

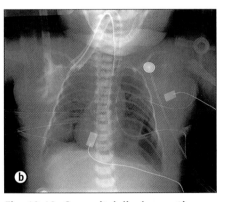

Fig. 13.40 *Congenital diaphragmatic hernia. (a) The stomach is seen to lie within the chest cavity. (b) After operation a degree of lung hypoplasia is evident as the left lung remains small.*

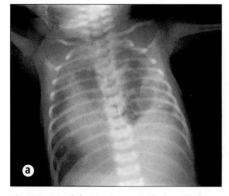

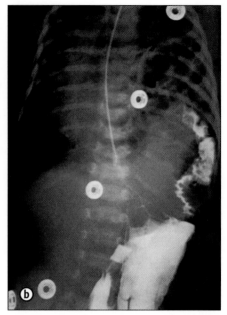

Fig. 13.41 *(a) Diaphragmatic hernia in an infant presenting with vomiting. (b) Bowel loops in the left chest are seen with contrast.*

chapter 14

Metabolic Disorders

There are probably more similarities in metabolism between infants, children and adults than there are differences. However, children and especially babies are more susceptible to hypoglycaemia than adults—perhaps because they have greater basal energy expenditure. The relative fluid composition of the body is also different (**Fig. 14.1**) and there are differences in the metabolism of many substances, particularly drugs.

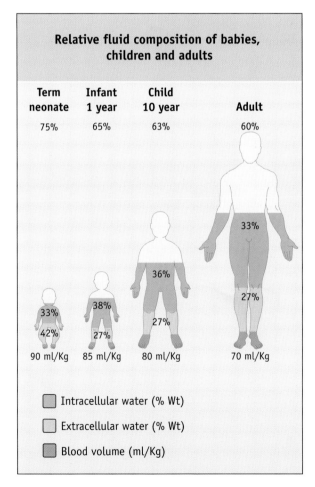

Relative fluid composition of babies, children and adults

Term neonate	Infant 1 year	Child 10 year	Adult
75%	65%	63%	60%
			33%
		36%	
			27%
33%	38%		
42%	27%	27%	
90 ml/Kg	85 ml/Kg	80 ml/Kg	70 ml/Kg

Intracellular water (% Wt)

Extracellular water (% Wt)

Blood volume (ml/Kg)

Fig. 14.1 *Relative fluid composition of babies, children and adults.*

HYPOGLYCAEMIA AND KETOSIS

All cells in the body use glucose to produce energy. The entry of glucose into cells is controlled by insulin, although neural cells are an important exception as their glucose

---

Causes of hypoglycaemia

Endocrine

Insulin mediated
- Endogenous—transient
    Infants of diabetic mothers
    SGA infants
    Beckwith–Wiedemann syndrome
- Endogenous—persistent
    Nesidioblastosis
    Insulinoma
- Exogenous
- Non-insulin-mediated (tumour producing IGF-I, IGF-II)

Deficiency
- Growth hormone—hypopituitarism
- ACTH/cortisol—hypopituitarism
- Cortisol—adrenal failure

Metabolic

Carbohydrate
- Defects of gluconeogenesis
- Glycogen storage diseases (types I, III, VI, IX)
- Galactosaemia
- Fructosaemia

Fatty acid
- Fatty acid oxidation defects
- Ketone-body utilization defects
- Respiratory chain defects

Organic acid
- Maple syrup urine disease
- Methylmalonic and propionic aciduria

Amino acid
- Tyrosinaemia

Other
Alcohol
Toxins
Liver failure

---

entry is independent of insulin and dependent instead on the blood glucose concentration. Thus brain function is particularly affected during hypoglycaemia.

Ketone bodies (acetone, beta-hydroxybutyric acid and aceto-acetic acid) are intermediate metabolites and represent a major source of energy. They are produced in the liver from the breakdown of fatty acids and are then transported and used by the peripheral tissues as an energy source. A small amount of glucose is also necessary to metabolize these ketones. Between meals (during fasting) there is a low level of insulin secretion to allow glucose entry into cells. The basal level of insulin also allows metabolic pathways which release stored energy to become active. In particular, fatty acids are metabolized and ketone bodies are released into the blood where they are rapidly cleared by the tissues. Glucose is also produced from other substrates—gluconeogenesis. During a meal, however, insulin is released and acts to clear glucose from the blood and inhibit fatty acid breakdown and gluconeogenesis.

In diabetes mellitus the absence of insulin means that glucose cannot enter the body's cells. The concentration of glucose in the blood rises and causes an osmotic diuresis leading to dehydration. Production of ketones is facilitated but they cannot be peripherally utilized without glucose. They are found in the urine and, because they are volatile, are also smelled on the breath. This is diabetic ketoacidosis.

Small or even moderate amounts of ketones can also be found in the urine of children who are unwell from infection as they are predominantly utilizing fat stores instead of carbohydrate for energy because they are not eating.

INSULIN-INDUCED HYPOGLYCAEMIA

A common cause of hypoglycaemia is the exogenous insulin taken by diabetics. As the blood glucose level falls, there is a compensatory release of stress hormones such as adrenaline, glucagon, growth hormone and cortisol in order to try to reverse the effects. This produces many of the adrenergic symptoms—pallor, sweating, shaking, tachycardia

Symptoms of hypoglycaemia

Autonomic
- Trembling
- Sweating
- Hunger
- Heart pounding
- Anxiety

Neuroglycopenic
- Drowsiness
- Confusion
- Incoordination
- Lack of concentration
- Difficulty with speech

Non-specific
- Nausea
- Tiredness
- Headache

and agitation. Cerebral dysfunction occurs as the brain is deprived of glucose, leading to loss of consciousness and possibly seizures.

KETOTIC HYPOGLYCAEMIA

Spontaneous hypoglycaemia is seen in young children, probably due to insufficient mobilization of carbohydrate stores between meals. The insulin levels are low and there are large amounts of ketones in the blood. It is still not clear why this happens but it may represent an accelerated form of the ketosis that is usually seen in starvation.

NEONATAL HYPOGLYCAEMIA

Hypoglycaemia is a particular problem in babies. Limited glycogen and fat reserves are major contributing factors in preterm infants and those babies who are small for gestational age. Intrapartum asphyxia consumes glycogen stores, and if the baby is also cold in the immediate postnatal period this can further divert energy reserves towards generating heat. There are often delays in establishing milk feeds.

An exact definition of hypoglycaemia has been difficult to establish but 2.6 mmol/l blood glucose has become a generally accepted threshold. Below this level, abnormalities on the electro-encephalogram and later neurodevelopmental problems have been noted.

NESIDIOBLASTOSIS

Nesidioblastosis is a developmental disorder of the islets of Langerhans in the pancreas (Fig. 14.2) which is particularly associated with the Beckwith–Wiedemann syndrome (Fig. 14.3). The mechanisms controlling the regulation of insulin secretion are lost and large quantities of insulin are released, resulting in profound hypoglycaemia. The hyperinsulinaemia also suppresses ketone production and this is particularly dangerous as the brain can therefore be starved of its alternative energy source. Glucose infusions, frequent high energy enteral feeds, steroids, diazoxide (an anti-hypertensive drug which also elevates blood glucose) and octreotide (a somatostatin analogue) are used but 95% subtotal pancreatectomy is usually required.

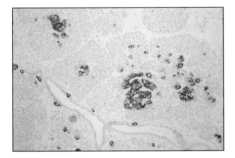

Fig. 14.2 Abnormal pancreatic islet formation in nesidioblastosis.

DIABETES MELLITUS

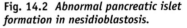

Diabetes mellitus is the most common endocrine disease in childhood with a prevalence of 1 in 350 children. In childhood almost all cases are insulin dependent (IDDM). Diabetes mellitus is more common in countries that lie further away from the equator, and there has been a definite increase in its incidence.

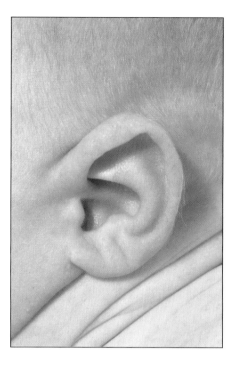

Fig. 14.3 *Ear creases in Beckwith–Wiedemann syndrome.*

The cause of insulin dependent diabetes mellitus is still not clear but genetic and environmental factors have been implicated. There is a strong association between HLA DR3 and DR4 and IDDM. In predisposed individuals autoantibodies directed against the islet cells are detectable in the blood. It is not clear whether these antibodies cause the disease or are a secondary phenomenon. Similarly, it is not clear whether viruses such as mumps are implicated in the pathogenesis of IDDM or merely reveal chronic insulin deficiency. Studies have indicated that there is a long prodromal phase before clinical signs develop (**Fig. 14.4**). Initially there may be autoantibodies and pancreatic damage but sufficient insulin production to meet the body's needs. With time, impaired insulin release from the beta cells causes impaired glucose tolerance and subtle signs of weight loss and fatigue. Later, insufficient insulin production or the stress of an infection produces polyuria and compensatory polydipsia. Eventually, progressive dehydration and accumulation of ketoacids leads to diabetic ketoacidosis. The breath smells of ketones, there is hyperventilation due to acidosis, and severe dehydration may result in coma.

Ketoacidosis is more common in younger children, with 50% of diabetic infants compared to 15% of older children presenting in this way. It is important for the clinician to be aware of the subtle presenting signs of diabetes. Hyperventilation should always lead to urine testing for glycosuria and weight loss, lethargy or malaise even in the absence of polyuria and polydipsia should require exclusion of diabetes. As many people cannot smell ketones these should be specifically tested for with urinary dip sticks.

HYPERGLYCAEMIA WITHOUT KETOACIDOSIS

Most new diabetics present with hyperglycaemia, weight loss and polyuria/polydipsia without ketoacidosis. They should be referred immediately to hospital for evaluation. For these families the initial priority is initiation of monitoring for the possible onset of

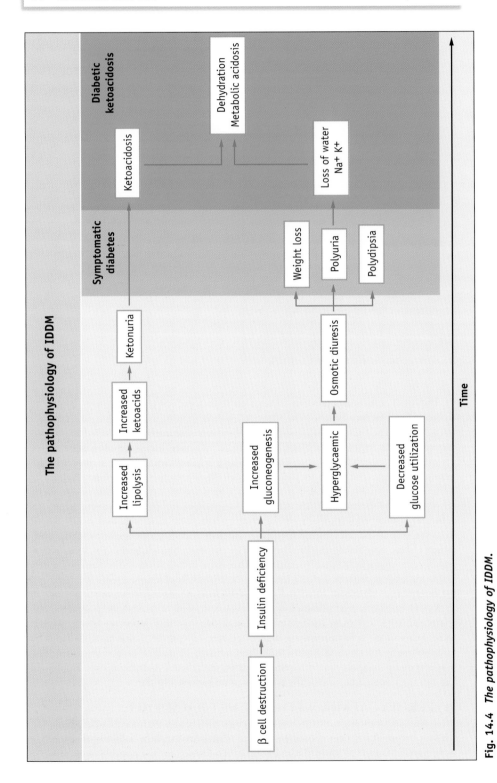

Fig. 14.4 The pathophysiology of IDDM.

Management of ketoacidosis

- The initial priority in treating diabetic ketoacidosis is recognition of hypovolaemic shock and replacement of the circulating volume with plasma or saline (**Fig. 14.5**). Acidosis, which is due to ketoacids and lactic acid, usually clears quickly once the circulation is restored, and sodium bicarbonate is rarely needed.
- Dehydration is corrected gradually; care must be taken, as too rapid fluid replacement can lead to cerebral oedema. A recent weight is often the best indicator of the degree of dehydration as weight loss in grams relates directly to millilitres of water. This volume, together with calculated maintenance fluid requirements, is given; two thirds in the first 24 hours and the last third in the second 24 hours.
- Insulin is provided as an infusion at 0.1 unit/kg/hour. This leads to a gradual reduction in the blood glucose level. Once the child is fully rehydrated and feeling much better, normal diet and twice daily subcutaneous insulin can be started and intravenous therapy stopped.
- Once the blood glucose level begins to fall, potassium also leaves the blood and enters the cells. It is important to monitor the plasma levels and provide extra potassium supplements once urine flow has been confirmed or serum potassium measured. Continuous ECG monitoring is used to monitor the T wave changes (**Fig. 14.6**) associated with hyperkalaemia and monitor for arrhythmias; frequent electrolyte measurements are performed.

ketoacidosis and education. Many hospitals arrange for admission for a few days to teach finger prick blood glucose testing and the technique of insulin injection. An increasing number of centres aim to manage the initial treatment and education on an outpatient basis or at home with community diabetic nurse specialists. It is usual to start with a very small dose of insulin twice daily and gradually increase the dose to bring blood glucose under control.

LONG-TERM MANAGEMENT
The aims of management are to maintain normoglycaemia, promote normal growth and development, and allow as normal a lifestyle as possible. It is now clear that good glycaemic control prevents the onset of complications. Traditionally diet, insulin and exercise formed the prescription for diabetic treatment.

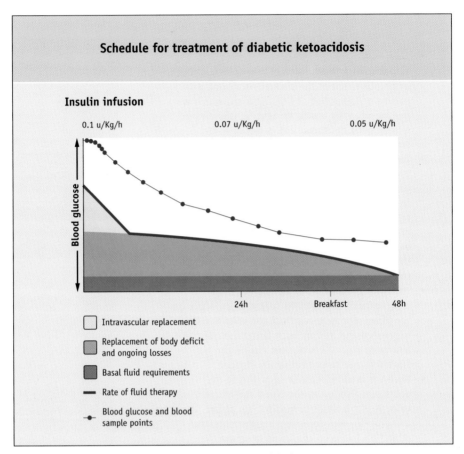

Fig. 14.5 *Schedule for treatment of diabetic ketoacidosis.*

Education

An important concept in the management of diabetes is that parents and children, when they are able, should make the daily decisions that the condition necessitates. To do this they must be taught about their disease, its practical aspects, and how to make decisions. The provision of a specialist clinic and diabetic team has been demonstrated to improve understanding and metabolic control. The banding of children into children's clinics and adolescent clinics has been an important improvement to the diabetic services. Joint clinics with adult diabetologists have also been beneficial—both in smoothing the transition to the adult clinic and improving paediatric diabetic management.

Organizations such as Diabetes UK, formerly the British Diabetic Association, are an important source of education and support. They have local meetings, provide information via a magazine, and also organize camps where children can meet other diabetics and learn to become more independent.

Diet

Diet forms one of the cornerstones of diabetic management, but undoubtedly causes a great deal of anxiety for families. The general aim is to provide sufficient nutrition for

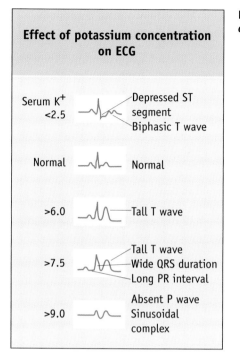

Fig. 14.6 *Effect of potassium concentration on ECG.*

normal growth and development in a form that prevents swings from hyperglycaemia to hypoglycaemia. The paediatric dietitian plays a fundamental role in this process. Fibre is of particular importance in diabetes as it smoothes the uptake of glucose from the gut. Sucrose, although usually avoided in diabetes, is part of childhood. Rather than a ban on sweets and chocolates, a reduction in amounts is more favourable, with encouragement to eat fruit instead. Children are no longer managed with exchanges of carbohydrate but are encouraged to take three normal meals and snacks in between with an emphasis on the use of complex carbohydrates that release glucose in a controlled prolonged fashion.

Exercise

In the presence of insulin, exercise reduces blood glucose because of consumption by muscle and enhances sensitivity to insulin. Regular exercise has been shown to reduce insulin requirements and improve glycaemic control. As well as the metabolic benefit, there is a psychological one as children with diabetes are not excluded from sport and team games. Sometimes extra calories are needed before exercise, and glucose should be available if there are symptoms of hypoglycaemia. Rarely, after hard exercise, late hypoglycaemia may occur due to depletion of glycogen reserves.

Insulin

There is now clear evidence that maintaining normal glucose levels prevents or prolongs the onset of diabetic complications; this is especially important in the paediatric group. Although the quantity of insulin each diabetic needs must be titrated against blood tests, in general 0.8 unit/kg/day is needed in childhood. In the period from 6 months to 1 year after diagnosis, residual insulin production means that less exogenous insulin (about

0.5 unit/kg/day) or sometimes none at all is needed. This is known as the honeymoon period. In adolescence up to 1.2 unit/kg/day may be needed.

The most common regimen is twice daily injections. Insulin, in proportions of one third rapid acting and two thirds moderately long acting, is injected subcutaneously. Two thirds of the total daily requirement is given before breakfast and the remaining third before the evening meal. The amount of insulin is altered depending on the pattern of the blood glucose reading. For example, if blood glucose is consistently high before lunch, the amount of morning fast acting insulin is increased; if blood glucose is high before the evening meal, the moderate acting insulin is increased. Fixed ratio insulin mixes are ideal for most children. In older children a long acting insulin can be used with additional injections of fast acting insulin before meals, allowing greater flexibility of lifestyle (Fig. 14.7). These insulins are available as premixed cartridges for use in injector pens (Fig. 14.8) which allow a dose to be dialled rather than drawn up, thus simplifying the process. Both these methods are highly effective if the family and child are motivated and prepared to make adjustments in dose themselves when the pattern of control, as judged on blood glucose stick testing, varies. It is not appropriate to wait months until the next outpatient clinic before making changes.

Monitoring and hypoglycaemia

The mainstay of monitoring is blood glucose stick testing. It is usual to perform a test each morning before breakfast and another test at a different time, for example again before lunch, the evening meal or at bedtime. By carrying out tests at different times a glucose profile can be obtained over a few days and the insulin dose adjusted accordingly. Some

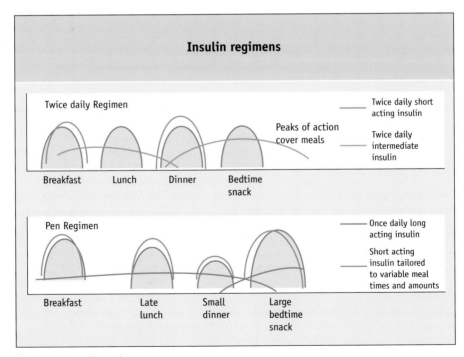

Fig. 14.7 *Insulin regimens.*

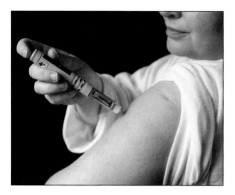

Fig. 14.8 *Injection of insulin using a pen injector. Injector pens are popular with children. They are easy to use and carry a very fine needle.*

families find that recording glucose levels more intensively over a complete 24 hour period a few times per week is equally acceptable. It is particularly important to carry out tests during symptoms which could be those of hypoglycaemia, and when unwell.

The degree of glucose binding to haemoglobin (HbA$_{1C}$) provides an objective indicator of average glucose levels over the preceding couple of months. A level below 8% is satisfactory in childhood.

Mild hypoglycaemic episodes are common and usually predictable. They occur when extra exercise or insufficient food is taken and respond quickly to carbohydrate. The symptoms may be vague, and complaints of feeling dizzy or unwell should lead to blood glucose testing to confirm hypoglycaemia. In severe episodes where there is loss of consciousness, a glucagon injection will temporarily raise blood glucose levels sufficiently to permit eating. Alternatively, glucose gel may be applied to be absorbed across the gums.

Nocturnal hypoglycaemia is feared by parents and children. It can present with paradoxical morning hyperglycaemia due to a compensatory release of stress hormones. This is known as the Somogyi effect and should prompt a reduction, rather than an increase, in insulin dosage.

Adolescence

Adolescence, with the physical and emotional transition to an independent adult, is a difficult time for any individual. For the diabetic there are also difficulties in control due to changing insulin and energy requirements. It must be emphasized that instability at this time has a physiological basis; for example, there is relative insulin resistance because of increased levels of growth hormone. However, it is also important to realize that some children may express their anxieties as poor glycaemic control. Thus, the help of a child psychologist may be needed for some, but meeting with other adolescents in a dedicated clinic is beneficial to most.

Complications

Complications of diabetes rarely occur before puberty and their onset is prevented by good blood glucose control. The main complication is growth failure, but good control prevents this. Although screening for complications does not form a large part of paediatric management, information with regards to diet, smoking, and care of injection sites should be part of general education. The site of insulin injection should be rotated to avoid lumps in one place. Although constant use of the same site reduces the discomfort of injection, the result is unsightly (**Fig. 14.9**) and leads to erratic insulin absorption. Diabetic nephropathy is heralded by microalbuminuria, and many clinics check for this at the yearly

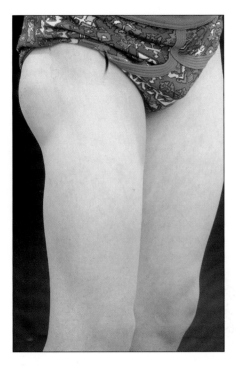

Fig. 14.9 *Lipodystrophy at injection sites.*

assessment visit beginning 5 years after initial diagnosis. It is sensible to check the fundi for congenital abnormalities that may be confused with pathological change in later life.

INBORN ERRORS OF METABOLISM

All the biochemical processes that provide energy and cellular growth are controlled by enzymes. Enzymes are catalytic proteins encoded by genes, and mutations or allelic variations of specific genes can therefore disrupt metabolism. Most disruptions, or errors, of metabolism are caused by a reduction in the amount of an enzyme due to a mutation inherited in an autosomal or X-linked recessive fashion (**Fig. 14.10**). If the reduction is mild, there may be no obvious effects or symptoms may only occur when under stress, such as with infection.

Severe disruption to important metabolic pathways is usually evident in the neonatal period and may result in neonatal death. All errors produce symptoms because of lack of an important product or excessive production of an alternative metabolite (**Fig. 14.11**).

PHENYLKETONURIA

Phenylketonuria is the most common inborn error of amino acid metabolism, with an incidence in the United Kingdom of about one in 12 000 live births. There are several enzyme deficiencies, leading to an inability to metabolize phenylalanine to tyrosine. The excess phenylalanine is then excreted in the urine as phenyl ketones. Many sufferers have blonde hair due to competitive inhibition of the enzyme tyrosinase, which is essential for melanin production from tyrosine (*see* **Fig. 14.11**).

Types of inborn errors of metabolism

Type	Examples
Carbohydrate metabolism	Galactosaemia, fructosuria
Lipoprotein metabolism	Hyperlipoproteinaemias
Organic acid metabolism	Maple syrup urine disease
Amino acid metabolism	Phenylketonuria, cystinuria
Urea cycle disorder	Hyperammonaemia
Mucopolysaccharidosis	Hurler syndrome

Fig. 14.10 *Types of inborn errors of metabolism.*

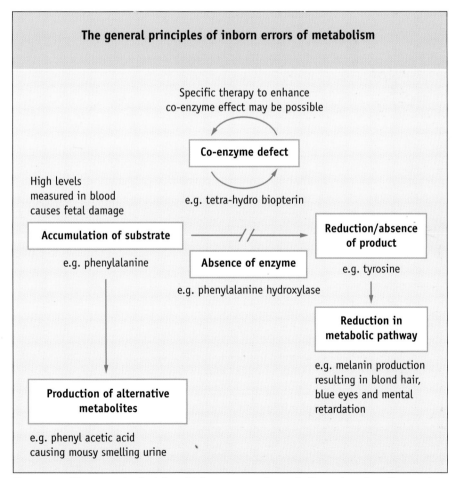

Fig. 14.11 *The general principles of inborn errors of metabolism using phenylketonuria as an example.*

Guthrie card

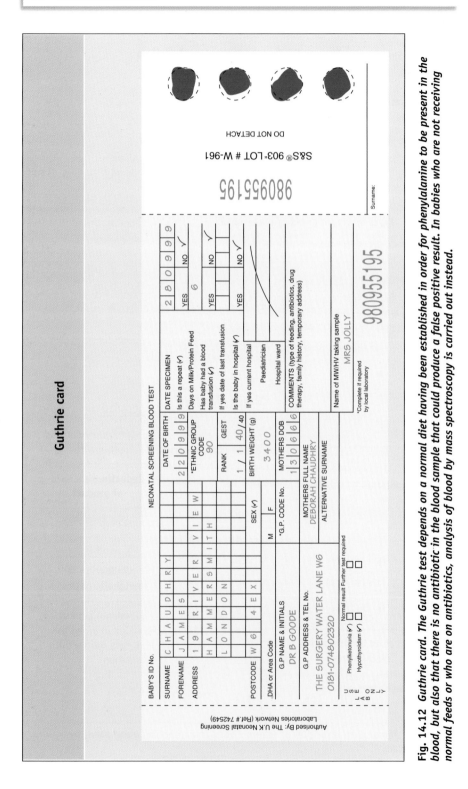

Fig. 14.12 Guthrie card. The Guthrie test depends on a normal diet having been established in order for phenylalanine to be present in the blood, but also that there is no antibiotic in the blood sample that could produce a false positive result. In babies who are not receiving normal feeds or who are on antibiotics, analysis of blood by mass spectroscopy is carried out instead.

Phenylketonuria is inherited like most metabolic disorders in an autosomal recessive fashion but because of the different enzyme deficiencies there may be a variable degree of disease. The fetus and infant are most susceptible to the effects of phenylalanine.

Babies born with phenylketonuria are normal at birth but if the condition is not diagnosed cerebral damage and mental retardation develop and, even if they can be halted, cannot be reversed after 6 months of age. Vomiting, microcephaly, seizures and abnormal movements are other features. In later childhood the dietary restriction can be relaxed although there is a risk of behavioural problems and neurological problems such as ataxia; increasing evidence suggests that dietary restriction should be lifelong.

Female sufferers must not become pregnant while taking a normal diet because even if the fetus is normal it will be damaged by the phenylalanine levels. Growth retardation, microcephaly and mental retardation are common features if spontaneous abortion does not occur. It has been suggested that women of childbearing age with phenylketonuria should remain on a strict diet or at least be on a diet before conception.

Screening

Neonatal screening for phenylketonuria has been very successful, and in countries where this operates it is the main diagnostic route before any neurological symptoms or signs occur. The Guthrie test is based on inhibition of bacterial growth by phenylalanine in blood (**Fig. 14.12**).

OTHER METABOLIC DISEASES

Over 2000 inborn errors of metabolism have been recognized in humans and the number of known conditions increases each year. They may affect the regulation of intermediate metabolism, such as carbohydrate, fat and protein homeostasis, or specific organelles within cells such as in the lysosomal storage diseases and peroxisomal disorders. Any part of the body may be affected by such disorders and thus presentation may be to a variety of paediatric specialists (**Fig. 14.13**). There is an increasing number of dysmorphic conditions that are caused by inborn errors of metabolism. It is important to consider metabolic disease as, if suspected, it is often easily diagnosed and treated and complications can be avoided. For some problems there are specific pharmacological and dietary therapies. Organ transplantation (liver, kidney and bone marrow) may help others. For many conditions there is, however, little apart from supportive measures that can be offered. Genetic counselling is an important part of the management of these families.

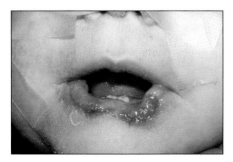

Fig. 14.13 *Self mutilation in the Lesch–Nyhan syndrome. Lesch–Nyhan syndrome is an X-linked disorder seen in boys. It is characterized by spasticity and self mutilation and diagnosed by a high serum level of uric acid.*

chapter 15

Endocrine Disorders

Growth and physical development are dependent on normal endocrine function. Early diagnosis and care in treating endocrine problems is important to avoid the physical and psychological effects of abnormal growth:

- Thyroxine is particularly important for brain development in infancy; deficiency causes cretinism. Hypothyroidism should always be excluded as a cause of short stature as it is also required for bone growth. Conversely, hyperthyroidism may produce a tall child.
- Growth hormone (GH) is not necessary for growth in fetal life or infancy but is the main regulator of growth after the age of 2 years (see Fig. 4.1).
- Sex steroids are notable because as well as accelerating skeletal growth they cause closure of the epiphyses. Excessive levels in childhood produce tall stature in childhood but eventual short stature in adulthood.

THYROID HORMONE PRODUCTION

Thyroxine (T4) is produced in response to thyroid stimulating hormone (TSH), which in turn is produced from the pituitary due to the action of hypothalamic thyroid releasing hormone (TRH). Thyroid hormones are regulated by a negative feedback loop in which the active hormones inhibit the release of TRH and TSH from the hypothalamus and pituitary respectively (**Fig. 15.1**).

The thyroid gland is active in the fetus from 20 weeks' gestation. Most of this thyroxine (T4) is converted to inactive reverse tri-iodothyronine (rT3), but after 30 weeks the levels of active T3 begin to rise. In addition, there is also a small transplacental passage of maternal T4. At birth there is a massive surge in TSH, peaking at 30 minutes, which stimulates T3 and T4 secretion. Re-equilibration of TSH to normal levels occurs a few days later and is in part due to maturation of the negative feedback mechanism but also to the increased conversion of T4 to active T3 (**Fig. 15.2**). Screening for neonatal hypothyroidism takes place at the end of the first week of life when levels of TSH and T4 have normalized.

CONGENITAL HYPOTHYROIDISM

Congenital hypothyroidism is usually caused by an abnormality of the thyroid gland and only rarely due to a problem with the pituitary or hypothalamus.

- The thyroid may fail to develop (agenesis).
- The normal embryological progression of the gland from the base of the tongue to the neck may be disrupted (thyroglossal cyst or ectopic thyroid).
- There may be an inborn error of thyroid hormone biosynthesis.
- Maternal and fetal iodine deficiency may be responsible for dyshormonogenesis.

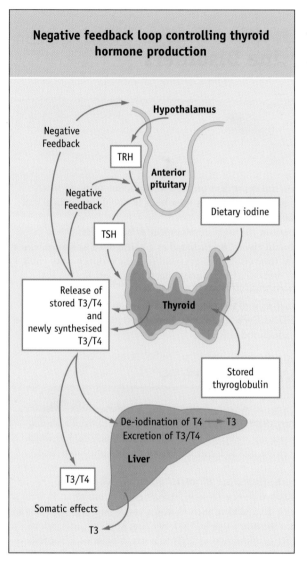

Fig. 15.1 *Negative feedback loop controlling thyroid hormone production.*

Congenital hypothyroidism can easily be missed because infants are asymptomatic at birth and the early signs are subtle. Initially there is normal growth and development. Symptoms only begin to appear after 3–6 months.

Neonatal screening programmes operate in most developed countries and are based on blood spot analysis for TSH or T4 taken at the end of the first week of life. One spot of blood on the card is used for the Guthrie test to identify babies with phenylketonuria, but extra spots allow for other neonatal screening programmes such as congenital hypothyroidism. T4, or more commonly TSH, can be assayed. Whilst the T4 assay will detect all babies with low levels of hormone, the finding of elevated TSH levels depends on release of the pituitary from negative feedback. This will not be seen where there are hypothalamic or pituitary abnormalities.

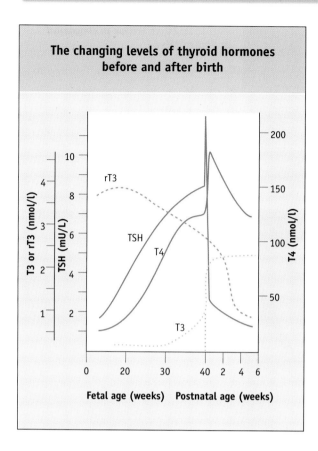

The changing levels of thyroid hormones before and after birth

Fetal age (weeks)   Postnatal age (weeks)

Fig. 15.2 *The changing levels of thyroid hormones before and after birth.*

Symptoms of hypothyroidism

- Poor feeding
- Prolonged jaundice
- Constipation
- Facial features may become coarse
- Large tongue (**Fig. 15.3**)
- Umbilical hernia (**Fig. 15.4**)
- Intellectual and developmental delay

Treatment of neonatal hypothyroidism is with lifelong thyroxine replacement therapy. The dose of thyroxine is adjusted to normalize TSH and T4 levels, as well as to provide a normal growth velocity for age.

NEONATAL HYPERTHYROIDISM

Neonatal hyperthyroidism is a rare but serious condition that is usually due to transplacental transfer of thyroid stimulating immunoglobulin (TSI) from a mother with active or inactive autoimmune thyroid disease (Graves' disease or Hashimoto's thyroiditis).

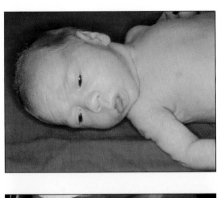

Fig. 15.3 *Large tongue in congenital hypothyroidism.*

Fig. 15.4 *Umbilical hernia in congenital hypothyroidism.*

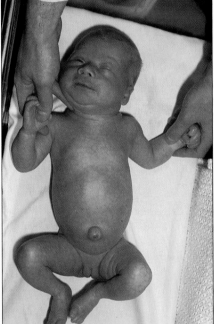

High output cardiac failure and cardiac arrhythmias can lead to the death of the baby. Prompt treatment with propranolol, carbimazole and potassium iodide is important to control symptoms and suppress thyroid hormone production. After 6 weeks the TSI has disappeared from the baby's circulation and the drugs can be cautiously withdrawn.

THYROID DYSFUNCTION IN OLDER CHILDREN
Symptoms of thyroid dysfunction
The role of thyroxine is to control the metabolic rate, thus explaining many of the clinical features of under- or over-secretion. It is essential for bone growth.

The clinical features of thyroid dysfunction usually have an insidious onset and can be missed for some time (**Fig. 15.5**). Hyperthyroidism in school age children often comes to

Symptoms and signs in hypothyroidism and hyperthyroidism

Hypothyroidism	Hyperthyroidism
Cold intolerance*	Heat intolerance (common)
Lethargy, reduced activity	Anxiety and restlessness (disruptive behaviour)
Constipation and weight gain	Increased appetite, weight loss and diarrhoea
Reduced growth velocity and delayed bone age, delayed puberty	Rapid growth and accelerated bone maturity
Bradycardia*, cold peripheries* and dry skin*	Tachycardia, tremor and hot sweaty hands
Slow relaxing reflexes*, sparse hair*, loss of eyebrows*	Eye signs—lid retraction and exophthalmos
Goitre	Goitre—often with bruit

* These symptoms are common in adults but very rare in childhood hypothyroidism.

Fig. 15.5 *Features of thyroid dysfunction.*

notice because of disruptive behaviour, but hypothyroidism is often missed for longer as the children are quiet and do not cause any trouble.

Hypothyroidism

Lack of thyroxine releases TSH from negative feedback control and stimulates hyperplasia of the thyroid gland. This goitre is often present before there is frank hypothyroidism. Rarely, the high levels of TSH may be associated with precocious puberty. Hypothyroid children are often not detected until there is growth failure with delayed bone age.

- Iodine deficiency is the commonest cause of hypothyroidism and goitre in childhood.
- Hashimoto's disease is an autoimmune thyroiditis in which autoantibodies eventually destroy all thyroid hormone production. As with other autoimmune disease, there is often a family history and girls are more frequently affected.
- Children with diabetes mellitus and Down syndrome are at increased risk of hypothyroidism and should be screened for hypothyroidism at intervals.
  Treatment for all these conditions is with thyroxine replacement therapy.

Hyperthyroidism

Hyperthyroidism in childhood is rare. It is mainly due to Graves' disease, but a few cases of Hashimoto's thyroiditis initially present in this way before hypothyroidism becomes established. The symptoms and signs are similar to those in adulthood. The blood levels of T3 and T4 are elevated and TSH is suppressed. Antibodies directed against the TSH receptor are also found.

Treatment is aimed at providing initial relief of symptoms and then establishing a euthyroid state. The distressing symptoms of hyperthyroidism are mediated by beta adrenergic pathways, and a beta blocker such as propranolol is useful for the first weeks. It is important to remember that beta blockers should be used with care in asthmatics (worsening bronchospasm) and in diabetics (the warning symptoms of hypoglycaemia are blocked).

Reduction of thyroid activity is generally achieved with propylthiouracil or carbimazole. These drugs can be titrated to normalize biochemistry or, more commonly, used to block endogenous thyroxine production completely so that full replacement doses of thyroxine can be given. This is an easier regimen to manage and may be more effective.

Transient rashes may occur with carbimazole but the most important side-effect is an idiosyncratic agranulocytosis. The white cell count must be checked if a child on carbimazole treatment develops a fever.

Treatment is maintained for 9–12 months, by which time remission is achieved in half of children. If remission is not achieved, then subtotal thyroidectomy or treatment with radio-iodine[131] are effective therapies. There do not seem to be any long-term risks of malignancy with radio-iodine treatment. After these interventions, follow-up for hypothyroidism should be undertaken.

HYPOPARATHYROIDISM

Parathyroid hormone is the key hormone in calcium and phosphate homeostasis.

Hypoparathyroidism is seen in the Di George syndrome (absent thymus, parathyroids and cardiac defects) but also in normal babies. It is especially common in babies born to mothers whose diets are deficient in calcium and vitamin D. As a result, the mothers have compensatory high PTH levels, but the fetal PTH production is suppressed. After birth the PTH remains low, resulting in low serum calcium levels and high serum phosphate levels which can produce tetany and seizures. The serum PTH level is not elevated, as it should be with hypocalcaemia, but is within the normal range or low. Treatment is with magnesium which allows release of PTH.

In pseudohypoparathyroidism the levels of PTH are normal but there is end organ resistance to the hormone. There are commonly short metacarpals (**Fig. 15.6**), hypoplastic tooth enamel and learning difficulties in these children. The hypocalcaemia is variable; children with dysmorphic features but normal bone chemistry are also seen within the same families.

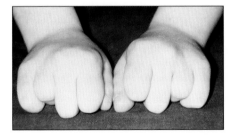

Fig. 15.6 *Short metacarpals in pseudohypoparathyroidism.*

GROWTH HORMONE DEFICIENCY

Complete deficiency of growth hormone (GH) may be congenital in origin and related to abnormalities of the hypothalamic–pituitary axis, such as the growth hormone deficiency seen with midline defects of the head. Deficiency may also be acquired because of tumours such as craniopharyngioma or after cranial irradiation for cancer.

Many children have a partial deficiency of growth hormone, either because of reduced pulsatility or quantity of released GH. There is also an interest in children who have short stature because of skeletal dysplasias as they may be helped to some degree by replacement therapy. This is particularly the case in Turner syndrome.

Investigations

Investigations for growth hormone deficiency are complicated and can be dangerous. As an initial screen, insulin-like growth factor binding protein 3 can be measured and, if normal, probably excludes GH deficiency; however, this is not generally available outside specialized centres. In practice there is no one perfect test to assess growth hormone production, and the experience of a specialist is desirable. Release of GH can be measured in response to insulin-induced hypoglycaemia. This test should only be performed in a specialist centre as over-vigorous correction of severe hypoglycaemia has caused cerebral oedema and death. Other agents include clonidine and glucagon.

Treatment for growth hormone deficiency is with regular subcutaneous injections of recombinant human growth hormone.

PUBERTY

The onset of normal puberty is preceded by several years of increasing pulsatile gonadotrophin release and increasing sex hormone levels. Gonadotrophin releasing factor (GnRF) is produced by the hypothalamus in a pulsatile manner and stimulates the release of follicle stimulating hormone (FSH) and luteinizing hormone (LH) from the anterior

---

Insulin tolerance test
(should only be done in specialist centres)

Use
Assessment of growth hormone deficiency
Assessment of hypothalamic–pituitary–adrenal axis

Contraindications
Epilepsy
Severe hypopituitarism

Dose
0.15 U/kg body weight soluble insulin intravenously

Aim
To produce adequate hypoglycaemia (signs of neuroglycopenia—tachycardia and sweating, and blood glucose less than 2.2 mmol/l: 40 mg/100 ml)

Blood samples
0, 30, 45, 60, 90, 120 minutes for growth hormone, blood glucose and plasma cortisol

Results
Normal: GH >20 mU/l
Normal: cortisol >550 nmol/l

pituitary. The pulsatile GnRF release is initially nocturnal but later occurs throughout the day. Sustained high levels of GnRF block secretion of LH and FSH, and a synthetic analogue can be used to block the changes in precocious puberty.

In boys, the Leydig cells produce testosterone which is peripherally converted to dihydrotestosterone and produces penile growth, pubic hair and deepening of the voice. The onset of puberty is marked clinically by an increase in testicular volume to 4 ml; this is due to an increase in the mass of Sertoli cells.

In girls, the first indication of puberty is breast formation which is largely driven by increasing oestrogen levels from the ovaries. The cyclical increase in FSH and LH levels leads to development of the follicles and maturation of the uterus, eventually culminating in the menarche. The appearance of pubic hair is due to androgens, mainly from the adrenal gland.

PRECOCIOUS PUBERTY

Puberty begins in 97% of girls after 8 years of age and in 97% of boys after 9 years. However puberty can, in healthy children, begin before these ages and it is usually unrewarding to investigate girls with onset of puberty before 6 years (or commencement of menses before 8 years). The orderly progression of puberty is known as consonance and indicates normality; abnormal progression, or dissonance, is worrying.

Precocious puberty in girls

Most girls with early onset to puberty will have a family history of early puberty and progress through the stages in an orderly way (consonance).

Sometimes an intracranial lesion may activate the hypothalamic–pituitary–gonadal axis. A hamartoma involving the hypothalamus, raised intracranial pressure or a tumour may be found and computed tomography or magnetic resonance imaging should always be performed (Fig. 15.7).

McCune–Albright syndrome is a rare cause of precocious puberty in girls and is suggested by the combination of irregularly edged brown skin macules, fibrous dysplasia of the skeleton and autonomous activity of the endocrine glands. There is also dissonance as vaginal bleeding occurs earlier than breast changes.

Hypothyroidism can be associated with precocious or delayed puberty, even if the child is clinically euthyroid.

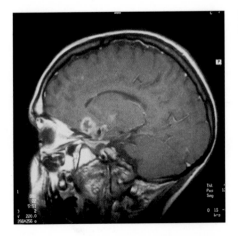

Fig. 15.7 *CT scan showing intracranial tumour responsible for precocious puberty.*

Precocious puberty in boys

In contrast to girls, an underlying abnormality is frequently found in boys with precocious puberty. Intracranial tumours are the most common cause and produce symmetrical enlargement of the testes and a normal pattern of development. Even if a lesion is not found on initial imaging, the child must be observed for some years to exclude an intracranial lesion.

Adrenarche and virilization

In both boys and girls the adrenal glands produce increasing levels of androgens (adrenarche) which coincides with puberty. The testicular production of androgens overshadows the adrenal production in boys and produces the masculine phenotype. In girls the adrenal amounts of androgens are insufficient to produce masculine effects. Small amounts of pubic hair may be found in mid-childhood and are caused by adrenal gland production of androgens.

Virilization in girls comprises enlargement of the clitoris and pubic hair development without breast changes (**Fig. 15.8**). At the time of birth the most likely cause is congenital adrenal hyperplasia (CAH) producing indeterminate genitalia. The presence of an androgen-secreting tumour should be sought in childhood, but CAH may also produce progressive virilization starting at this time. Virilization can also occur in boys (penile enlargement and pubic hair), but the testes remain small. The source of androgens may be an adrenal tumour. Sometimes there is a tumour within the testes, in which case one testis is enlarged by the tumour.

Premature thelarche

Breast development in female infants may occur as an isolated feature. The enlargement is usually transient, cyclical and asymmetrical. There is no evidence of puberty, and

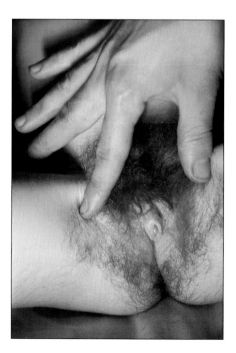

Fig. 15.8 *Virilization.*

ultrasound scanning shows that although there are follicles within the ovaries the uterus remains small. No treatment is required except for reassurance of the parents.

General management of precocious puberty

The most important effect of excessive androgens and precocious puberty is the acceleration in osseous maturation. Although this initially produces increased height for age, the acceleration produces early fusion of the epiphyses and final short stature. Early diagnosis is essential to minimize this effect. The hormonal effects of early puberty also produce psychological and behavioural difficulties for children and families, and specific help and support must be directed at this problem.

Gonadotrophin releasing hormone (GnRH) analogues are now the treatment of choice and act by inhibiting the hypothalamic release of GnRH. This does not reverse secondary sex characteristics to any great degree but halts the pubertal process until a more appropriate age. Cyproterone acetate can be used to block sex steroid production, but it also reduces the adrenal response in stress and additional corticosteroids will be needed at such times.

DELAYED PUBERTY

Delayed puberty is diagnosed if breast stage 2 is not present in a girl at 14 years of age, or if a boy's testicular volume is still less than 4 ml at 16 years of age. However, these children are usually seen because of relative short stature as their peers enjoy the pubertal growth spurt.

There are two groups of disorder: hypogonadotrophic hypogonadism, where the pituitary/hypothalamic release of luteinizing hormone and follicle stimulating hormone does not occur, and hypergonadotrophic hypogonadism, where the gonads fail to respond despite high levels of gonadotrophins.

Hypogonadotrophic hypogonadism

Hypogonadotrophic hypogonadism is usually a temporary phenomenon. Reassurance that puberty is about to commence may be sufficient therapy for the family. However, the use of a low dose of anabolic steroid or low dose depot androgen may be important in producing a growth spurt in boys. Oestrogens can similarly be used to promote a growth spurt in girls.

- Constitutional growth delay is the commonest cause of hypogonadotrophic hypogonadism and delayed puberty. There is a history of short stature in the child, and other members of the family have entered into puberty late. The bone age is delayed appropriately for the child's height.
- Children with chronic illness such as cystic fibrosis, inflammatory bowel disease or chronic renal failure often have late onset of puberty.
- Excessive exercise, stress, emotional distress, malnutrition and anorexia nervosa are all similarly associated with late puberty.
- Permanent failure of pituitary function (idiopathic, associated with midline cerebral defects or anatomical malformations) requires treatment with replacement hormones.

Hypergonadotrophic hypogonadism

Appropriate sex hormone replacement therapy is used to induce puberty and support secondary sexual characteristics in children with failure of the hypothalamic–pituitary–gonadal axis:

- Gonadal dysgenesis in association with chromosomal disorders such as Turner syndrome (XO) and Klinefelter syndrome (XXY).

- Gonadal damage from irradiation and some chemotheraputic agents.
- Testicular feminization syndrome. There is an enzyme block in the conversion of testosterone to dihydrotestosterone or insensitivity of the target tissues. The external genitalia remain female in appearance as there is no androgen effect on the genitalia and there will be no progression at the time of puberty.

INDETERMINATE GENITALIA

In humans, genetic sex is determined by the presence of the Y chromosome which carries the testis-determining gene (TDG) and causes the fetal gonad to differentiate into a testis; in its absence ovaries develop (gonadal sex). The testicular Sertoli cells produce müllerian inhibiting factor (MIF) which causes regression of the müllerian ducts and prevents the development of internal female genitalia (**Fig. 15.9**). The external genitalia, which initially

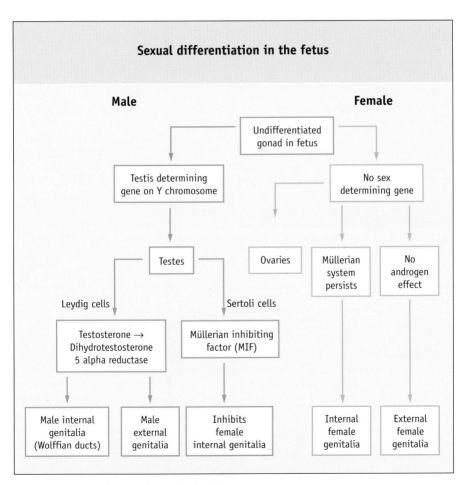

Fig. 15.9 *Sexual differentiation in the fetus.*

appear female, are masculinized by the direct effects of dihydrotestosterone causing phallic enlargement and scrotal formation (phenotypic sex) occurring between 4 and 14 weeks' gestation. The most common cause of indeterminate genitalia is congenital adrenal hyperplasia which produces virilization of the female. Undescended testes and hypospadias may cause confusion over gender assignment (**Fig. 15.10**).

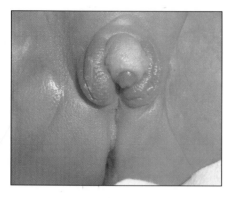

Fig. 15.10 *Undescended testes and hypospadias with shawl scrotum.*

MANAGEMENT OF INDETERMINATE GENITALIA

When a baby is born, one of the first questions relates to its sex, which will dictate the way family, society and the individual view his or her sexuality. If the gender is not immediately clear it is essential not to give a male or female label to the baby until the abnormalities have been investigated. It is also important to diagnose infants with congenital adrenal hyperplasia as they may be at risk of a salt-losing crisis.

- Gonadal sex should be determined by the presence of testes or ovaries. Abdominal ultrasound may be required to search for testes.
- Phenotypic sex is based on identification of internal female organs and the external genitalia, in particular the size of the phallus.
- Genetic sex is determined by a rapid karyotype.

On the basis of these findings a decision is made on the gender to which to assign the baby. An acceptable penis may be difficult to produce if the phallus is very small, and surgery to produce female external genitalia may be more successful.

CONGENITAL ADRENAL HYPERPLASIA

Congenital adrenal hyperplasia (CAH) is due to an inborn error in cortisol biosynthesis and occurs in 1 in 10 000 live births. The commonest defect is the 21-hydroxylase defect. The deficiency of 21-hydroxylase, or more rarely 11-β-hydroxylase, prevents formation of aldosterone and cortisol. Lack of cortisol stimulates more ACTH production, driving the formation of testosterone which then produces virilization (**Fig. 15.11**).

Girls are virilized at birth, with marked clitoral enlargement and some degree of labial fusion. In boys, the physical signs of penile enlargement and increased scrotal pigmentation may be missed at birth, but progressive virilization (enlarging penis, pubic hair and accelerated growth but small testes) occurs with time.

Girls are relatively safe from salt-losing crises as they are readily identified. However, boys may not be identified at birth, and the weight loss, vomiting and dehydration of a salt-losing crisis may be confused with other causes of failure to thrive, such as urinary tract infection or pyloric stenosis. Electrolyte determination in dehydrated salt losers will

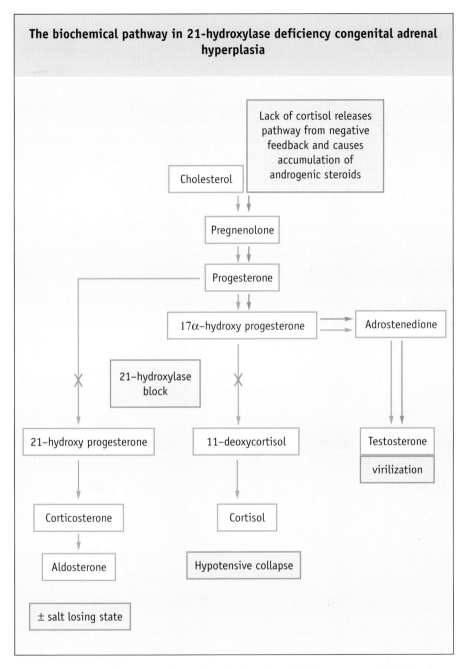

Fig. 15.11 *The biochemical pathway in 21-hydroxylase deficiency congenital adrenal hyperplasia.*

show hyponatraemia, hyperkalaemia and elevated urea. The level of 17-hydroxyprogesterone is elevated in all infants with 21-hydroxylase deficiency.

Initial resuscitation with saline and correction of electrolytes may be necessary for salt-losing babies. DOCA is a mineralocorticoid that can be given parenterally with hydrocortisone until oral fludrocortisone and hydrocortisone can be tolerated. Progress is monitored by 17-hydroxyprogesterone levels and appropriate growth. Lifelong replacement therapy is necessary and hydrocortisone should be increased during times of stress (illness or operation). There should also be free access to salt.

Surgery is required in girls to recess the clitoris and fashion a vagina. The internal organs and fertility are normal in both sexes.

Prenatal diagnosis for the families of previously affected children is important as there is a 1 in 4 risk of recurrence. Mothers take dexamethasone as soon as they are pregnant as the critical time of male external genital development occurs early in gestation. Identification of restriction fragment length polymorphisms (RFLPs) after chorionic biopsy or measurement of 17-hydroxyprogesterone in amniotic fluid is performed. If the child is male or unaffected, the corticosteroids can be stopped. This treatment reduces the severity of virilization in girls. At birth, steroid assays are performed to confirm that the baby is affected and replacement mineralocorticoids and glucocorticoids are given.

CUSHING SYNDROME

Adrenal and pituitary tumours are rare in childhood. The well-recognized side-effects of corticosteroids usually occur as a result of therapeutic doses in children with life-threatening disorders such as asthma, renal disease and as immunosuppression (**Figs 15.12, 15.13**).

HYPOADRENALISM

Hypoadrenalism is also seen in various congenital defects affecting the midline of the head. Other hypothalamic–pituitary functions are disturbed and there is usually lack of gonadotrophins and hypothyroidism. The features of hypoadrenalism are part of congenital adrenal hyperplasia.

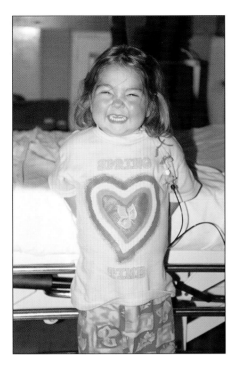

Fig. 15.12 *Cushingoid facies.*

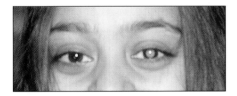

Fig. 15.13 *Steroid cataract.*

chapter 16

The Urinary System

The majority of children have no problems with their urinary system. Some have trivial congenital abnormalities that require no intervention, such as a minor hypospadias. A minority of children have severe abnormalities requiring investigation and treatment. These congenital abnormalities are often associated with others in a syndrome (**Figs 16.1–16.5**), and are often diagnosed on antenatal ultrasound scan. The important points in assessing congenital lesions are the quantity of functional renal tissue and the presence of obstruction in the draining system. Urinary tract infection and ureteric reflux are important conditions commonly encountered by general paediatricians.

Common renal malformations	
Potter sequence (oligohydramnios sequence)	The amniotic fluid volume is maintained by urine produced by the fetus. Bilateral non-functioning kidneys lead to oligohydramnios and the fetus becomes squashed in appearance and has contractures of the joints. Normal formation of the lungs is also dependent on the presence of amniotic fluid, and oligohydramnios in the second trimester is often associated with lung hypoplasia. The degree of pulmonary insufficiency is the important factor governing the immediate survival of these babies as nowadays renal dialysis can be provided for neonates.
The disappearing kidney	Antenatal ultrasound scanning sometimes shows a small or absent kidney. These unilateral dysplastic kidneys are generally non-functioning and often involute in the first years of life. It is important to evaluate fully these babies as one third to one half of remaining kidneys are dysplastic or exhibit ureteric reflux. If the solitary kidney and its drainage system is normal then regular urinalysis (checking for proteinuria) and assessment of blood pressure are all that is required.
Adult polycystic disease	Progressive cyst formation in the kidneys destroys normal renal tissue causing hypertension and renal insufficiency in early adult life. Cysts also occur in the liver, pancreas and ovaries but rarely cause symptoms. In some families there is an association with aneurysms in the cerebral circulation and subarachnoid haemorrhage. Two genes have now been identified; there is autosomal dominant inheritance.

Fig. 16.1 *Common renal malformations.*

Common renal malformations (continued)

Infantile polycystic disease	The cysts in infantile polycystic disease are less than 2 mm in diameter and cannot be identified on ultrasound scanning. Instead the kidneys have increased echogenicity (brightness) and appear larger than normal due to the bulk of cysts. The liver also contains cysts; hepatic failure and portal hypertension, as well as chronic renal failure, are problems that occur in childhood. This condition is due to a single gene with autosomal recessive inheritance.
Duplex systems	In a duplex system there are two ureters draining the kidney. Ureteric reflux and obstruction are important problems which can reduce functioning renal tissue and predispose to infection.
Horseshoe kidneys	The kidneys are fused in the midline; there are few clinical consequences.
Pelviceal-ureteric junction (PUJ) obstruction	Obstruction of the proximal ureter produces dilatation of the renal pelvis—hydronephrosis. Most cases are idiopathic and may be familial.
Posterior urethral valves	This is a common cause of bilateral renal obstruction in male children. It is usually diagnosed on antenatal ultrasound scanning but can present after birth when there is a poor urinary stream in an infant with a distended bladder or with a urinary tract infection. Following birth the bladder is temporarily drained with a suprapubic catheter before the diagnosis is confirmed with a cystogram and the membrane is removed by diathermy.
Prune belly sequence	Prune belly sequence occurs only in boys. The name describes the combination of deficient abdominal muscles, undescended testes and complex genito-urinary anomalies. The condition is thought to be due to obstruction of the fetal urinary system which subsequently clears. The cause is not known but may be a temporary obstruction to urinary flow producing massive hydronephrosis and disruption to abdominal muscle formation.

Fig. 16.1 *Common renal malformations (continued).*

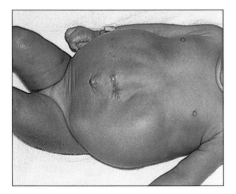

Fig. 16.2 *Prune belly sequence.*

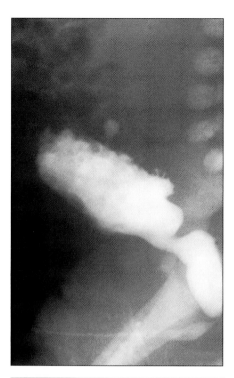

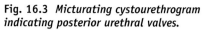

Fig. 16.3 *Micturating cystourethrogram indicating posterior urethral valves.*

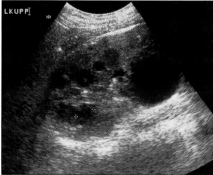

Fig. 16.4 *Ultrasound scan showing large cysts in adult-type autosomal dominant polycystic kidney disease.*

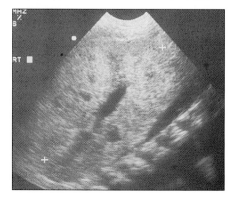

Fig. 16.5 *Ultrasound scan showing typical 'bright' appearances of infantile or autosomal recessive polycystic kidney disease.*

POLYDIPSIA AND THE TUBULAR DISORDERS

Most abnormalities of the renal tubule are rare and involve specific or generalized abnormalities of amino acid transport across the renal tubule (**Fig. 16.6**). However, a more common clinical problem is a child who drinks and urinates excessively. As an initial screen, it is helpful to collect the first urine specimen after waking in the morning to check for glycosuria, which will exclude diabetes mellitus, and measure the osmolarity. If the urine is concentrated above $600\,\mu mol/kgH_2O$, the concentrating ability of the kidney is normal and the polydipsia is a behavioural problem.

If the urine fails to concentrate (less than $600\,\mu mol/kgH_2O$), diabetes insipidus is likely. In diabetes insipidus the collecting tubules do not re-absorb water, the urine remains dilute, and the child must therefore drink to keep up with the obligatory urinary losses. Diabetes

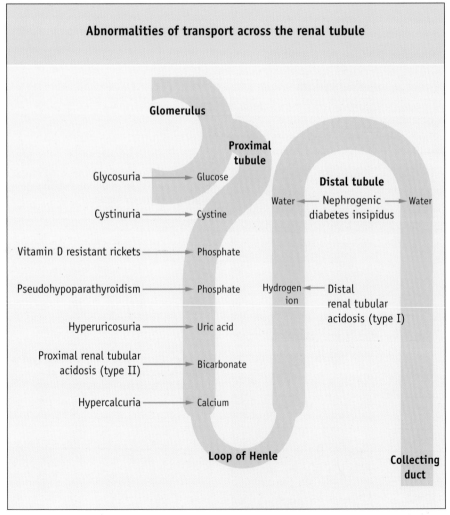

Abnormalities of transport across the renal tubule

Glomerulus

Proximal tubule

Glycosuria ⟶ Glucose

Distal tubule

Water ⟵ Nephrogenic ⟶ Water
diabetes insipidus

Cystinuria ⟶ Cystine

Vitamin D resistant rickets ⟶ Phosphate

Pseudohypoparathyroidism ⟶ Phosphate

Hydrogen ⟵ Distal
ion　　renal tubular
acidosis (type I)

Hyperuricosuria ⟶ Uric acid

Proximal renal tubular
acidosis (type II) ⟶ Bicarbonate

Hypercalcuria ⟶ Calcium

Loop of Henle

Collecting duct

Fig. 16.6 *Abnormalities of transport across the renal tubule.*

insipidus may be due either to a lack of production of antidiuretic hormone (ADH) by the posterior pituitary (cranial DI) or to a renal tubular insensitivity to the hormone (nephrogenic DI). Intranasal desmopressin spray can be given to determine whether the collecting ducts are sensitive to ADH and identify cranial diabetes insipidus.

Sometimes the morning urine osmolarity is equivocal. In such cases a water deprivation test is carried out. Fluid intake is restricted and the urine volume and osmolality is measured as well as the plasma osmolality. This is a dangerous test which must be stopped if there is excessive weight loss.

URINARY TRACT INFECTIONS

Urinary tract infection (UTI) is common in childhood. The sex incidence of UTI is equal in babies but in older children is much higher in girls (2–3%) than in boys (1%).

The usual definition of infection is a pure growth of more than 10^5 bacterial colonies per ml of urine, but the criterion of greater than 10^4 per ml is often used in boys. The usual organisms are *E. coli* (**Fig. 16.7**), *Proteus* spp. (especially boys), and *Pseudomonas* spp. (especially if there is a structural abnormality).

Diagnosis

It is important to make an accurate diagnosis and identify children with predisposing abnormalities of the urinary tract such as congenital malformations and refluxing ureteric systems as undiagnosed infection can lead to renal scarring, functional impairment and hypertension in later life.

Whilst older children are more likely to have frequency and dysuria, it is often hard to diagnose urinary tract infection in infants and babies as the presentation can be non-specific. Prolonged jaundice, poor weight gain, irritability, and diarrhoea and vomiting are common presentations, as is generalized septicaemia. In practice, any child with a fever should be considered for UTI and appropriate measures taken to exclude it properly.

Collection of urine in a plastic bag attached to the perineum is a method commonly used in babies, but is much less satisfactory than a clean catheter specimen. Urine bag specimens are useful to exclude urinary tract infection if the urine is sterile. Positive identification can be effective if the skin is properly cleaned to remove contaminating

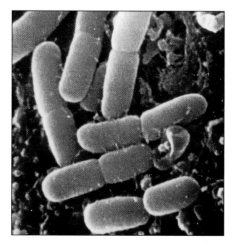

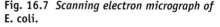

Fig. 16.7 *Scanning electron micrograph of E. coli.*

bacteria (**Fig. 16.8**). The urinary stream from boys can also be collected into a sterile container by a patient parent. In a septicaemic infant, when therapy needs to be started immediately, suprapubic aspiration or urethral catheterization may be used to collect urine.

Microscopy of fresh urine is helpful. Although white cells are often seen in any pyrexial illness, the presence of white cells and bacteria is suggestive of infection. Dip sticks for nitrite (produced by bacteria) and white cell esterase are also helpful in diagnosis. Urine is always cultured to identify the organism and its sensitivities. A mixed growth usually indicates contamination.

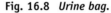

Fig. 16.8 *Urine bag.*

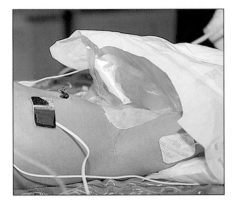

Treatment

Treatment with trimethoprim or an oral cephalosporin is the usual initial therapy for a relatively well child until the bacteria are identified and sensitivities known. In babies or an ill child an intravenous cephalosporin, possibly with gentamicin, would be given. There should be rapid recovery once antibiotics have been administered. After a 7 day course the urine is re-checked for bacteria but the child should remain on a night-time prophylactic antibiotic dose, which prevents urinary tract infection, until the renal tract has been evaluated. If there is evidence of reflux, prophylactic antibiotics are continued until the age of 5 when the risk of forming new scars diminishes.

Evaluation of the renal tract

The investigations required after a proven UTI remain a topic for debate but the principles are simple (**Fig. 16.9**):

- The renal tract should be demonstrated to be structurally normal; this is done with ultrasound scanning (**Fig. 16.10**). Older children (over the age of 8) probably need not have further imaging if the initial ultrasound scan is normal.
- The presence of scars in the kidney parenchyma should be sought. This is less important in older children as the tendency to form new scars diminishes after the age of 4 or 5 years. Scars are visualized with a DMSA isotope scan, which should be deferred for some weeks after the acute infection as the appearances of resolving acute infection can be confused with permanent scarring (**Fig. 16.11**).
- The presence of ureteric reflux (urine washing back to the kidneys on micturition) is more difficult to ascertain as there is some controversy about which children need a formal micturating cystogram. In this investigation infants are catheterized and X-ray contrast passed into the bladder until it is full. Then, during spontaneous micturition, the ureters are visualized with X-ray screening (**Fig. 16.12**). An indirect micturating

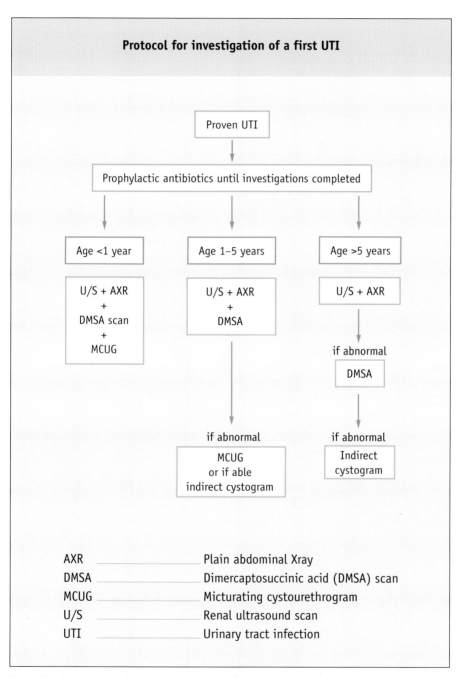

Protocol for investigation of a first UTI

Proven UTI

Prophylactic antibiotics until investigations completed

Age <1 year

Age 1–5 years

Age >5 years

U/S + AXR
+
DMSA scan
+
MCUG

U/S + AXR
+
DMSA

U/S + AXR

if abnormal

DMSA

if abnormal

MCUG
or if able
indirect cystogram

if abnormal

Indirect
cystogram

AXR	Plain abdominal Xray
DMSA	Dimercaptosuccinic acid (DMSA) scan
MCUG	Micturating cystourethrogram
U/S	Renal ultrasound scan
UTI	Urinary tract infection

Fig. 16.9 *Protocol for the investigation of a first UTI.*

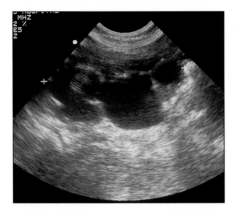

Fig. 16.10 *Ultrasound scan showing calyceal dilatation due to pelviceal-ureteric junction obstruction.*

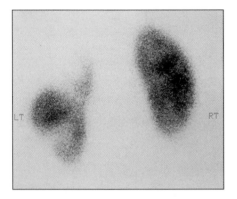

Fig. 16.11 *DMSA scan showing scars in left renal cortex.*

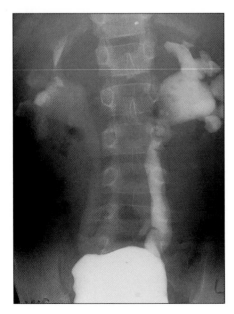

Fig. 16.12 *Micturating cystourethrogram showing reflux of contrast to the kidneys with ureteric dilatation.*

cystogram can be used in older children if they can pass urine voluntarily. A radioisotope, MAG 3, is injected into a vein and the radioactivity detected with a gamma camera. It has a rapid early renogram phase, allowing visualization of the renal parenchyma and detection of most scars. As it passes through the parenchyma an estimation of differential renal function is possible. Reflux can be detected when the bladder is emptied.

HYDRONEPHROSIS

Hydronephrosis is an abnormal dilatation of the renal pelvis which renders the kidney susceptible to infection because of stasis (*see* Fig. 16.10). Identification of hydronephrosis depends on the urinary flow rate. It may be missed in obstructed urinary systems if there is low urinary flow and suspected in normal kidneys with a high flow.

It has been shown that many children with urinary tract infection associated with ureteric reflux also have large renal pelvices. This has led to antenatal screening in an attempt to identify persistent renal pelviceal dilatation and thus protect those at risk of reflux before any scarring has occurred. Infants with antenatally recognized enlarged renal pelvices are carefully followed by serial ultrasound scans while receiving antibiotic prophylaxis. If the pelvices remain enlarged with respect to the size of the growing kidney, an isotope scan and micturating cystogram are carried out to identify ureteric reflux.

DUPLEX KIDNEYS

In a duplex system there are two ureters—one draining the upper kidney pole and the other draining the lower pole (**Figs 16.13, 16.14**). The ureter draining the lower pole may enter the upper part of the bladder and allow urine to reflux. The ureter draining the upper pole may form a ureterocele in the bladder or, in girls, may drain ectopically into the vagina causing persistent dribbling.

HAEMATURIA

Blood in the urine may be visible to the naked eye (macroscopic) or visible only with a microscope (microscopic). Discoloured urine may, however, be due to other pigments such as beetroot, myoglobin or haemoglobin. Concentrated urine may appear red due to the presence of urate; this is often encountered in the nappies of newborn babies.

A pragmatic approach to the investigation of haematuria is adopted and investigations are not usually carried out unless haematuria is gross or recurrent. In general, if there is haematuria without proteinuria, then there is usually little benefit from investigations (**Fig. 16.15**). The important exception to this is nephroblastoma (Wilms tumour).

PROTEINURIA

Protein in the urine is an important symptom of renal disease. Heavy proteinuria is seen in nephrotic syndrome, and moderate amounts can also be seen in nephritic syndrome (**Fig. 16.16**). However, the presence of protein in the urine can be frequently misleading;

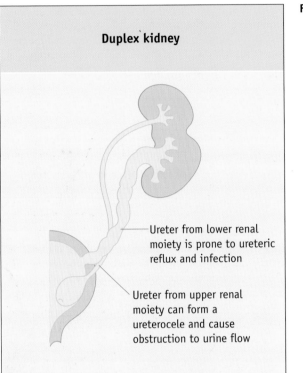

Fig. 16.13 *Duplex kidney.*

Duplex kidney

Ureter from lower renal moiety is prone to ureteric reflux and infection

Ureter from upper renal moiety can form a ureterocele and cause obstruction to urine flow

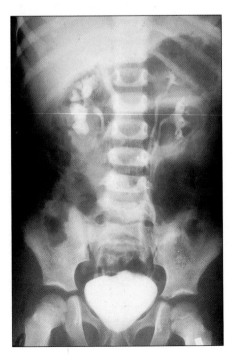

Fig. 16.14 *Intravenous pyelogram (IVP) showing left duplex system and stone in left renal pelvis.*

Causes of haematuria

Diagnosis	Key features	Investigations
Nephroblastoma	Abdominal mass	Ultrasound
Urinary tract infection*	Dysuria, frequency although signs may be subtle in the very young	Urine microscopy and culture
Nephritic syndrome*	May be accompanied by hypertension and acute renal failure	Evidence of streptococcal infection and, if atypical features, renal biopsy
Alport syndrome	Family history of renal disease or deafness. X-linked inheritance	Typical onion skin appearance to the glomerular basement membrane on renal biopsy (usually not required)
Vasculitis*	Other features of Henoch–Schönlein purpura	Special investigations usually not required
Drugs	Cyclophosphamide	Prophylactic mesna is usually given
IgA nephropathy	Associated with viral infections	Not progressive and investigations not usually required
Exercise (march haematuria)	Long distance running	History
Renal stones	Renal colic	Ultrasound, intravenous urogram (IVU)
Munchausen syndrome	Inconsistency in signs and symptoms	Can be a difficult diagnosis

*Conditions which have protein as well as blood in the urine.

Fig. 16.15 *Causes of haematuria.*

Nephrotic and nephritic syndromes

	Nephrotic syndrome	Nephritic syndrome
Features	• Significant proteinuria • Hypoalbuminaemia • Oedema • Hyperlipidaemia	• Haematuria • Oedema • Hypertension • Acute renal impairment
Common causes	• Minimal change disease • Membranous nephrotic syndrome	• Post-streptococcal glomerulonephritis • Henoch–Schönlein nephritis • Autoimmune vasculitis

Fig. 16.16 *Nephrotic and nephritic syndromes.*

231

for example, transient proteinuria occurs during exercise, and any pyrexial illness can be associated with proteinuria.

NEPHROTIC SYNDROME

The loss of large amounts of protein across the glomerulus leads to hypoalbuminaemia and a fall in the oncotic pressure of the blood. There is also fluid retention because of activation of the renin–angiotensin system. Fluid begins to pass into the tissues, accumulating initially in lax tissues in the dependent areas. For example, periorbital swelling upon waking in the morning is often the first sign (**Fig. 16.17**). Later, the genitalia

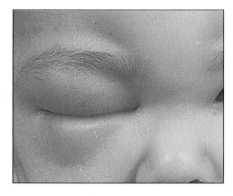

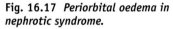
Fig. 16.17 *Periorbital oedema in nephrotic syndrome.*

become oedematous, the lower limbs are affected, and eventually ascites and pleural effusions collect. These shifts of fluid from the intravascular compartment into the tissues can leave a child in hypovolaemic shock despite having too much fluid in the body as a whole. This requires emergency restoration of the circulating volume with albumin solution. Diuretics such as frusemide may be given with albumin to treat symptomatic oedema (e.g. painful scrotal swelling, abdominal pain from tense ascites or dyspnoea from pleural effusions).

The nephrotic syndrome is also associated with a hypercoagulable circulation due to loss of natural antithrombins. Cerebral and renal thromboses may occur. There are also low levels of immunoglobulins in nephrotic syndrome, placing the child at risk of bacterial infections. Prophylactic penicillin is given until the plasma protein levels are normalized.

In childhood, almost all cases of nephrotic syndrome are caused by minimal change nephropathy (**Figs 16.18, 16.19**). If there are no unusual features (normal renal function, blood pressure, complement and no haematuria in a child under 10 years) then the condition is likely to be steroid responsive. Prednisolone is usually given at 60 mg/m²/day for four weeks and then tailed off over the following two weeks. A renal biopsy is only required if there is no response or if atypical features are present.

Most children recover completely or have infrequent relapses, often after viral infections. Up to a third may have frequent relapses and need corticosteroids on a regular alternate-day basis.

NEPHRITIC SYNDROME

Nephritic syndrome is inflammation of the glomerulus. It is characterized by the presence of large numbers of red cells, white cells and granular casts in the urine. Hypertension occurs when there is fluid overload due to impairment of renal function.

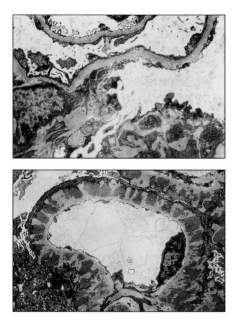

Fig. 16.18 *Electron micrograph of minimal change nephropathy with characteristic fusion of foot processes.*

Fig. 16.19 *Electron micrograph of membranous nephropathy.*

A number of rare diseases of the glomerular apparatus may be diagnosed on renal biopsy (**Fig. 16.20**), but the most common cause is post-streptococcal glomerulonephritis.

Post-streptococcal glomerulonephritis

Post-streptococcal glomerulonephritis is caused by an immunological mechanism which is usually provoked by a preceding group A beta haemolytic streptococcal infection involving the throat or skin. Rarely, other bacteria or viruses may provoke the same illness. Children present with the features of nephritic syndrome, often accompanied by headache, lethargy, malaise or abdominal pain.

The diagnosis is suggested by the combination of a recent streptococcal infection, confirmed by rising ASO or antiDNA-ase B titres, and reduced C3 complement levels. Autoantibodies should be tested to exclude systemic disorders such as systemic lupus erythematosus.

Although the streptococcal infection has resolved, it is usual to treat with a course of penicillin. The general management is the same as for acute renal failure and the condition is usually self-limiting with 95% of children recovering completely.

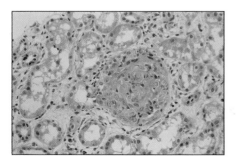

Fig. 16.20 *Focal segmental glomerulonephritis.*

ACUTE RENAL FAILURE

The sudden loss of kidney function is rare in children and usually occurs in those with acute life-threatening conditions following trauma, septicaemia or major surgery. The causes can be divided into three groups of conditions:

Pre-renal
Ischaemic injury (acute tubular necrosis) occurs following a period of reduced perfusion to the kidneys due to hypovolaemia or hypotension. In general, the tubules recover if perfusion is restored.

Renal
Haemolytic-uraemic syndrome (see below) and post-streptococcal glomerulonephritis (see above) are two common causes of renal failure due to disease within the kidneys.

Post-renal
Obstruction to the drainage of urine is an uncommon but important cause of renal failure as it can be quickly corrected and renal function preserved. To cause clinical renal failure the obstruction must be bilateral, as for example in congenital abnormalities such as posterior urethral valves. Loss of kidney function may be accelerated if there is coincident infection.

HAEMOLYTIC-URAEMIC SYNDROME
Haemolytic-uraemic syndrome (HUS) is a very common cause of acute renal failure in children; it typically follows a bout of diarrhoea. There is a typical triad of acute renal failure, thrombocytopenia, and microangiopathic haemolytic anaemia. The condition is believed to be caused by bacteria such as *E. coli* 0157 (*see* Fig. 16.7) which produces verotoxin. HUS seems to follow on from endothelial cell dysfunction and neutrophil activation. Cerebral irritation, fits, stroke and pancreatitis are well recognized features of the illness, and a high white cell count is associated with cerebral involvement, long-term renal problems and death.

There is an atypical form of HUS which is not associated with diarrhoea. It affects younger children, often occurs within families, and has a high mortality.

There is no specific treatment for HUS and general management is as for acute renal failure.

MANAGEMENT OF ACUTE RENAL FAILURE
Despite the many different causes of acute renal failure, the principles of management are simple and directed at managing the electrolyte and fluid homeostatic functions of the kidney while waiting for a spontaneous return of function.

Management of acute renal failure

- All children with ARF need an urgent renal ultrasound to exclude obstruction to urine flow and to identify underlying abnormalities.
- Hypotension, hypovolaemia and shock should be treated with colloidal solutions and inotropes if necessary to ensure adequate renal perfusion. A dopamine infusion may be used to improve renal blood flow.
- Careful fluid management is important to prevent fluid overload and hypertension. For example, dextrose solution is used to replace insensible fluid losses occurring across the skin and respiratory tract and any additional urine is also replaced with dextrose solution. It is usual to try to invoke a diuresis by a large dose of diuretic such as frusemide. The best way to monitor fluid balance is with a strict in–out fluid chart and frequent weighings.
- The major electrolyte problem in acute renal failure is hyperkalaemia, especially if there has been surgery or infection, as high levels can cause fatal arrhythmias. It is usual to reduce potassium intake to a minimum but, if elevated concentrations are encountered, an intravenous salbutamol infusion or a dextrose infusion with insulin can be used to move potassium into the intracellular compartment. In an emergency calcium can be used to oppose the effects of hyperkalaemia on the heart. Calcium resonium, an ion exchange resin, can be given orally or rectally to sequestrate potassium from the body but dialysis should be started.
- Metabolic acidosis occurs because the kidney is not able to excrete the acids produced from the breakdown of amino acids. Compensatory hyperventilation can be distressing and require treatment with sodium bicarbonate.

MANAGEMENT OF CHRONIC RENAL FAILURE

Most chronic renal problems only progress to symptomatic renal failure in adulthood. The main causes of chronic renal failure (CRF) in childhood are congenital abnormalities, endstage glomerulonephritis, HUS and rare inherited kidney disease (**Fig. 16.21**).

Causes of chronic renal failure	
Cause	**Percentage of cases**
Structural malformation	40
Glomerulonephritis	25
Hereditary nephropathy	20
Systemic disease	10
Miscellaneous/unknown	5

Fig. 16.21 *Causes of chronic renal failure.*

The most important difference between children and adults with CRF is that children are still capable of growth. This means that most protein is diverted to growth rather than being broken down for metabolism. Children only become symptomatic when renal function has diminished by 60–80% from normal (**Fig. 16.22**). After this, symptoms of lethargy, poor appetite and diminished growth are common findings. Growth also assumes importance in children with renal failure because transplantation is easier in larger children. A regular diet providing 130% of the nutrition of a normal child is supplied. This intake can be difficult to achieve because children with CRF have diminished sense of taste and altered gastrointestinal motility predisposing to gastro-oesophageal reflux; they also fail to gain weight because of the chronic disease process. Feeds often need to be given via a gastrostomy (**Fig. 16.23**).

Symptoms of chronic renal failure and their management

Problem	Cause	Treatment
Growth failure	Poor calorie intake	• Calorific supplements
		• Protein supplements
	Acidosis	• Sodium bicarbonate
	Deranged biochemistry	• Sodium chloride supplements
Renal osteodystrophy (renal rickets)	Phosphate retention	• Restrict dietary phosphate
		• Calcium carbonate as phosphate binder
	Defective vitamin D metabolism	• 1α-cholecalciferol
Anaemia	Reduced erythropoietin	• Erythropoietin
	Nutritional deficit	• Supplements if deficient in folic acid or iron
Hypertension	Sodium retention	• Sodium restriction/diuretics
	Renin release	• ACE inhibitors/nephrectomy

Fig. 16.22 *Symptoms of chronic renal failure and their management.*

Fig. 16.23 *Button gastrostomy.*

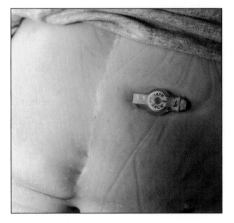

Polyuria is common in CRF and is due to a urinary concentrating defect. There may be an obligatory salt loss in some children which requires ready access to water and sodium supplementation. Hyperphosphataemia is also common, due to lack of renal phosphate excretion, and can result in a reduction in calcium levels and elevation in parathyroid hormone release. This secondary hyperparathyroidism mobilizes calcium and phosphate from bone, further increasing phosphate levels and producing renal metabolic bone disease. To overcome this problem calcium carbonate is given to bind phosphate in the gut and vitamin D is provided as 1α-cholecalciferol. Anaemia responds well to recombinant human erythropoietin injections, and hypertension is treated by conventional agents such as nifedipine.

RENAL REPLACEMENT THERAPY

When renal function has diminished to a level at which medical measures are insufficient, dialysis or transplantation is needed. The preferred method is peritoneal dialysis. Fluid is placed within the peritoneal cavity and then drained out at intervals (**Fig. 16.24**). Fluid and electrolyte imbalances can be gradually corrected by varying the hypertonicity and electrolyte composition of the dialysate. Older children and adults can change the peritoneal fluid 3–4 times per day (continuous ambulatory peritoneal dialysis, CAPD). The main problem with peritoneal dialysis is peritoneal infection. In small children more cycles are needed and the dialysis is performed overnight by a machine which fills and drains the peritoneal cavity automatically while the child is asleep (continuous cycling peritoneal dialysis, CCPD—**Fig. 16.25**). As only one connection to the peritoneal catheter is required each night this method is associated with fewer peritoneal infections.

Haemofiltration is a slow but gentle method of renal replacement therapy used in sick and haemodynamically unstable children, usually in the intensive care unit. Blood is continuously removed from the child (**Fig. 16.26**), ultrafiltered (**Fig. 16.27**) and returned to the body. Haemodialysis is a more efficient and rapid method that also requires good venous access. It is used when there are severe disturbances of homeostasis or if the peritoneum is unavailable, for example after abdominal surgery or because of peritoneal infections. Haemodialysis is carried out in hospital three times a week for 3–4 hours. It is expensive and limiting for the child because the child has a restricted fluid intake as well as having to visit the hospital.

The best option is a kidney transplant and this is now possible in all but the smallest infants. However, there is a lack of small cadaveric organs for children and so a single kidney from live relative is sometimes used. There is a higher rate of success with kidneys donated by family members but even so the 5 year success rate for transplantation is about 70%. As with any transplantation process there may be problems with acute and chronic rejection, and lifelong immunosuppressive therapy is needed. Transplanted kidneys do not last indefinitely and may be subject to recurrent disease or need replacement.

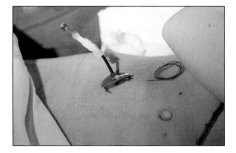

Fig. 16.24 *Peritoneal dialysis catheter.*

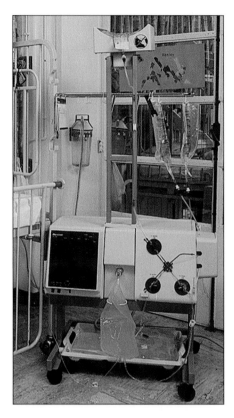

Fig. 16.25 *Continuous cycling peritoneal dialysis machine.*

Fig. 16.26 *Venous access for haemofiltration.*

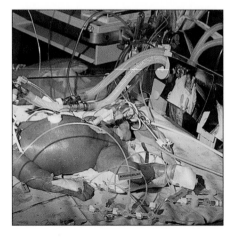

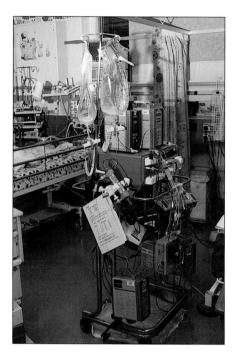

Fig. 16.27 *Haemofiltration machine.*

chapter 17

Dermatology

The main role of the skin is to protect the body from physical, chemical and biological environmental insults. This is achieved by the keratinized horny layer of the skin which also reduces evaporation of water into the atmosphere. Epidermal melanocytes produce melanin and protect the body from the damaging effects of ultraviolet radiation. In regulating body temperature, blood can be diverted away from the skin surface to conserve heat, or towards the surface to lose heat. Sweating and evaporation of the moisture is another important way in which the skin reduces body temperature. There are numerous sensory appendages in the skin sensing pain, temperature and touch. The production of vitamin D also takes place within the skin (**Fig. 17.1**).

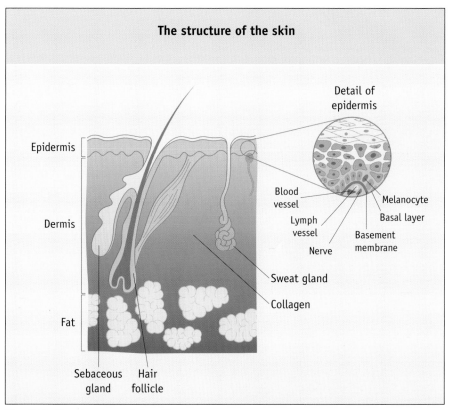

The structure of the skin

Epidermis

Detail of epidermis

Blood vessel

Melanocyte

Basal layer

Dermis

Lymph vessel

Basement membrane

Nerve

Sweat gland

Collagen

Fat

Sebaceous gland   Hair follicle

Fig. 17.1 *The structure of the skin.*

NEONATAL RASHES

Skin begins to develop in the third week of fetal life; there is a basal layer which eventually forms the dermis and epidermis, and an outer periderm which is shed during gestation.

The sweat glands only reach the skin surface after a few days in term babies, and effective sweating may not be possible for some weeks; this may hamper the diagnosis of cystic fibrosis. Sweat rash (miliaria) (**Fig. 17.2**) is commonly seen and is due to the accumulation of sweat within sweat ducts of the dermis. Accumulation of sebum and keratin can also form cysts called milia which are commonly seen on the face of newborn babies.

Baby rash, or erythema toxicum neonatorum, is seen on the trunk and limbs in up to 50% of babies (**Fig. 17.3**). It usually begins within a few days of birth and lasts for a few days. The cause is unknown but the lesions contain eosinophils. The appearances are

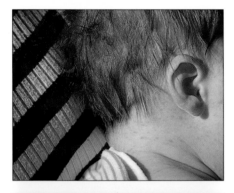

Fig. 17.2 *Miliaria or sweat rash has a typical appearance with pinhead sized papules and vesicles.*

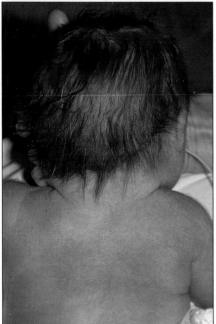

Fig. 17.3 *Erythema toxicum neonatorum.*

characteristic but occasionally can be confused with a staphylococcal infection. In general, rash within the first three days is due to erythema toxicum and a rash beginning after this time will be due to infection. Microscopy of a bacteriological swab will differentiate the two conditions.

Superficial skin infections with staphylococci and streptococci are not uncommon and usually originate from passage through the birth canal. The infection may appear as a red rash that is more prominent in the axillae and groin folds (**Fig. 17.4**). The infection usually localizes to form pustules, or as blisters. In many cases the infection resolves without treatment but oral flucloxacillin is useful if the lesions are clearly not resolving quickly.

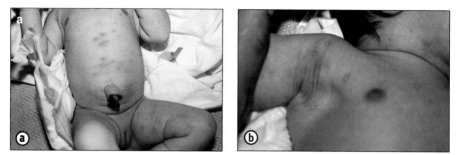

Fig. 17.4 *(a) Staphylococcal infection causing pustules on the skin; (b) staphylococcal pustules are commonly found in the skin folds.*

NAPKIN RASHES

There are four main causes of napkin rash which can be distinguished by their classical appearances.

Ammoniacal dermatitis (**Fig. 17.5**) — This is caused by prolonged contact with ammonia which is produced by bacterial action on urine. The rash can be severe with the

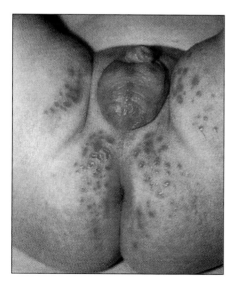

Fig. 17.5 *Ammoniacal napkin rash with typical sparing of the flexures.*

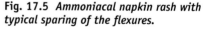

development of raw areas. Areas that do not come into contact with the urine are unaffected. This characteristic sparing of flexures allows differentiation from candidal infection. Rapid resolution can be obtained by exposure of the skin to air and the use of barrier creams such as zinc oxide. Modern disposable nappies draw urine away from the skin and cause fewer problems.

Candida albicans — *Candida albicans* causes an erythematous rash involving the flexures and often demonstrating satellite lesions within the napkin area (**Fig. 17.6**). A clinical diagnosis suffices in most cases but, if necessary, a bacterial swab will identify the fungal elements. Nystatin cream is an effective treatment, but the rash often recurs on stopping as the rectum can act as a reservoir of infection. Oral nystatin suspension, which is not absorbed, should therefore be given to clear the rectum. Candida can also affect the mouth and can be distinguished from adherent milk curd as candidal lesions tend to affect the buccal membranes and milk curd the tongue. Candidal lesions also leave a raw surface if gently scraped away with a finger nail.

Seborrhoeic dermatitis — Seborrhoeic dermatitis is an erythematous rash with distinctive greasy scales and involves the seborrhoeic areas such as the groin (**Fig. 17.7**), ears and forehead. It commonly occurs on the scalp where it is known as cradle cap (**Fig. 17.8**).

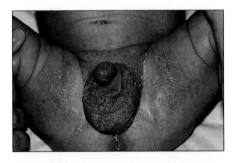

Fig. 17.6 *Candidal napkin rash.*

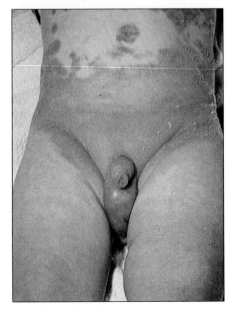

Fig. 17.7 *Seborrhoeic dermatitis can affect the napkin area. The appearances are similar to napkin psoriasis.*

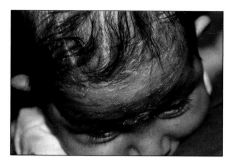

Fig. 17.8 *Cradle cap. Mild cases of cradle cap respond well to liberal use of aqueous cream but in resistant cases there is a rapid response to 0.1% hydrocortisone.*

Atopic eczema — This can also affect the napkin area in babies and often becomes secondarily infected.

BIRTH MARKS

MELANOCYTIC NAEVI

Congenital melanocytic naevi are present at birth and can vary considerably in size, larger ones often having a garment-like distribution. There is a risk of transformation to malignant melanoma which probably occurs in around 5% of cases. This usually occurs after adolescence, but large naevi can transform in childhood. Itching, bleeding or rapid growth suggest the possibility of malignancy.

Melanocytic naevi, also known as moles, appear in infancy and usually persist throughout life (**Fig. 17.9**). Malignant change should be suspected if they itch, bleed, enlarge or spill pigment into the surrounding skin.

Café-au-lait spots are particular macules seen in neurofibromatosis and tuberous sclerosis (**Fig. 17.10**).

Babies belonging to dark-skinned races are often relatively pale at birth. Mongolian blue spots are blue-black pigmented marks commonly seen in such infants; the mark is due to a collection of spindle shaped melanocytes deep within the dermis (**Fig. 17.11**). These spots become less noticeable as the rest of the skin darkens, but often persist as a slate grey discoloration. They are of no pathological significance but are sometimes confused with bruises.

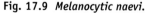

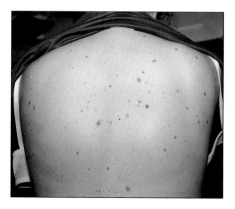

Fig. 17.9 *Melanocytic naevi.*

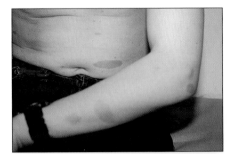

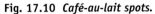

Fig. 17.10 *Café-au-lait spots.*

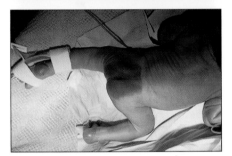

Fig. 17.11 *A particularly distinct Mongolian spot in an African baby.*

HAEMANGIOMAS

Haemangiomas are tumours composed of blood vessels. The most common lesion encountered is the stork mark or naevus simplex (**Fig. 17.12**). These are fine networks of capillaries found at birth on the nape of the neck, around the brow, upper eyelid and upper lip. They occur in up to 50% of newborn infants. The stork mark affecting the face fades before the end of the first year but the marks on the nape of the neck often persist.

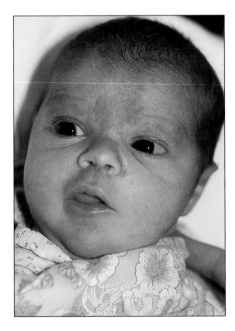

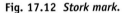

Fig. 17.12 *Stork mark.*

A port wine stain (naevus flammeus) is a dense confluent collection of dilated capillaries within the dermis that can occur anywhere on the body and does not fade with time (**Fig. 17.13**). They usually only pose a cosmetic problem but in the Sturge–Weber syndrome there is a capillary-venous malformation in one cerebral hemisphere associated with a facial naevus. Underlying cortical dysplasia may result in seizures, hemiplegia and mental retardation.

Capillary haemangiomas or strawberry naevi are elevated lesions that appear soon after birth initially as an area of pallor which then becomes red and elevated, appearing like a ripe strawberry (**Fig. 17.14**). They continue to enlarge in size until they outgrow their blood supply and the centre of the tumour infarcts, secondary infection sometimes occurring as they involute. Regression and healing without scarring has usually occurred well before 5 years of age. If the airway or eyesight is compromised injections of corticosteroids can be used which lead to faster resolution.

Cavernous or deep haemangiomas are often present at birth and grow with the infant. The overlying skin is often bluish in colour and the lesions are often mistaken for bruises (**Fig. 17.15**). Although they often resolve they can persist and sometimes enlarge. Large lesions may have feeding vessels which can be embolized.

Fig. 17.13 *Port wine stain.*

Fig. 17.14 *Strawberry naevus.*

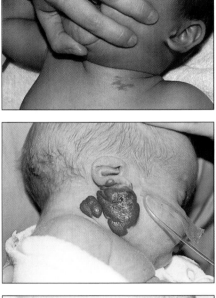

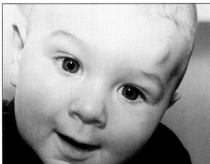

Fig. 17.15 *A cavernous haemangioma. Dermoids can appear in this position on the face, but they are hard to palpation whilst haemangiomas are soft.*

RED AND SCALY RASHES IN CHILDHOOD

ECZEMA

The rash of eczema is red, scaly and very itchy. Patches affect the face and extensor surfaces in infants but predominantly the flexor surfaces of older children (**Fig. 17.16**). Sufferers also tend to have generally dry skin and are usually atopic. With chronicity and scratching, patches become thickened (lichenification).

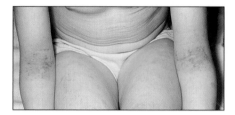

Fig. 17.16 *Eczema.*

The onset is in infancy but the condition usually clears before adulthood in all but the severest cases. In some children there is a history of the rash beginning when cow's milk was first introduced, and more severe cases of eczema not responding well to topical therapy can be tried on diets that exclude cow's milk protein. In practice this is hard to do correctly and requires the help of a dietitian to ensure that milk products are not inadvertently ingested. There is some evidence to suggest a reduction in the incidence of eczema if cow's milk protein is avoided until 6 months of age.

Management of eczema is otherwise symptomatic. When the rash is dry and scaly, emulsifying ointments are used liberally to moisturize the skin. Soap, detergents and other astringents are avoided. Wool is very irritant to the skin but cotton and polyester are well tolerated.

Topical corticosteroids can be used to control the inflammatory process. Weak hydrocortisone is used sparingly on the face but stronger fluorinated steroids can be used on the skin of the body. Wrapping in moist occlusive dressings is useful in severe cases as they increase skin hydration and steroid absorption. Oral steroids are avoided in acute treatment as they produce a rebound of the rash on stopping therapy; long-term use of systemic steroids produces Cushingoid side-effects (*see* **Fig. 15.12**).

Exacerbations of eczema are usually associated with infection and it is usual to prescribe a course of flucloxacillin or erythromycin to treat the usual mixed infection of staphylococci and streptococci.

Itching is a major problem, especially during the night when the child is asleep, and antihistamines such as trimeprazine or chlorpheniramine are useful for short periods.

Herpes simplex infection is dangerous for children with severe eczema as it can produce a serious disseminated infection known as Kaposi's varicelliform eruption.

PSORIASIS

Psoriasis usually begins in children of school age and is seen as a red scaling rash, often confined to the extensor surfaces (**Fig. 17.17**). Removal of the silver flakes reveals pinpoint haemorrhages that confirm the diagnosis. A more diffuse rash of discrete lesions may be seen after an upper respiratory viral infection.

Treatment is with coal tar and salicylic acid preparations which are applied to the lesions. Other treatments commonly used in adults, such as retinoic acid derivatives and

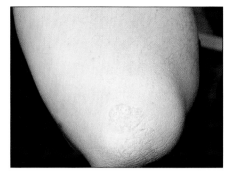

Fig. 17.17 *Psoriasis.*

psoralens with ultraviolet A radiation (PUVA), are avoided in childhood as the long-term effects are unclear.

SKIN INFECTIONS IN CHILDHOOD

VIRAL WARTS

Warts are benign tumours due to papilloma viruses. They are common in children and occur on the hands (**Fig. 17.18**) and often the face. If present on the soles of the feet (verruca) they may cause discomfort on walking. Although they resolve with time, salicylic acid can be applied; in resistant cases cryotherapy with liquid nitrogen is effective.

Genital warts (**Fig. 17.19**) have been regarded as suggestive of sexual abuse, but it is increasingly apparent that this is not always the case.

HERPES SIMPLEX INFECTION

Herpes simplex virus type 1 is often contracted by children after being kissed by a relative with cold sores. A subclinical or limited infection can occur but sometimes a generalized gingivostomatitis results with blisters on the gums and buccal membranes at the front of the mouth (**Fig. 17.20a**). Erosions have often formed by the time of presentation, and antiviral therapy with acyclovir will not hasten recovery. Analgesia is important as the lesions are painful, and often intravenous fluids may be required if the child cannot be tempted to drink (**Fig. 17.20b**). Secondary bacterial infection is uncommon.

Herpes virus can also be introduced into abrasions on the skin and cause recurrent infections. Herpes simplex virus type 2 is responsible for genital herpes infection in adults.

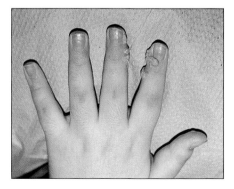

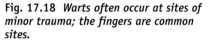

Fig. 17.18 *Warts often occur at sites of minor trauma; the fingers are common sites.*

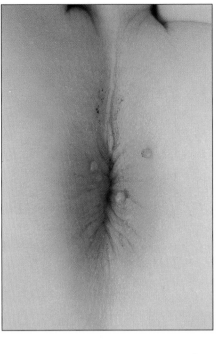

Fig. 17.19 *Anal warts.*

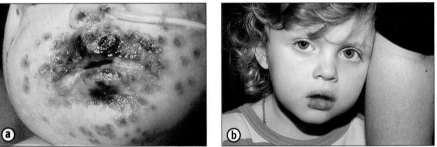

Fig. 17.20 *(a) Herpes gingivostomatitis; (b) refusal to drink from a bottle in mild herpes gingivostomatitis.*

Mothers with primary infections during delivery may infect their babies but recurrent lesions carry a low risk. Herpes encephalitis is uncommon and usually there is no accompanying rash.

Herpes zoster is due to reactivation of herpes zoster virus after chickenpox and occurs in childhood, especially in immunosuppressed individuals; acyclovir can be used to limit the severity of the attack.

MOLLUSCUM CONTAGIOSUM

Molluscum contagiosum is a poxvirus infection. Although the condition is self limiting, the typical discrete umbilicated lesions can be cleared by puncturing the centre with an orange stick dipped in phenol. Most parents opt to leave the lesions to resolve on their own.

IMPETIGO

Impetigo is a superficial infection of the skin characterized by golden crusting (**Fig. 17.21**) and is usually due to a combination of group A streptococci and staphylococci. It is commonly seen on the face, often complicates eczema, and is highly contagious. Topical antibiotics such as fusidic acid are used to treat localized impetigo, but in an extensive infection systemic anti-staphylococcal drugs such as flucloxacillin or erythromycin are required.

ERYSIPELAS

Erysipelas is a group A streptococcal infection of the dermis causing erythema, induration and swelling of the skin with a rapidly spreading but clearly demarcated edge (**Fig. 17.22**). Toxic epidermal necrolysis or staphylococcal scalded skin syndrome is caused by staphylococci carrying phage type 71 which produces an epidermolytic toxin. There is erythema and pain followed by peeling of the skin.

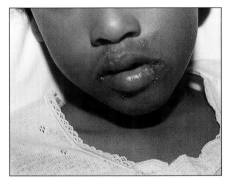

Fig. 17.21 *Perioral impetigo.*

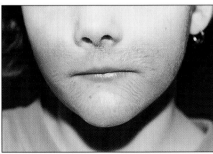

Fig. 17.22 *Erysipelas.*

ALOPECIA

Disease of the scalp often leads to hair loss.

Alopecia areata is an autoimmune process in which patches of hair fall out. Residual hairs have an appearance like an exclamation mark. It is usually self limiting; in severe cases high dose corticosteroids can allow regrowth although relapse usually occurs on stopping. The condition can involve the whole scalp (alopecia totalis) or whole body (alopecia universalis). Psychological problems may occur as a result.

Hair loss due to breakage of the hair shaft occurs in dermatophyte fungal infections of the scalp, contracted from cats and dogs. There is a characteristic patchy alopecia with an annular scaling lesion exhibiting central clearing (ringworm). The infected hairs fluoresce green under ultraviolet light and the fungal hyphae can be identified with a microscope. Treatment is with topical imidazole cream or systemic antifungal drugs.

Infants often have hair loss due to friction from rubbing the back of the head on bed sheets (**Fig. 17.23**). This also affects children with cerebral palsy who spend most of their time in a supine position. Habitual hair pulling or tightly arranged hair styles can produce a similar effect in older children.

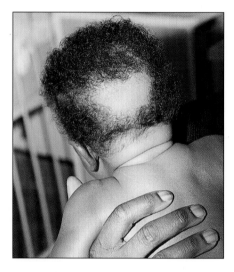

Fig. 17.23 *Occipital alopecia due to head rubbing in a normal healthy infant.*

INFESTATIONS

Children often suffer from infestations, usually passed on at school. Such infections do not reflect poor hygiene.

Infestation with head lice or pediculosis capitis is extremely common in school children (*see* Fig. 9.1). Itching of the scalp and the presence of minute white egg capsules is usually sufficient to make the diagnosis. An overnight application of malathion kills the lice.

Scabies is caused by the mite *Sarcoptes scabei*. The mite burrows into skin folds and around the waist, genitalia and buttocks. In babies the burrows may occur on the palms of the hands. Although the mite and larvae can be identified under the microscope a clinical diagnosis is sufficient to treat the child and all close contacts with permethrin.

Erythematous papules on exposed skin commonly are due to a hypersensitivity reaction to the bites from fleas carried on family pets (**Fig. 17.24**). Treatment is directed at the pets.

NEURODERMATOSES

Neurofibromatosis, tuberous sclerosis and the Sturge–Weber syndrome have characteristic dermal appearances with important involvement of other body systems, especially the central nervous system.

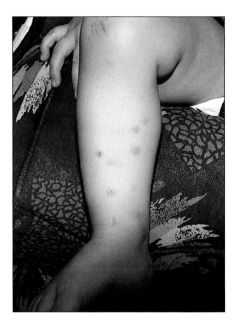

Fig. 17.24 *Erythematous papules due to flea bites.*

NEUROFIBROMATOSIS

There are two forms of neurofibromatosis, both characterized by the appearance of multiple large smooth edged brown macules (café-au-lait spots) with increasing age (*see* **Fig. 17.10**). The presence of more than 5 café-au-lait spots is almost pathognomonic of neurofibromatosis. Peripheral neurofibromatosis appears in childhood and is due to a failure of neural crest cell migration (**Fig. 17.25**). Other features are axillary freckling, which only occurs at around the time of puberty (**Fig. 17.26**) and plexiform neurofibromas in adult life which may undergo malignant change. The central form appears in young

Features of peripheral neurofibromatosis	
Café-au-lait spots	More than 5 spots, greater than 1.5 cm in diameter, are diagnostic. They are best seen under ultraviolet light
Axillary freckling	Occurs in later childhood
Subcutaneous plexiform neurofibromas	Derive from the sheaths of peripheral nerves
Tumours of cranial nerves	Schwannomas and gliomas
Dumbbell tumours of intravertebral foramina	Produce scoliosis and compression of emerging nerve roots (can become malignant)
Renal artery stenosis and pulmonary valve stenosis	Systemic hypertension

Fig. 17.25 *Features of peripheral neurofibromatosis.*

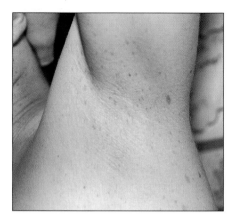

Fig. 17.26 *Axillary freckling in neurofibromatosis.*

adults and is associated with acoustic neuromas and gliomas on the cranial nerves. There is no incidence of malignant change in the central form, but pressure effects and nerve palsies due to tumours may require surgical intervention. Genetic counselling is important in both types of neurofibromatosis as they have an autosomal dominant inheritance, but there is a 50% new mutation rate.

TUBEROUS SCLEROSIS

Tuberous sclerosis is also an autosomal dominant disorder which occurs in 80% of cases as a new mutation. However, a family history is often overlooked as members may be apparently unaffected and it is important to check for evidence of skin stigmata or cerebral tubers. The characteristic feature of the disease is the presence of cells, with the appearance of a neuroblast, which can form multiple gliomas or a diffuse gliosis within the brain. There is accompanying sclerosis due to astrocyte fibrils.

There is a variety of skin manifestations of tuberous sclerosis, many of which only become evident in later childhood (**Fig. 17.27**). For example, adenoma sebaceum (**Fig. 17.28**), the characteristic facial rash caused by multiple angiofibromas occurring in a butterfly distribution over the cheeks and nose, does not usually occur before school age. Neurological problems, however, are often heralded by poor developmental progress or

Dermal features of tuberous sclerosis	
Adenoma sebaceum	Red-yellow warty lesions over the cheeks and nose due to hyperkeratosis and blockage of sebaceous glands
Depigmented patches	Revealed with Wood's light
Shagreen patches	Thickened rough patches of skin on the back
Café-au-lait patches	Best seen with a Wood's light
Subungual fibromata	Small tumours occurring below the nails
Phakomata	Dense white patches on the retina

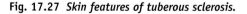

Fig. 17.27 *Skin features of tuberous sclerosis.*

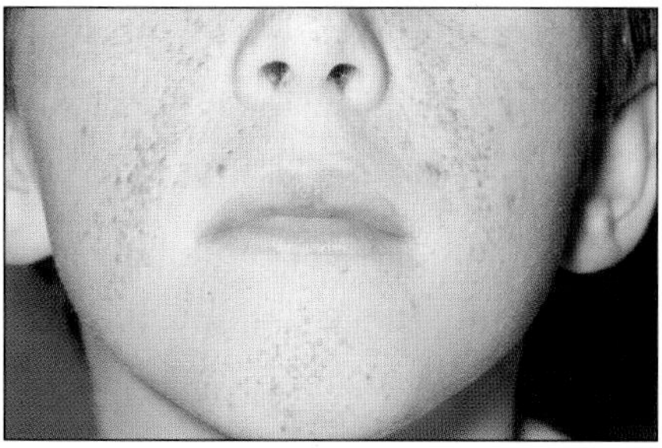

Fig. 17.28 *Adenoma sebaceum.*

delay in infancy and, commonly, infantile spasms. These severely affected children go on to have intellectual impairment and learning difficulties.

Management mainly involves control of seizures and optimizing neurodevelopmental progress. Genetic counselling is important in view of the high spontaneous mutation rate and the high frequency of asymptomatic parents.

chapter 18

Rheumatology

ACUTE ARTHRITIS

Arthralgia, pain without local signs, is a common feature of many viral illnesses. However, the combination of a painful and swollen joint, often associated with an effusion, suggests an inflammatory process. Although older children will complain specifically about such symptoms, small children often present with an unwillingness to use a limb (**Fig. 18.1**). The most important diagnosis to exclude is pyogenic infection as early treatment will prevent destruction of the articular surfaces.

SEPTIC ARTHRITIS

A red, hot and swollen joint in a pyrexial child raises the question of pyogenic infection. The organism responsible is usually *Staphylococcus aureus*, but *Streptococcus pyogenes*,

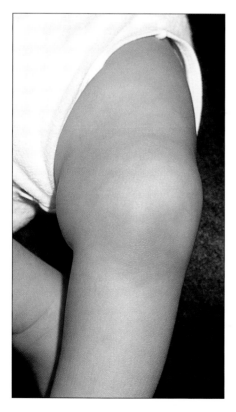

Fig. 18.1 *Arthritis presenting as reluctance to walk.*

Escherichia coli or *Salmonella* spp. may be responsible. Children being treated with immunosuppressive drugs or those with sickle cell disease (hyposplenism) are at increased risk of infections with these organisms. *Haemophilus influenzae* type b is now a rare pathogen due to widespread vaccination.

Management

X-ray changes in the joint are a late feature of infection, and ultrasound is the imaging method of choice. Whenever possible, aspiration of the joint should be carried out and a cell count, Gram stain and culture performed. The blood film commonly shows a neutrophilia and a rapidly progressive anaemia may be seen. Erythrocyte sedimentation rate (ESR) and C reactive protein (CRP) are raised and blood cultures may reveal the causative organism.

Flucloxacillin with ampicillin, or cefuroxime alone are suitable antibiotics and should produce a rapid improvement. However, antibiotics are continued for up to three weeks.

The long-term prognosis is good if treatment is started early, but damaged joints may have early onset of osteoarthritis. Delay in treatment, irrespective of the site of infection, results in rapid and progressive destruction of cartilage and bone.

JUVENILE CHRONIC ARTHRITIS

Juvenile chronic arthritis (JCA) is defined as chronic inflammation of the joints which lasts for more than 3 months in a child aged less than 16 years. There are three forms that are unique to children and are classified according to the type of onset in the first 3 months of disease: systemic, pauci-articular and polyarticular JCA. In addition, children may also suffer from early onset of adult diseases such as ankylosing spondylitis, rheumatoid arthritis or SLE.

PAUCI-ARTICULAR ARTHRITIS

Pauci-articular arthritis mainly affects girls under the age of 6, with a peak incidence at 3 years of age. Fewer than five joints are involved (**Fig. 18.2**) in an asymmetrical pattern but, apart from mild anaemia, systemic upset is minimal. There are no diagnostic tests and rheumatoid factor is negative. Some children have chronic iridocyclitis which, in 90% of cases, is associated with anti-nuclear antibodies. Regular ophthalmic review is essential if sight is to be preserved. Asymmetrical limb growth is a problem in uncontrolled disease due to asymmetrical inflammation and hyperaemia to the growth plate (**Fig. 18.3**).

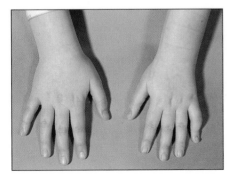

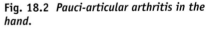

Fig. 18.2 *Pauci-articular arthritis in the hand.*

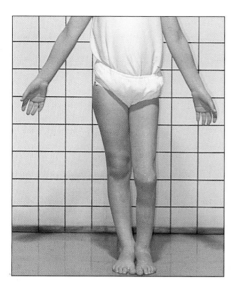

Fig. 18.3 *Unequal leg lengths following asymmetrical arthritis in infancy.*

Older children presenting with pauci-articular JCA tend to have a variety of underlying causes which include early onset of the adult disease.

POLYARTICULAR ARTHRITIS

Polyarticular arthritis tends to occur in older children, mainly girls, with a peak age of 9 years. Systemic upset is mild and the arthritis is symmetrical, involving both large and small joints. Involvement of the temporomandibular joint is a specific feature and may lead to micrognathism. There are no definitive tests as these children are typically negative for rheumatoid factor and other autoantibodies, and the diagnosis remains a clinical one.

SYSTEMIC JCA (STILL'S DISEASE)

Systemic JCA is a systemic disease; generalized arthritis is the main, but not usually the presenting, feature. The initial illness consists of a high remitting fever and malaise accompanied by a salmon pink macular rash that often appears at the height of the fever and fades afterwards (**Fig. 18.4**). Anaemia, lymphadenopathy and hepatosplenomegaly are common findings. Rheumatoid factor and autoantibodies are not found but normocytic, normochromic anaemia is a usual finding. The non-specific features and enlargement of lymphoid tissues often suggest other conditions that may be associated with arthritis, such as neuroblastoma and leukaemia.

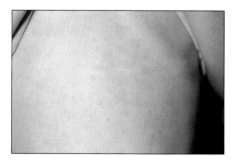
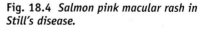

Fig. 18.4 *Salmon pink macular rash in Still's disease.*

OTHER CHRONIC ARTHRITIDES

Ankylosing spondylitis

An asymmetrical arthritis affecting the lower limbs, often associated with heel pain due to inflammation of the Achilles tendon insertion, is seen predominantly in boys with HLA B27 and represents early onset of ankylosing spondylitis. Older boys presenting after puberty may have back pain as a result of involvement of the sacroiliac joints.

Inflammatory bowel disease, cystic fibrosis and psoriasis can all feature polyarthritis as part of the disease process.

Juvenile rheumatoid arthritis

Juvenile rheumatoid arthritis is seen in teenage girls and represents early onset of adult disease. In contrast to the other types of JCA, rheumatoid factor is positive.

MANAGEMENT OF CHRONIC ARTHRITIS

A multidisciplinary approach is vital in the management of JCA. Specialist rheumatologist as well as general paediatric support is required, together with physiotherapy and occupational therapy. Clinical and educational psychologists may need to address the emotional needs of the child and family.

Physiotherapy is of paramount importance to prevent contractures forming; regular passive stretching by parents is the main method. Night splints are essential to prevent wrist and knee contractures (**Fig. 18.5**). Hydrotherapy allows active movement of joints in a weightless environment but is not widely available (**Fig. 18.6**). Activities to maintain muscle strength are encouraged as disuse and corticosteroids can rapidly produce wasting.

Symptomatic relief is afforded by NSAIDs, often in high doses, and it is hoped that in time the conditions may burn out. There is a greater realization now that arthritis lingers on, and there is the possibility that early aggressive treatment with drugs such as

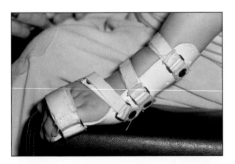

Fig. 18.5 *Night splint.*

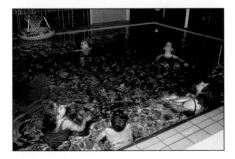

Fig. 18.6 *Hydrotherapy.*

methotrexate will alter the natural history of the disease. Inflamed joints respond well to corticosteroid injections: therapy with systemic corticosteroids, methotrexate or chloroquine is tried if symptoms are not controlled with NSAIDs.

Surgery may be needed occasionally to release soft tissue contractures and restore function, but this can be avoided by early physiotherapy. Joint replacement is deferred for as long as possible (**Fig. 18.7**).

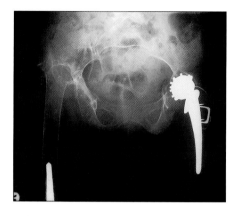

Fig. 18.7 *Hip and knee joint replacement after juvenile chronic arthritis.*

chapter 19

Neurology

DEVELOPMENT OF THE BRAIN IN INFANCY

Many disorders in paediatric neurology occur as a consequence of disruption to the normal development of the brain. In general, the earlier the insult the more severe the disruption. For example, failure to close off the anterior end of the neural tube leads to anencephaly—an absence of the cerebral structures above the brain stem (**Fig. 19.1**). Later, abnormalities in cellular relations and gyral patterns can occur, such as migration defects (**Figs 19.2, 19.3**); these are often associated with seizures and developmental delay. Glial multiplication, synapse formation and myelination continue in the first years of life and are important in learning and development. In early life the brain exhibits a degree of plasticity, and if an area of cerebral cortex is disrupted other parts can take over. Later this becomes more difficult as the cortex is dedicated to specific functions.

PERIVENTRICULAR HAEMORRHAGE AND LEUKOMALACIA

Preterm infants below 32 weeks' gestation have rich but frail capillary beds lining the lateral ventricles. In response to swings in acidaemia, oxygenation or perfusion these vessels may rupture and bleed. These problems are easily detected and followed by serial cranial ultrasound scans (**Fig. 19.4**). Little damage may be done if bleeding is confined to

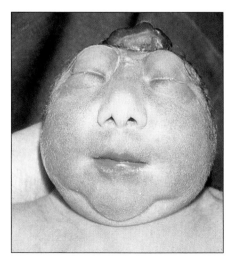

Fig. 19.1 *Anencephaly.*

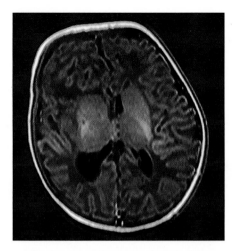

Fig. 19.2 *MR scan showing migration defects involving both hemispheres. There is a double layer of cortical mantle in the left temporal region and an absence of occipital gyral folds on the right.*

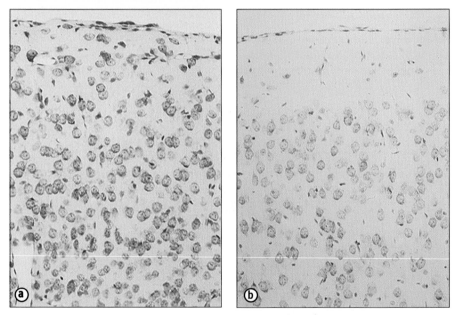

Fig. 19.3 *Section of brain showing (a) abnormal migration of neurones and (b) normal appearances.*

the ventricles, but permanent deficits may result if there is distension of the ventricles or extension of blood into brain parenchyma (**Fig. 19.5**). Hypoxia and ischaemia to the brain in the preterm infant may result in poor perfusion to the watershed areas lying between the anterior and middle cerebral artery distributions. Resulting infarction or haemorrhage (periventricular haemorrhage) often leads to the later formation of periventricular leukomalacia (**Fig. 19.6**) or porencephalic cysts. Apart from the avoidance of preterm labour and ensuring a smooth passage through neonatal intensive care there are no proven methods to prevent such injuries.

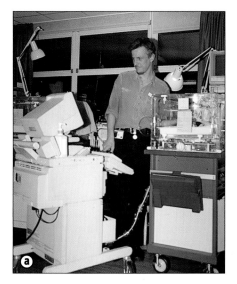

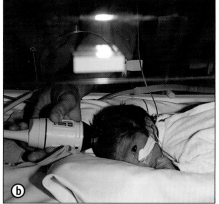

Fig. 19.4 *(a,b) Cranial ultrasound scanning; (b) the anterior fontanelle provides a window for the ultrasound probe.*

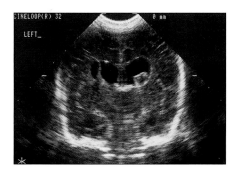

Fig. 19.5 *Ultrasound scan in a preterm infant revealing resolving blood clots within the lateral ventricles and an area of parenchymal breakdown above the right ventricle.*

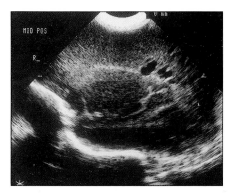

Fig. 19.6 *Periventricular leukomalacia.*

HYPOXIC ISCHAEMIC ENCEPHALOPATHY

The newborn infant brain is able to weather an insult which in later life would be devastating; this is even more true of the preterm infant. However, severe hypoxaemia and poor perfusion to the brain may result in hypoxic ischaemic encephalopathy (HIE) with fits and coma leading to death or severe disability. Magnetic resonance imaging can be used to visualize the damage, and magnetic resonance spectroscopy can measure metabolic components such as lactate which are associated with cerebral damage (*see* Chapter 7 Newborn).

HYDROCEPHALUS

Cerebrospinal fluid (CSF) is produced by the choroid plexus and circulates through the ventricular system and around the spinal cord before being re-absorbed by the arachnoid granulations lying over the cerebral hemispheres. Interruption of this normal circulation causes a build-up of CSF and dilatation of the ventricles or subarachnoid space—hydrocephalus. This may be congenital in origin, e.g. stenosis of the aqueduct of Sylvius, or acquired after haemorrhage or infection, or caused by a tumour. Compensatory hydrocephalus is an increased volume of CSF occurring following cerebral atrophy.

In babies there may be no symptoms, or general irritability and vomiting may be accompanied by widening of the cranial sutures, bulging fontanelle, and an increase in head circumference. The scalp veins become prominent as hydrocephalus progresses and there is eyelid retraction allowing extra sclera to be seen. This sign is called sunsetting (**Fig. 19.7**).

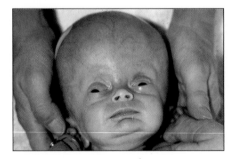

Fig. 19.7 *Sunsetting is a late sign in hydrocephalus.*

Older children with fused cranial sutures will present with features of raised intracranial pressure if there is a rapid increase in CSF (effortless vomiting, headache, papilloedema and vertigo), but may have more insidious personality and behavioural changes and intermittent early morning headache if there is a slower build-up of fluid.

Post-haemorrhagic hydrocephalus (**Fig. 19.8**) usually resolves as the clots blocking the circulation of CSF are broken down. Acetazolamide and frusemide may control production of CSF while this happens, but a ventriculo-peritoneal shunt will be required to drain a persisting fluid collection. CT and MR scanning are important investigations as they demonstrate the site and cause of obstruction and allow accurate planning of neurosurgical procedures.

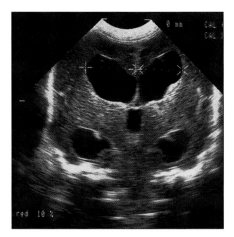

Fig. 19.8 *Cranial ultrasound can demonstrate enlarged ventricular spaces, as in this preterm infant with post-haemorrhagic hydrocephalus.*

INFECTIONS OF THE CENTRAL NERVOUS SYSTEM

MENINGITIS

Bacterial infection, viral infection and leukaemic infiltration are important causes of inflammation of the meninges. Older children complain of photophobia, headache and vomiting, and show neck stiffness but this is not usually present in babies under 16 months, and they may be non-specifically unwell. The very young may present with irritability, a high-pitched cry, poor feeding, vomiting or drowsiness, and fever.

Meningism is the presence of signs of meningitis without actual infection of the meninges. Viral infections, tense cervical lymphadenitis and apical pneumonia are common causes.

Bacterial meningitis

Bacterial meningitis is largely a disease of childhood and is particularly common in the first year of life. The common organisms in childhood are *Streptococcus pneumoniae* and *Neisseria meningitidis*. *Haemophilus influenzae* (Hib) is now uncommon since the advent of routine vaccination. In the newborn, Group B *streptococcus* and *E. coli* predominate. The key to diagnosing meningitis is a high index of suspicion, especially in the very young, and a low threshold to perform a lumbar puncture (**Fig. 19.9**). If the child is very ill and there is concern about raised intracranial pressure, deranged clotting, or infective lesions over the lumbar spine, antibiotics should be started and CSF obtained when the situation

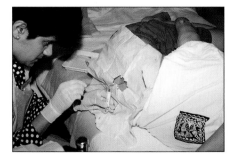

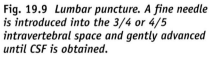

Fig. 19.9 *Lumbar puncture. A fine needle is introduced into the 3/4 or 4/5 intravertebral space and gently advanced until CSF is obtained.*

267

improves. A retrospective diagnosis can sometimes be made by immunofluorescence for antigens to the common organisms.

The cell counts and biochemistry of CSF give an indication of the cause of meningitis (**Fig. 19.10**). In the neonatal period, values for cell counts and protein levels are much higher than in later life; for example, up to 30 cells/mm^3 and 1.5 g/l of protein may be normal.

A third generation cephalosporin, such as cefotaxime, is the favoured treatment for infection with these organisms, although many doctors still consider benzyl penicillin to be the optimal choice in pneumococcal and meningococcal meningitis if the organisms are sensitive. Fluid restriction is important during treatment of meningitis, as inappropriate secretion of anti-diuretic hormone (ADH) can lead to hyponatraemia and convulsions. Dexamethasone is advocated for *Haemophilus* and pneumococcal meningitis as it may reduce the incidence of late sequelae, in particular deafness. About 10% of survivors have problems such as convulsions, deafness, cerebral palsy, mental handicap or more subtle learning difficulties. Hearing is tested 4–6 weeks after recovery.

Viral meningitis

Coxsackie and ECHO viruses are often implicated in viral meningitis, and mumps commonly causes a lymphocytic meningitis as part of an encephalitis. Although it may be difficult to differentiate viral from bacterial meningitis on clinical grounds, the absence of neutrophilia in the blood and a marked lymphocytosis with normal glucose concentration in the CSF (**Fig. 19.11**) should allow diagnosis. There are usually no sequelae.

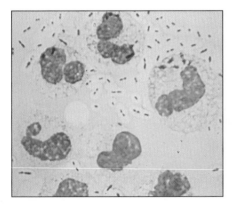

Fig. 19.10 *Bacteria and neutrophils within the CSF.*

Interpretation of CSF results in meningitis

	Normal	Bacterial	Viral	Tuberculous
Appearance	Clear	Cloudy	Clear	Opaque
Cell count/mm^3	0–5	10–10 000	20–1000	200–500
Type of cell	Lymphocytes	Polymorphs	Lymphocytes	Lymphocytes
Protein g/l	0.2–0.4	0.5–5.0	0.2–1.0	0.5–5.0
Glucose mmol/l	>2/3 of blood	Low	Normal	Very low

Fig. 19.11 *Interpretation of CSF results in meningitis.*

Tuberculous meningitis

Although tuberculous meningitis is rare in industrialized countries, it should be considered whenever an apparently sterile meningitis is encountered. The children usually have a focus on chest X-ray and a positive skin test to tuberculin purified protein derivative (PPD). Treatment is with conventional anti-tuberculous drugs together with corticosteroids to prevent inflammatory complications such as hydrocephalus.

ENCEPHALOPATHY AND ENCEPHALITIS

Encephalopathy is a non-specific term that indicates disruption of the brain. The presentation involves clouding of consciousness, coma and focal neurological signs. Lead, other toxins, hepatic failure, Reye syndrome and inborn errors of metabolism may be responsible for encephalopathy. However, most cases of encephalopathy are due to viral infection:

- Herpes simplex encephalitis is important as it is treatable with acyclovir. Focal seizures and signs suggesting a temporal lobe lesion are features of the disease, but it is important to note that a herpetic skin rash is often missing. CT scanning and EEG demonstrate an encephalitic process confined to the temporal lobes.
- Chickenpox can produce an acute self-limiting encephalitis manifest as ataxia.
- Measles can be accompanied by an encephalitis which may have serious consequences.
- Subacute sclerosing panencephalitis is a late complication of measles infection in which persistence of the virus leads to slow but progressive degeneration of the brain; the electroencephalogram is diagnostic (**Fig. 19.12**).

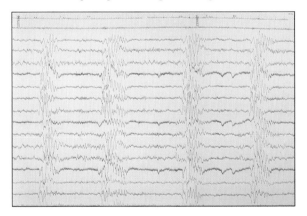

Fig. 19.12 *Alternating periods of burst and suppression activity on the EEG are diagnostic of subacute sclerosing panencephalitis.*

HEADACHE

The most common cause of headache is tension in the temporalis and frontal muscles due to psychological stress. Abdominal pain may also be found, but there are usually no additional symptoms. The headache typically occurs at the end of the day or in association with a stressful event. Rest or simple analgesics provide relief. These headaches can be disruptive; a sympathetic approach, often with a diary of headaches and daily happenings, will help to improve matters.

Migraine is a severe headache which is often unilateral and sometimes preceded by visual disturbances. Nausea and photophobia are common accompanying features. Medication can be taken with each attack if attacks are infrequent (paracetamol for pain and metoclopramide for nausea). If there are frequent attacks, drugs such as propranolol or pizotifen may help and dietary exclusion of provoking factors such as cheese or chocolate may be useful.

The headache of raised intracranial pressure is distinctive. It is worst on waking and often associated with vomiting. Coughing and straining make it worse and there is little relief with simple analgesics. Investigation to detect an underlying cause is essential.

Benign intracranial hypertension is a term used for an isolated increase in intracranial pressure without an obvious cause. Associations with corticosteroid or antibiotic use have been suggested. The condition eventually tends to remit spontaneously but optic nerve damage can result from chronic elevated CSF pressure. Visual field assessment and repeated lumbar punctures to control CSF pressure may be necessary.

Other causes of intermittent headache are refractive errors leading to eye strain, and pain from teeth or sinuses.

CONVULSIONS

FEBRILE CONVULSIONS

Five per cent of children between the ages of 6 months and 5 years will suffer short-lived generalized convulsions during pyrexial illnesses. These children are developmentally normal but often have a family history of febrile convulsions. It is thought that a rapid rise in temperature or viraemia affects the developing brain which has a relatively low convulsive threshold. It is not uncommon for a repeat convulsion to occur in the same illness and a third of children have a further convulsion in the next few years. This is not epilepsy: remarkably few children go on to suffer from non-febrile seizures. Children with unusual seizures that are either long or focal in nature, or that are provoked by a temperature of less than 38.5°C may actually be demonstrating an epileptic tendency revealed by the temperature.

The diagnosis is made on clinical grounds by eliciting a classical history. It is important to ensure that serious infections such as meningitis, encephalitis or urinary tract infection (UTI) are not missed. In infants older than 1 year this can be done by thorough examination with frequent reassessments. If no serious infective focus is found on clinical examination and a viral infection is suspected no other investigations are usually required, except perhaps a urine culture. In infants below 1 year of age it can be difficult to exclude meningitis, and lumbar puncture should generally be performed.

There is little, apart from early use of paracetamol, that can be done to prevent further febrile fits. Rectal diazepam can be prescribed if the seizures are frequent or prolonged. There seems to be little risk of mesangial temporal sclerosis unless the seizures are very long — over 30 minutes.

EPILEPSY

Epilepsy is a disorder of the brain characterized by episodic electrical discharges leading to recurrent seizures (fits or convulsions). A number of conditions associated with loss of consciousness or apparent abnormal movements are seen in children; the importance of correct diagnosis lies in the vastly different prognosis and treatment compared to epilepsy (Fig. 19.13). Partial and generalized seizures are differentiated by the loss of consciousness.

Partial seizures

Simple partial seizures — These originate from the primary sensory or motor cortex. Motor seizures involve twitching of a limb or the face and may spread along one side of the body (Jacksonian march), during which consciousness is preserved. Sensory or psychic symptoms may also occur if discharges arise in the relevant part of the cerebral cortex. *Complex partial seizures* — These arise from the temporal lobes and lead to altered consciousness, complex and stereotyped semi-purposeful movements, or strange sensations. There is no recollection of events and the child may be unable to describe the initial sensory manifestations. An EEG may show discharges originating from the temporal lobe (**Fig. 19.14**).

Events mimicking seizures	
Breath-holding attacks	Common in toddlers and associated with sudden upset or rage. The child stops breathing and rapidly becomes quite cyanosed, often losing consciousness and perhaps even having a tonic-clonic convulsion. An important feature in the story is that attacks can usually be averted if the child is distracted.
Reflex anoxic seizures	Similar to breath-holding attacks in that they occur with upset but the child becomes pale and limp. They are due to increased vagal responsiveness.
Faint	Teenagers often faint and the children report fading consciousness during the episode rather than an abrupt loss of consciousness as in generalized seizures.
Rhythmical movements	In small children these may be due to masturbation or tics which are paroxysmal involuntary movements.
Night terrors and myoclonic jerks	Non-epileptic events associated with sleep.
Pseudoseizures	Apparent convulsions, often in a child known to have epilepsy. Such children often have underlying psychological difficulties.

Fig. 19.13 *Events mimicking seizures.*

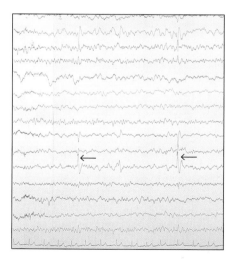

Fig. 19.14 *Epileptiform focus in the temporal lobe producing spiked discharges on the EEG (arrowed).*

Any of the above partial seizures may spread over the cortex and become a generalized tonic-clonic seizure. Unless a careful history is taken it may be easy to miss the focal beginning to these fits.

Generalized seizures

Absence or petit mal epilepsy — This is a common epilepsy beginning between 3 and 10 years of age. There is a loss of awareness but no collapse or other movements—the child stops what it is doing and looks blank for some seconds before continuing. The EEG shows the characteristic 3 per second spike and wave pattern which can be induced by hyperventilation or flashing lights (**Fig. 19.15**). Children usually grow out of these convulsions before puberty.

Tonic-clonic seizures — These seizures are characterized by loss of consciousness with a period of rigidity which involves cessation of respiration. A phase of generalized jerking then follows during which faecal and urinary incontinence may occur. In this latter clonic phase irregular respiration occurs and salivation appears as foaming at the mouth.

Myoclonic seizures — These are sudden shock-like spasms, often involving the whole body, which cause violent extension or flexion and may cause injury. They are usually associated with other forms of epilepsy and usually represent serious neurological conditions. There are more benign forms, for example juvenile myoclonic epilepsy.

Infantile spasm — This is a specific form of myoclonic epilepsy found mainly in infants under 1 year of age. The violent flexion is often described as 'a jack-knife convulsion' but frequently is not recognized as being abnormal for some time, often being mistaken for colic or playing with toes. The myoclonic jerks occur in bursts accompanied by a cry or colour change. A halt or regression in development and responsiveness often accompanies their onset. The EEG shows hypsarrhythmia—chaotic asymmetrical high amplitude polyspike and wave activity (**Fig. 19.16**). Many children will have no identifiable causative lesion, but it is important to search for a cause as truly idiopathic cases have a better prognosis overall (**Fig. 19.17**). Treatment is usually with corticosteroids although the Cushingoid side-effects are troublesome. Benzodiazepines such as clonazepam have been used, and newer drugs such as vigabatrin and lamotrigine are effective.

Management of seizures

When a child presents with a seizure, the first consideration is the immediate safety and resuscitation of the child by control of the airway, oxygen and assistance of ventilation. If

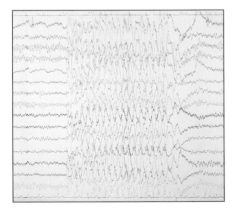

Fig. 19.15 *Petit mal provoked by flashing lights.*

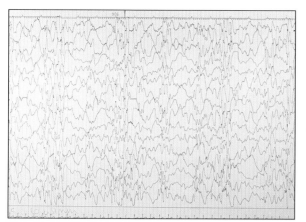

Fig. 19.16
Hypsarrhythmia.

Causes and investigation of infantile spasms

Cause	Investigation
Idiopathic	Exclusion of other causes
Cerebral malformation, e.g. migration defects	MRI
Cerebral catastrophe, e.g. intracranial bleed or hypoxic damage	MRI, clotting screen; consider non-accidental injury
Tuberous sclerosis	Wood's light, MR scan, examine family
Chromosomal abnormalities, e.g. trisomy 13	Karyotype
Congenital infection, e.g. toxoplasmosis, CMV, rubella	Serology of infant and mother
Encephalitis and meningitis	Screen for infection and lumbar puncture
Metabolic disorders	Organic and amino acids, ammonia and lactate

Fig. 19.17 *Causes of infantile spasms.*

there is prolonged fitting this is stopped initially by rectal diazepam or, if this fails, paraldehyde or intravenous diazepam. If the child is pyrexial or there is any suggestion of infection a full infection screen including lumbar puncture is performed and antibiotics to cover meningitis are started. It is usual to exclude hypoglycaemia and to check electrolytes, magnesium and calcium levels.

There are two elements to diagnosis: firstly the confirmation that a fit has taken place and secondly the search for an underlying cause if necessary. A seizure is diagnosed on the basis of a good clinical history as the paroxysmal nature means that the clinician may not witness an event. It is usual to perform an EEG, which is a recording of the electrical activity over the surface of the brain. It is important to note that a few children without seizures will have an apparently abnormal EEG, and that some with epilepsy will have normal records. The EEG is performed some weeks after the seizure as the record is disordered in the postictal phase and focal discharges can be missed. Photic stimulation, hyperventilation and sleep can all enhance the appearance of an abnormal focus. MRI is the preferred imaging modality when searching for focal abnormalities. A lateral skull X-ray is useful if congenital infection is suspected as calcium deposits are not seen on MRI.

Drug therapy

When medication is started the dosage is increased until control of seizures is attained or side-effects ensue (**Fig. 19.18**). Drug levels may help to decide whether a dosage reduction or change to another drug is necessary if there appear to be side-effects. Levels are often taken following a seizure to check compliance.

Children are advised to avoid dangerous situations, for example swimming alone, climbing tall trees, or cycling in traffic. The bathroom door should never be locked. Some epilepsies are provoked by photic stimulation and it is sensible to avoid flickering video screens.

It is usual to try to produce a seizure-free period of 1–2 years before slowly withdrawing medication. Rarely, surgical removal of an epileptic focus or even hemispherectomy may help to control intractable seizures.

Prognosis

Well controlled epilepsy may have little impact on family life. However, when there is difficulty in seizure control and developmental delay, there is often increased family stress and problems with schooling. There is a general increase in mortality with epilepsy: deaths occur during the seizures, from underlying conditions, and also from accidents.

Drug therapy for epilepsy		
Drug	**Indication**	**Side-effects**
Sodium valproate	Absence and other generalized seizures	Nausea or obesity. Idiosyncratic hepatotoxicity
Carbamazepine	Especially partial epilepsy, also generalized epilepsies	Rashes and ataxia
Phenytoin	Partial and generalized epilepsies	Hirsutism, gum hypertrophy
Phenobarbitone	Generalized and partial seizures, especially in neonates	Sedation, overactive behaviour
Ethosuxamide	Absences	Gastrointestinal upset
ACTH and prednisolone	Infantile spasms	Cushingoid habitus, hypertension and glycosuria
GABA transaminase inhibitors (vigabatrin and lamotrigine)	Especially effective in infantile spasms and resistant generalized and partial seizures	Agitation or sedation in high doses
Paraldehyde	Acute treatment of seizures	Prolonged contact dissolves plastic syringes
Diazepam	Acute treatment of seizures	Respiratory depression

Fig. 19.18 *Drug therapy for epilepsy.*

DISORDERS OF THE SPINAL CORD AND PERIPHERAL NERVES

SPINA BIFIDA

The neural tube closes by the fourth week after fertilization. Failure of closure may be due to a number of causes such as irradiation, sodium valproate, folic acid deficiency, or an autosomal dominant process. The marked fall in the incidence of neural tube defects seems to be independent of interventions such as screening by ultrasound and alpha-fetoprotein estimation. Multivitamin and folate supplements are now advocated prior to conception to reduce the risk of neural tube defects.

Spina bifida occulta (**Fig. 19.19a**) is a local failure of formation of the vertebral arches. There may be an overlying cutaneous lesion such as a tuft of hair or a pigmented patch;

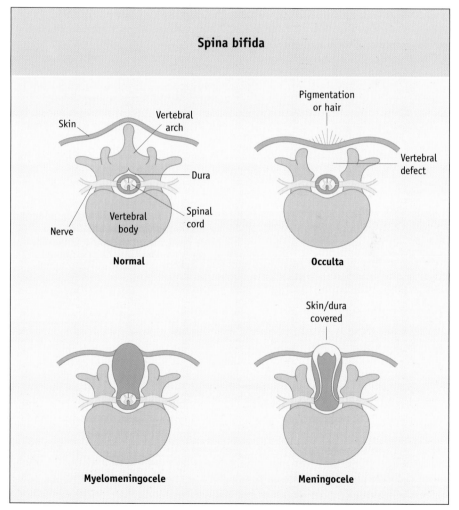

Fig. 19.19 *Spina bifida: (a) occulta, (b) myelomeningocele and (c) meningocele.*

the bony defect may be an incidental X-ray finding. The lesion rarely poses any problems but accompanying bony spurs tethering the spinal cord (diastematomyelia) can cause toe walking and incontinence during growth.

Spina bifida meningocele (**Fig. 19.19b**) also has a relatively good prognosis as the spinal cord itself is unaffected.

In myelomeningocele (**Figs 19.19b, 19.20**) disruption of the cord produces paresis and muscle imbalance below the level of the defect. Apart from the risk of infection ascending into the central nervous system the degree of neurological impairment in myelomeningocele is related to the degree of cord disruption. Incontinence and weakness or paresis below the lesion, dislocation of the hips, and talipes are common findings. If the lesion is closed surgically or by spontaneous epithelialization a build-up of CSF usually takes place and hydrocephalus develops, requiring a ventriculo-peritoneal shunt.

Pits are commonly seen on the skin overlying the lower spine (**Fig. 19.21**). The lower dermal pits over the coccyx are always blind-ending but higher sacral pits may communicate with the dura and lead to meningitis. Sacral pits should be carefully inspected to ensure that they are blind-ending. Ultrasound or magnetic resonance scanning can be performed if there is doubt.

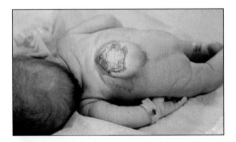

Fig. 19.20 *Meningocele has a relatively good prognosis as the spinal cord itself is unaffected. In myelomeningocele disruption of the cord produces paresis and muscle imbalance below the level of the defect.*

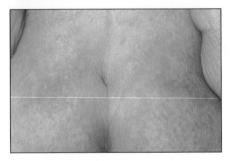

Fig. 19.21 *Sacral pits should be inspected to ensure that they are blind-ending. If there is doubt, ultrasound or magnetic resonance imaging can be performed.*

SPINAL MUSCULAR ATROPHY

Degeneration of the anterior horn cells leads to hypotonia, weakness and fasciculation in the muscles. Fasciculation is most easily seen in the tongue, and there is superimposed noise on the electrocardiogram due to skeletal muscle activity.

There is a range of presentations from a weak and hypotonic baby (**Fig. 19.22**), to an infant unable to progress past sitting, to a child with a waddling gait and difficulty climbing stairs because of pelvic girdle weakness. As a group, these children are intelligent and alert. They rely on the diaphragm for breathing as the intercostal, as well as skeletal muscles are affected. With time, scoliosis and contractures develop and death during a

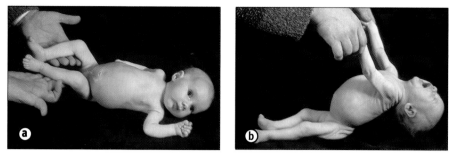

Fig. 19.22 *Spinal muscular atrophy: (a) infant with spinal muscular atrophy; (b) hypotonia.*

respiratory infection is common. The diagnosis is made on muscle biopsy and with electromyography (EMG); a gene defect on chromosome 5 is responsible.

PERIPHERAL NERVE LESIONS

Traction on the brachial plexus at the time of birth, often associated with shoulder dystocia, may result in an Erb's palsy (*see* Fig. 7.10). Forceps blades may put pressure on the facial nerve and cause facial asymmetry and incomplete eye closure (*see* Fig. 7.11).

Bell's palsy is an acute para-infectious mononeuritis of the VIIth cranial nerve that follows a viral infection (often mumps). Demyelination or compression of the nerve as it exits through the sternomastoid canal causes paralysis of the facial muscles on one side of the face. The involvement of the forehead differentiates this from an upper motor neurone lesion. Tears overflow, and speech and eating are impaired. The problem resolves within weeks in the majority of cases. Corticosteroids may have a beneficial effect if given in the first 48 hours. However, a VIIth cranial nerve paresis may also be due to leukaemic infiltration, a brain stem tumour, herpes simplex virus infection in the middle ear, Lyme disease or hypertension. A careful clinical examination, full blood count, blood pressure and audiometry are essential before starting steroids as they could worsen viral infection or induce partial remission from leukaemia with inevitable relapse which has a poor prognosis.

GUILLAIN–BARRÉ SYNDROME (POST-INFECTIOUS POLYNEURITIS)

Autoimmune-mediated demyelination of the peripheral nerves may occur following a viral infection; this is clinically manifest as an ascending paralysis. Pain in the limbs or meningism may dominate the presentation. Children of school age are most frequently seen and the diagnosis is suggested by an accompanying elevation of CSF protein in the presence of a normal CSF white cell count. The paralysis ascends but sphincter control is maintained and after a week the weakness starts to recede. Occasionally bulbar muscles may be involved with facial paresis and difficulty in swallowing; a close watch on respiratory function with peak flow and pulse oximetry will warn of impending respiratory failure which may need mechanical support. In severe cases plasmapheresis is used to remove antibodies and treat the weakness.

THE NEUROMUSCULAR JUNCTION—THE MYASTHENIAS

Myasthenia gravis is a disease of older children and adults in which the acetylcholine receptor of the neuromuscular junction is attacked by IgG antibodies leading to the almost pathognomonic finding of fatigability—increasing weakness with use of a muscle. This illness is more common in females and associated with other autoimmune diseases, for example diabetes mellitus. Transient neonatal myasthenia occurs in babies born to mothers with myasthenia gravis. Even in the absence of overt symptoms in the mother, transplacental passage of the IgG antibody can cause weakness, feeding difficulties and ptosis (**Fig. 19.23**) in the baby. This transient neonatal myasthenia eventually resolves over the following weeks.

A distinctly different entity is congenital myasthenia, in which there is an abnormality of the acetylcholine receptor. This condition is inherited in an autosomal recessive manner; symptoms are often milder and may not be recognized for many years.

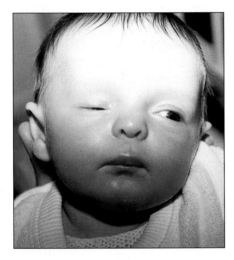

Fig. 19.23 *Bilateral ptosis in neonatal myasthenia.*

Diagnosis

The commonest reason for missing a diagnosis of myasthenia is because the possibility is not considered. Direct questioning reveals facial drooping, ptosis or squint occurring at the end of the day, and often difficulty in chewing through a long meal. Electromyography shows fatigue of muscle on repetitive nerve stimulation which may not be clinically apparent. An injection of edrophonium, a short-acting cholinesterase inhibitor, often demonstrates a dramatic improvement in muscle function, although in congenital myasthenia a longer therapeutic trial of pyridostigmine may be needed to produce a small improvement.

The mainstay of treatment is pyridostigmine given in divided doses throughout the day. Thymectomy may improve symptoms in autoimmune myasthenia gravis but has no role in the neonatal or congenital forms.

DISORDERS OF MUSCLE

THE MUSCULAR DYSTROPHIES

Congenital muscular dystrophy

The commonest cause of arthrogryposis (**Fig. 19.24**) due to muscle disease is congenital muscular dystrophy. This is probably a group of muscle disorders with similar clinical features. The diagnosis is made by examination of a muscle biopsy (**Fig. 19.25**). The clinical presentation ranges from severe arthrogryposis, to hypotonia and weakness with respiratory failure. Some children are initially hypotonic, but eventually manage to walk. Scoliosis and nocturnal hypoventilation are common problems in survivors.

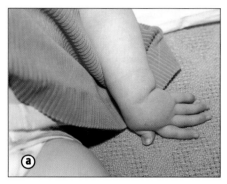
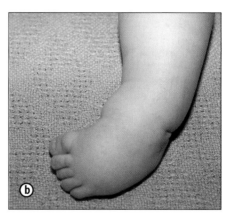

Fig. 19.24 *(a,b)* *Arthrogryposis.*

Duchenne muscular dystrophy

One in 3000 male children will suffer from this degenerative disease of muscle. There is absence of dystrophin (**Fig. 19.26**), a protein necessary for muscle cell well-being, due to an interruption of the gene at Xp21. Boys come to attention in the preschool years with frequent falls, difficulty with stairs, a waddling gait or inability to run. Gower's manoeuvre is employed to get up from the floor (**Fig. 19.27**). Pseudohypertrophy of the calves is seen, and shortening of the Achilles tendon often leads to toe walking (**Fig. 19.28**). The progression of weakness means that these boys are all wheelchair bound by their teens. Scoliosis easily develops once the child is in a permanent sitting position and there is a reduction in vital capacity of the lungs. Although the heart muscle is affected, problems are not usually apparent.

Many boys are already known to hospital services at the time of diagnosis as there are accompanying effects on the central nervous system that may result in speech delay and reduced intelligence. A useful screening test is creatine phosphokinase (CPK); the enzyme leaks from damaged muscle. Muscle biopsy and staining for dystrophin, as well as genetic studies of the gene at Xp21, confirm the diagnosis.

The aim of therapy is to maintain quality of life. Exercise and physiotherapy prevent contractures and maintain function. While the boys are walking there is rarely any scoliosis as the back muscles are exercised and keep the spine straight.

Callipers and percutaneous Achilles tendon tenotomy prolong standing, even though there may be no functional walking ability, as this delays scoliosis and positively improves

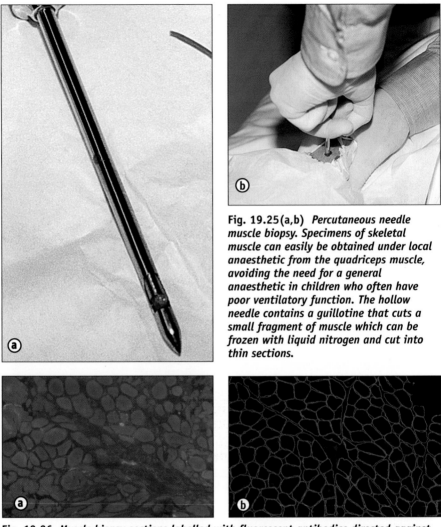

Fig. 19.25(a,b) *Percutaneous needle muscle biopsy. Specimens of skeletal muscle can easily be obtained under local anaesthetic from the quadriceps muscle, avoiding the need for a general anaesthetic in children who often have poor ventilatory function. The hollow needle contains a guillotine that cuts a small fragment of muscle which can be frozen with liquid nitrogen and cut into thin sections.*

Fig. 19.26 *Muscle biopsy sections labelled with fluorescent antibodies directed against dystrophin. (a) There is no positive staining in a boy with Duchenne muscular dystrophy. A normal biopsy is shown for comparison (b).*

quality of life. Respiratory compromise is inevitable and nocturnal hypoventilation due to chest deformity may be seen.

Becker muscular dystrophy

Becker muscular dystrophy is an allelic variant of Duchenne muscular dystrophy. Presentation is in later childhood, progression is slower, and patchy dystrophin is seen in the muscle. Intelligence and speech seem to be normal. Although there is a spectrum of disease severity, boys with Becker dystrophy are still able to stand at the age of 16 while Duchenne boys are usually in a wheelchair by 12. Becker dystrophy is associated with a cardiomyopathy which is rarely of clinical significance.

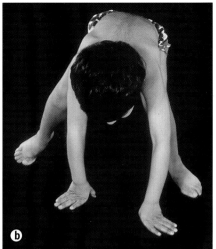

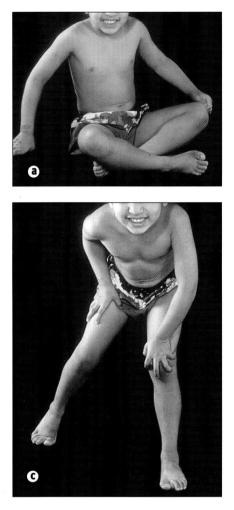

Fig. 19.27 (a–c) *Gower's manoeuvre. From sitting (a), the child pushes up from the floor to straighten his legs (b), then climbs up his legs to be fully standing (c).*

Myotonic dystrophy

Myotonic dystrophy is inherited in an autosomal dominant fashion. Affected males are bald with cataracts and testicular atrophy, and they exhibit myotonia—failure of muscle relaxation after a muscle contraction—which is often worse in the cold. Many affected females may be regarded as having mild rheumatism and the diagnosis missed. Affected mothers (even if asymptomatic) can give birth to weak, floppy infants with respiratory compromise and swallowing problems. These problems improve with time so that most children eventually walk unaided, but there are usually learning difficulties. The diagnosis is suspected on finding a failure of relaxation when shaking the mother's hand, but a myotonic notch seen on tapping the side of the tongue is a more sensitive test. Myotonia can be demonstrated on a maternal EMG, and muscle biopsy of the child helps to exclude other diagnoses. Surgery may be hazardous in myotonic dystrophy as the effect of muscle relaxant drugs may fail to reverse and malignant hyperpyrexia ensue.

281

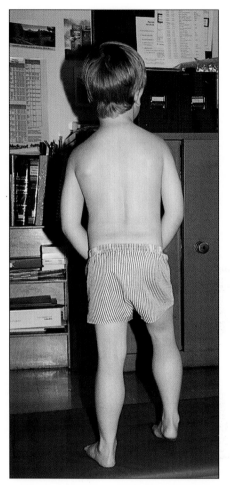

Fig. 19.28 *Prominent calves, shortening of the right Achilles tendon and lumbar lordosis in Duchenne muscular dystrophy.*

OTHER MYOPATHIC DISORDERS

There are a number of muscle disorders that are rarely seen. Some produce floppiness and weakness in the neonatal period and others cause progressive problems in later childhood.

Myotonia congenita — In myotonia congenita children demonstrate failure of muscle relaxation without dystrophy. The symptoms are worst upon waking or after inactivity but the degree of myotonia reduces with recurrent muscle use. The disease is inherited in autosomal dominant and recessive forms.

Myotubular myopathy — This condition presents in the neonatal period and the muscle biopsy shows that the muscle has not developed beyond a primitive myotubule stage.

Type V glycogen storage disease (**Fig. 19.29**) (McArdle disease) is due to a lack of muscle phosphorylase activity. In later childhood severe cramps after exercise suggest failure to mobilize muscle glycogen.

Pompe disease is due to lack of acid maltase and presents in the neonatal period with weakness, a cardiomyopathy and a large, glycogen-loaded liver.

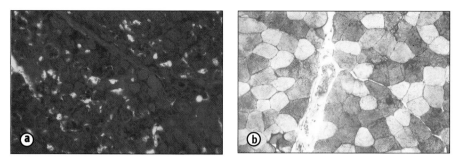

Fig. 19.29 *Abundant glycogen in type IV glycogen storage disease (a). A normal muscle biopsy (b).*

INFLAMMATORY MUSCLE DISEASE—DERMATOMYOSITIS

Dermatomyositis is a chronic inflammatory disorder of muscle often associated with a violaceous facial rash. The rash typically involves the eyelids, knuckles and other bony prominences. In acute cases there may be no rash but pronounced general weakness, muscle pain and misery. Contractures progress quickly as the muscles waste and become fibrosed. Subcutaneous calcification also occurs.

Muscle biopsy will demonstrate the perivascular inflammatory changes, and CPK and ESR can be used to follow the course of the disease. It is important to treat the disease early, even if this means delaying a confirmatory muscle biopsy. Steroids are the main treatment and should be tailed off very slowly to ensure that there is no relapse; azathioprine or cyclosporin can be added in resistant cases. Physiotherapy is of paramount importance to relieve contractures and prevent wasting of muscles.

ATAXIA

Ataxia denotes conditions in which there is incoordination of limb movement, gait and fine movement due to a disorder of the sensory proprioceptive nerves or dysfunction of the cerebellum. Ataxia of acute onset may be seen with the cerebellar post-infectious encephalitis of chickenpox, with cerebellar tumours or following drug ingestion, e.g. alcohol or anticonvulsants such as carbamazepine. There are many longstanding or degenerative conditions where this is a key feature, e.g. ataxia with cerebral palsy, Friedreich's ataxia and ataxia telangiectasia.

DEGENERATIVE CONDITIONS

There are many rare situations in which a child's normal developmental progress is interrupted and regression occurs. In many, an inborn error of metabolism has been found; in many more the cause remains idiopathic, for example:
Rett syndrome is an uncommon condition found in girls where normal development takes place for the first 6 months to 2 years, followed by regression in skills and withdrawal into an autistic-like state. Microcephaly, ataxia and stereotypic hand wringing movements occur; the diagnosis is confirmed by a typical EEG. The underlying cause is not clear.

283

Adrenoleukodystrophy is of X-linked recessive inheritance and only affects boys. There is an enzyme defect that prevents the breakdown of very long chain fatty acids which accumulate in the body. These boys begin to fail in their education during the primary school years, and progressive psychomotor retardation occurs with loss of hearing and vision. The diagnosis is made by finding excess very long chain fatty acids in plasma fibroblasts.

chapter 20

Children and Disability

Children with disability are an important patient group as they consume a disproportionate amount of health care resources. They often have additional medical problems which have a major effect on overall function. The multidisciplinary team has evolved to meet the needs of such children which are outside the expertise of any one specialist.

Recognition of disability is often delayed until the handicap is obvious. Screening for visual, hearing and general developmental problems helps to a large extent but it is always important to listen to the concerns of parents as they are often correct.

Most impairments in childhood are present at birth and unchanging, although as development progresses there may be changing needs (**Fig. 20.1**). Progressive, degenerative disorders are uncommon but, in addition to the changing needs of the child, the eventual outcome of death requires extra support. A particular example is muscular dystrophy (*see* Chapter 19).

PHYSICAL DISABILITY

Some children are physically disabled. Most are limited by a neurological or neuromuscular condition but others are compromised by problems such as cardiorespiratory disease, chronic arthritis and congenital limb anomalies.

Cerebral palsy is a general term for a disorder of movement and posture caused by a non-progressive insult to the immature brain. Although the lesion itself is non-progressive, its effects may change with the child's growth and development. An alternative term, central motor deficit, describes all non-progressive abnormalities of motor control, function and development in childhood, but specifically excludes disorders of the spinal cord, peripheral nerves and muscles. The causes of cerebral palsy can be categorized as pre-, peri- or postnatal in onset, but the time of the insult and recognition of its effects may not be the same; for example, birth asphyxia may not indicate hypoxia during the perinatal period but represent the effects of an insult earlier in the pregnancy (**Fig. 20.2**).

Although there is a variety of different causes of motor deficit, only a few patterns of disability are produced.

TYPES OF CEREBRAL PALSY

The spastic forms of cerebral palsy are upper motor neurone lesions characterized by hypertonicity, exaggerated reflexes, and an up-going plantar response.

Spastic hemiplegia

Spastic hemiplegia is the commonest form of spastic cerebral palsy. Two thirds of cases are prenatal in origin and the hemiplegia occurs more commonly on the right side. There may

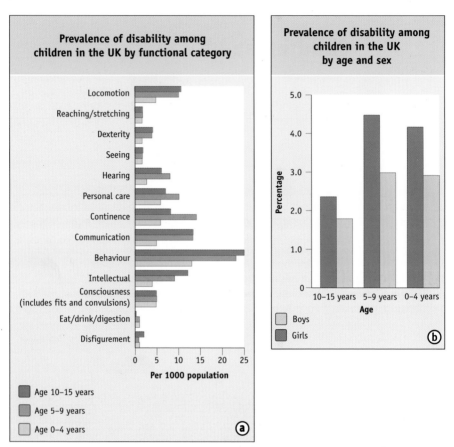

Fig. 20.1 *Prevalence of disability among children in the UK, 1985–1988: (a) by functional category; (b) by age and sex. Data from Bone M & Melzer H 1989 The prevalence of disability among children. OPCS Surveys of disability in Great Britain. Report 3. HMSO, London.*

be minimal facial weakness and the arm is less severely affected than the leg. Sometimes the residual effects may be sufficiently slight to be apparent only as a weakness or clumsiness on the affected side.

Spastic diplegia
Spastic diplegia is associated with preterm infants. The legs are affected with a typical internally rotated and flexed attitude. The upper limbs are only minimally affected. Intellectual impairment is not associated with this group.

Spastic quadriplegia
Children with spastic quadriplegia have severe spasticity in all limbs (**Fig. 20.3**) and generally are intellectually impaired and have other medical problems. This form of spasticity is caused by severe cerebral damage.

Causes of cerebral palsy

Abnormalities of brain development	• Neuronal migration defects • Hydrocephalus
Hypoxic ischaemic damage and cerebrovascular accidents	• Parenchymal damage after bleeding in preterm infants • Cerebrovascular accidents and hemiplegia • Hypoxic ischaemic encephalopathy (HIE)
Cerebral infection	• Congenital infection (CMV and toxoplasmosis) • Meningitis and encephalitis • HIV encephalopathy
Cerebral metabolic disorders	• Spastic quadriplegia
Obstetric causes	• Very low birth weight (<1500 g) • Multiple birth • Intrauterine growth retardation
Trauma and toxins	• Following head injury • Fetal alcohol syndrome • Crack cocaine
Genetic disorders	• Congenital ataxia

Fig. 20.2 *Causes of cerebral palsy.*

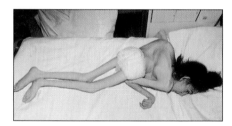

Fig. 20.3 *Severe spastic quadriplegia.*

Dyskinesia

Abnormalities of movement may occur in isolation or in association with spasticity. Hypoxic damage to the basal ganglia is associated with dystonia. There is often initial hypotonia in infancy before the disorders of movement are apparent.

- Athetoid movements are infrequent worm-like movements of whole limbs.
- Chorea describes frequent fleeting localized movements.
- Dystonic spasms are prolonged abnormalities of posture.
- Ataxia commonly accompanies spastic diplegia.

MANAGEMENT OF CEREBRAL PALSY

A variety of approaches involving intensive physiotherapy are aimed at improving the motor function of children with cerebral palsy. They seem to be beneficial but it is not clear whether the techniques themselves or the intensive support of the family are the key elements. The main role of conventional physiotherapy is to prevent contractures in affected limbs. A variety of aids are available to help children minimize their disability (**Fig. 20.4**).

Increased muscle tone is a major problem in children with cerebral palsy:

- Drug therapy with benzodiazepines or the muscle relaxant baclofen is often used.
- Injected botulinum toxin blocks activation of the motor endplate on the muscle and is very effective in reducing spasms for long periods.
- Surgical release of tendons may sometimes be necessary.
- Computerized gait analysis is sometimes used to analyze the pattern of walking and to plan surgery.

AUDITORY DISTURBANCE

The early recognition of impaired hearing is of great importance if adequate communication skills are to develop. The most common cause of deafness is the fluctuating conductive loss due to glue ear. Most sensorineural deafness is genetic in origin and accounts for greater than 40% of all cases of deafness (**Fig. 20.5**). Much of the inherited sensorineural deafness occurs sporadically and because there are no genetic prenatal tests for deafness, it is very difficult to give accurate genetic counselling to families. Deafness due to congenital rubella or postnatal infection with mumps is rare due to widespread vaccination. Meningitis remains an important cause of acquired deafness; all survivors of meningitis, whether viral or bacterial, should have audiometry in the weeks after discharge from hospital.

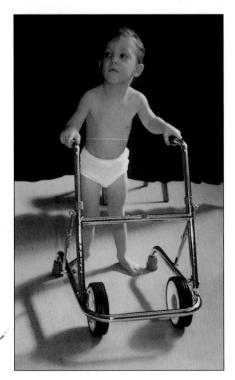

Fig. 20.4 *Rotary walking frame.*

Causes of deafness	
Genetic	
Single gene	• Autosomal recessive • Autosomal dominant
As part of a syndrome	• Down syndrome • CHARGE (Ear)
Non-genetic	
Glue ear	• Common
Intrauterine infection	• Rubella • Cytomegalovirus
Perinatal insults	• Hypoxic-ischaemic encephalopathy • Preterm infants and neonatal intensive care
Childhood infection	• Meningitis • Mumps

Fig. 20.5 *Causes of deafness.*

Preterm infants are more susceptible to the effects of hyperbilirubinaemia and are often treated with aminoglycosides. Although hearing loss in preterm infants is often attributed to these factors, the true cause is probably episodes of hypoxia.

SCREENING FOR DEAFNESS

The benefit of screening for deafness lies in early diagnosis and provision of rehabilitation measures before the child's development is compromised. Parents with concerns about their children's hearing should never be ignored as they are usually correct. Similarly, babies at high risk (family history of deafness, craniofacial abnormalities such as cleft palate and those involving the ear, prenatal infection, graduates of the neonatal intensive care unit, and those with hypoxic insults) should be tested in the neonatal period. Brain stem auditory evoked responses can be used to map the functioning of the auditory nerves and auditory cerebral cortex (**Fig. 20.6**).

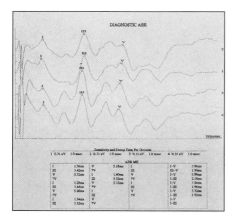
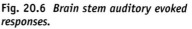

Fig. 20.6 *Brain stem auditory evoked responses.*

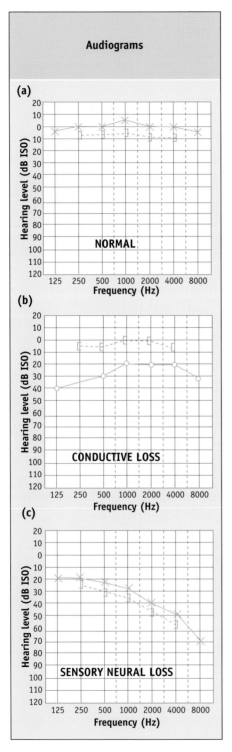

Fig. 20.7 *Audiograms. (a) Normal; (b) conductive deafness; (c) sensorineural deafness. Air conduction: 0, right ear; X, left ear. Bone conduction: [, right ear;], left ear.*

Most infants are screened by the distraction test at 6–9 months of age (*see* Fig. 3.9). Older children can be tested by pure tone audiometry (**Fig. 20.7**). For younger children it is useful to incorporate testing into a game, such as removing pegs from a board or pressing a button when they hear tone.

HEARING AIDS

Children with impaired hearing are assessed to see if a hearing aid will maximize their residual function and minimize their disability. Small aids worn behind the ear (**Fig. 20.8**) are available for the smallest of infants although they may need new earmoulds on a monthly basis because of growth. A bone conduction aid can be used if there is an abnormality of the external or middle ear (**Fig. 20.9**). Cochlear implants provide electrical stimulus directly to the cochlea to create the sensation of hearing (**Fig. 20.10**).

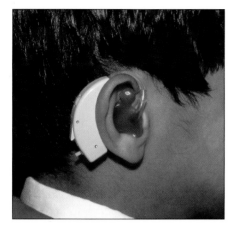

Fig. 20.8 *Hearing aid.*

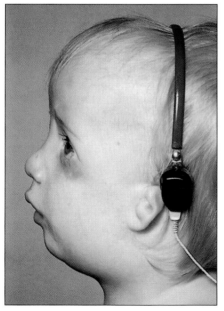

Fig. 20.9 *Bone conduction device.*

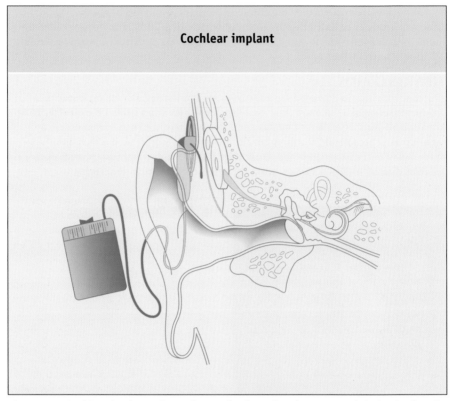

Cochlear implant

Fig. 20.10 *Cochlear implant. Electrodes are implanted and an external device is placed over the intact skin to detect and transmit sound. An extensive programme of training is required to gain maximal benefit from this device.*

VISUAL DISTURBANCE

The incidence of partial sight and blindness is about one in 1000 children, but clear definitions are not available. Genetic causes (retinal dystrophies, cataract, albinism) account for up to 60% of all severe visual impairment, and more than half of these children have additional disabilities or diseases. Seven per cent of children attending schools for severe learning difficulties have marked visual impairment.

Vision is the key sense in humans and underpins the development of all other senses. It is reasonably well developed at birth, and babies that are held in their parents' arms are able to focus on their faces. The visual system matures so that binocular vision becomes established after 6 weeks. Disruption of the visual signal during this critical time can lead to permanent amblyopia.

CONGENITAL VISUAL ABNORMALITIES IN THE NEWBORN

Examination of the eyes is probably the most important part of the first-day check. Abnormalities of the external eye or nystagmus (particularly if vertical or rotary) suggest a problem with vision. Congenital glaucoma (**Fig. 20.11**) may be noted due to clouding of

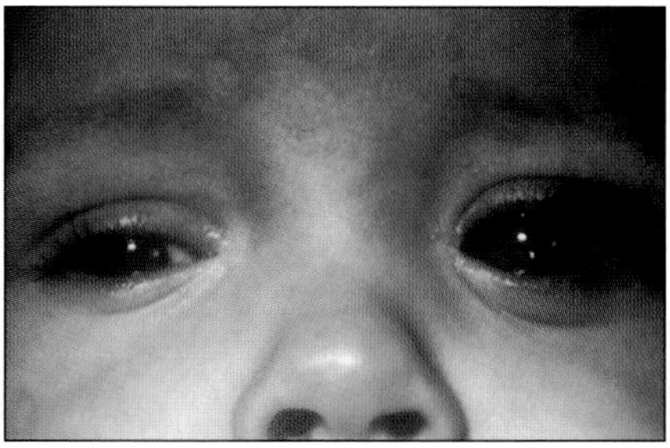

Fig. 20.11 *Congenital glaucoma.*

the cornea. Black specks in the red corneal reflex suggest an abnormality in the visual axis such as a cataract or retinoblastoma. Retinopathy of prematurity (*see* Fig. 7.36) is an important cause in preterm babies and is associated with high inspired oxygen concentrations. Minor degrees are quite common but fortunately often regress spontaneously. Cryocautery is an effective treatment for progressive disease. Other causes of severe visual impairment are associated with neurological syndromes, intrauterine infection and asphyxia.

GENERAL MANAGEMENT OF VISUAL DISABILITY

Specific therapy is directed at the cause of visual impairment but correction of minor refractive errors is important to maximize the available vision and ensure that other senses are optimized. As development is dependent on vision, parents must be taught to play with their babies to compensate for the lack of visual stimulation. Peripatetic teachers are available in many countries. Most children can be taught in mainstream education if additional help is available, and the use of tactile communication and sound is important.

The combination of visual and auditory impairment is devastating to the child's development; intensive training is required to overcome these problems.

SQUINTS

Squints are a source of anxiety for many parents and occur in up to 3% of children. Divergent squints in the first weeks of life are common and generally resolve, but convergent squints are usually abnormal. Examination of the fundus, lens, external ocular muscles, visual acuity (**Fig. 20.12**) and ocular reflexes should be performed as well as the light reflection test and cover test (**Fig. 20.13**). Prominent epicanthic folds may create the appearance of a convergent squint. It is always important to evaluate fully the eyes of any infant presenting with a possible squint to exclude treatable conditions that can interfere with normal development, such as cataract, glaucoma, severe refractive errors or retinoblastoma.

Once a squint is confirmed, any underlying pathology should be dealt with. Amblyopia may be corrected by occlusion of the good eye. Occlusion and later surgery to adjust the external ocular muscles may allow alternating vision and a good cosmetic result although true stereoscopic vision may never develop.

LANGUAGE DISTURBANCE

Language is an interactive system of symbols used for communication. There are different elements to language. It is used internally as a medium for thought and this can be noted

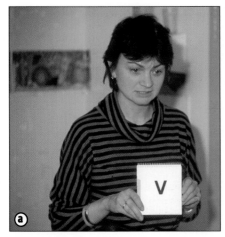

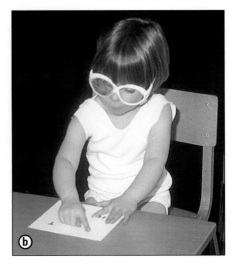

Fig. 20.12(a,b) *Visual acuity testing by matching letters.*

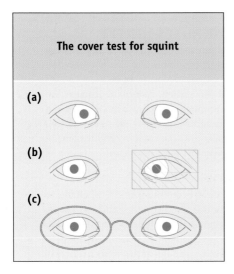

The cover test for squint

(a)

(b)

(c)

Fig. 20.13 *The cover test for squint. When the fixing eye is covered, the squinting eye takes up fixation. The diagram illustrates a right convergent squint (b).*
(c) Correction of a refractive error will produce a normal visual axis.

before any other means of communication has developed, for example by the way children use cups and other utensils for their correct purposes. Verbal comprehension develops alongside inner thought and reinforces the association between object and label. Expressive language occurs later. Initially, words are used without grammar but in context. The rules of grammar and the use of language in a social and interactive and abstract way develop with time.

The development of communication skills is dependent on vision, hearing and an appropriate environment. Early detection of difficulties is therefore important (**Fig. 20.14**). Although language is much more difficult to assess than vision and hearing, the absence of words by 2 years, or an unintelligible child at 3 years of age are general guidelines for speech therapy assessment.

Incidence of speech disorders	
1 in 1000	Have severe difficulties in acquiring spoken language
1 in 100	Have difficulties that seriously affect their education
1 in 100	Children stammer
1 in 10	Will have a problem with speech that interferes with their education at some point in their lives
1 in 2	Of children with mental handicap have speech or language difficulty

Fig. 20.14 *Incidence of speech disorders*

LEARNING DIFFICULTIES AND LANGUAGE

Specific language problems may be missed if children have learning difficulties, and conversely language difficulties in these groups can severely limit developmental progress. A particularly important example is children with Down's syndrome who may be limited due to cognitive and auditory impairment.

STAMMERING (DYSFLUENCY)

Almost everyone stammers when tired or under stress and many children go through a period, when aged about 3 or 4 years, when the fluent production of language is disturbed. This developmental non-fluency consists of repetition of a whole word and does not upset the child. However, other children suffer a permanent non-fluency around this time, characterized by having difficulty with parts of words and struggling to get words out. An initial assessment by a speech therapist is required.

MANAGEMENT OF LANGUAGE DISORDERS

In many children the cause of their speech difficulties can not be determined. However, they usually have recognizable patterns of difficulty, for example with expression of words, grammar or syntax. Most children will have a temporary and immaturity of language development and gain rapid benefit from speech therapy. Other children have greater problems with acquiring language, have distorted language patterns, and experience problems with their peers and education as a result. They require more intensive speech therapy and form a group with a poorer prognosis.

There is no single cure for stammering. Whilst there are techniques that can improve the flow of words, an important part of therapy is to help the child cope with and understand the condition. For instance, many children have difficulties with social interaction which may need specific psychological support.

Sometimes, for example in profoundly deaf children, it is not possible to gain speech and signing languages are taught instead.

ASSOCIATED MEDICAL CONDITIONS

Children with motor deficits commonly suffer other medical problems in addition to language, hearing and visual impairment. They may need the services of a hospital-based paediatrician, orthopaedic surgeons, dental surgeons, ophthalmologists, ENT surgeons, speech therapists, physiotherapists and occupational therapists. Child development centres were created to act as a central resource where different professionals could visit the child rather than the child attending many different hospitals. This concept has not succeeded and the current pattern of care is based around the community-based paediatrician who takes overall responsibility for the child and seeks opinions and treatment from relevant specialists.

EPILEPSY

Epilepsy is particularly common in children with cerebral palsy, especially those with spastic quadriplegia. All seizure types may occur and infantile spasms may herald later physical disability. The diagnostic principles are the same as with any child (*see* Chapter 19) although the confusion of convulsions with dyskinetic movements often occurs. Treatment is along conventional lines but combination therapy is often needed and continued indefinitely. Sedation and behavioural changes are common and important side-effects of drug therapy.

FEEDING PROBLEMS

Feeding problems are especially common in cerebral palsy due to persistence of primitive reflexes and oropharyngeal incoordination. If weight gain is poor it may be necessary to resort to nasogastric feeding or a gastrostomy. Gastro-oesophageal reflux and constipation are other common problems.

MENTAL RETARDATION

About one third of children with cerebral palsy have severe mental retardation which requires special schooling. Many others have less severe learning difficulties that can be dealt with by extra resources in mainstream education. In the United Kingdom a formal assessment of a disabled child's special educational needs must be made from the age of 2. This is known as an educational statement.

SOCIAL SUPPORT

Caring for a handicapped child is stressful, and social workers, medical and paramedical specialists have to provide emotional support for the carers in addition to their conventional roles. Respite care for severely handicapped children is important; rapid admission to hospital for apparently minor problems can avert much greater problems in coping.

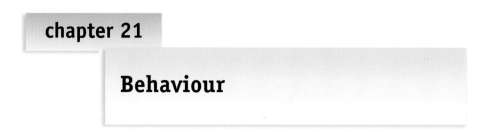

chapter 21

Behaviour

Children's behaviour depends on their stage of development. For example, in the neonatal period the sleep–wake cycle is closely linked with feeding, and breast-fed babies tend to sleep through the night at a later age than bottle-fed ones. Similarly, violent outbursts of crying are a means of signalling needs or displeasure before effective communication is established. Regression in behaviour, such as a return to bed wetting or disturbed sleep, often accompanies acute illness.

TEMPER TANTRUMS

Almost half of all 5-year-olds have regular outbursts of anger, especially when tired or hungry (**Fig. 21.1**). They are a normal part of early childhood when communication and social skills are undeveloped. As the child matures, sulking and brooding often become more common until eventually understanding and compromise supersede. Persisting tantrums and aggressive behaviour are more common in children with social disadvantage, communication difficulties, or general behavioural and developmental problems.

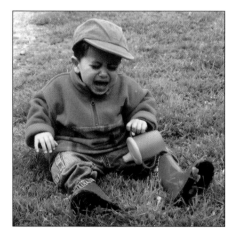

Fig. 21.1 *Temper tantrum*

SLEEP DISTURBANCE

At any one time a quarter of all preschool children are not sleeping well. Most infants do not need to wake during the night for a feed after they are 2 months old and after this time they wake because of a behavioural disturbance.

A bedtime routine is helpful for all children. It signals a series of events such as a bath, night-time drink, tooth brushing and story which then lead to bed and sleep. The familiarity of the routine allows calmness rather than excitement to prevail. A daytime nap is frequently found to be beneficial; if it is missed the overtired child can be difficult to get to sleep.

It is important to realize that children, like adults, require different amounts of sleep and often wake in the night. A problem only arises if they wake and demand attention, disrupting the rest of the household. Sedatives are not satisfactory for these problems. The child's behaviour must be modified to allow him or her to wake and be able to go back to sleep, alone. There are two main ways to modify the behaviour. The rapid way is to let the child cry in the night and not attend to it at all. The parents must be sure there are no other needs and be strong enough to put up with a few nights of misery. Most parents opt for a gradual approach of going to the child and soothing before leaving him or her to go back to sleep alone. The time spent and the amount of physical contact with the child is then gradually reduced.

Children commonly wake in the night after having bad dreams, but a rare but important condition is night terrors. These are different from nightmares and other forms of sleep disturbance and are frequently more worrying for parents than for the child. They usually occur at the same time during the night during slow wave sleep and are accompanied by autonomic disturbance (sweating, pallor and tachycardia) and an apparent terror for which the child afterwards has no recollection. A sleep EEG may be needed to exclude nocturnal epilepsy. Management is aimed at avoiding over-stimulation before sleep and relaxation after stressful events. Waking the child as symptoms begin to be exhibited can prevent an attack occurring.

EATING DISORDERS

Food fads are very common in toddlers and are best managed by gentle perseverance rather than a battle of wills. A particular problem in this age group are the children who will only drink milk and then risk iron deficiency anaemia. They must be limited in their milk intake and given foods that they are likely to eat.

Throughout the rest of childhood picky eaters distress their parents who worry about insufficient nutrition. Careful clinical evaluation, dietary assessment, and plotting of serial growth data is an important first step; with this information it is possible to identify the minority with medical problems. For the remainder, who eat sufficiently but are fussy, management involves a routine at mealtimes. For example, the family sits down to meals together without other distractions, such as television. Food is presented for a set period such as 20 minutes; although positive encouragement to eat can be given there should be no coercion or threats. The food is then to be removed, even if not finished, but no snacks or treats should be offered between meals.

ANOREXIA NERVOSA

Anorexia nervosa is a serious neurosis characterized by a persistent active refusal to eat and marked loss of weight (more than 25%). Important features are a disturbance of body image and fear of fatness.

The cause is unknown, and although it usually affects girls at the time of puberty it is becoming increasingly common in boys. In about half the cases a precipitating stress such as teasing (especially over physical appearance), parental discord, pubertal and sexual conflicts can be found.

Management

Treatment of anorexia is difficult and is based on behavioural strategies to increase weight, with psychotherapy and family therapy to resolve underlying conflicts. For those with severe problems treatment may need to be carried out as an inpatient with supervision of eating and target weights. The short-term results are good. Fifty per cent can be said to have fully recovered whilst 25% have improved. A further 20% have persisting problems with weight and menstruation. The mortality of anorexia is less than 5%; half of these deaths are due to suicide.

Anorexia nervosa—diagnostic criteria

- Weight loss: at least 25% of original body weight, or weight 25% below normal for age/height
- Avoidance of 'fattening' foods
- Amenorrhoea for at least 3 months
- Disturbance of body image: the patient sees herself as fat even when underweight

---

HYPERKINESIS AND ATTENTION DEFICIT DISORDER (HADD)

Children vary greatly in the amount of energy they have and the sleep they need. At one end of the spectrum is a group whose continuous activity is a problem for their parents. Exclusion diets are often tried in these hyperactive children, but they are not very successful. Hyperactivity, together with poor attention span and distractibility, is labelled 'the hyperkinetic syndrome' or 'attention deficit disorder'. Drug therapy is disappointing although Ritalin is useful in some children. Psychotherapy is aimed at improving parents' coping skills.

SUICIDE AND PARASUICIDE

Suicide is an act of deliberate self harm resulting in death. It is rare before puberty and usually involves male adolescents. The methods used are usually violent, such as hanging or jumping from high places, and the act seems to be precipitated by an immediate emotional crisis, for example a family dispute or a humiliating or disappointing experience. The children involved are often socially isolated. Another group are those who imitate the deaths of their role models, such as pop and film stars.

Parasuicide is the act of self injury which, whilst the intention was present, did not result in death. It should be regarded as a symptom of distress. It is mostly confined to adolescent girls who act impulsively after arguments with parents or friends. Ingestion of tablets and/or alcohol is the usual method and most immediately regret their actions.

However, half the children involved in parasuicide have symptoms of reactive depression, chronic psychiatric or behavioural problems. Violent methods such as self mutilation and hanging are very worrying and may be more suggestive of an underlying psychosis such as depression or schizophrenia.

Management

In all cases of self-inflicted harm an assessment of continuing self risk and the possibility of psychiatric disease must be made by a qualified person—usually a child psychiatrist. An overnight admission to hospital is usually needed for medical reasons and is often important as it removes the child from any provoking stress.

NOCTURNAL ENURESIS

The development of nocturnal bladder control is dependent on maturation of the nervous system, which is achieved in 95% of children by the age of 7 years. Twenty per cent of the remainder become dry at night each year thereafter, but in some families control develops later—even up to 16 years. Although primary enuresis is not caused by an emotional disturbance, family stress often follows and is best managed by an understanding paediatric community nurse. It is important to address the emotional issues for the child and family and the practical problems and cost of extra laundry.

Secondary enuresis is a return to bed wetting in a previously dry child. It may occur at times of illness or stress in some children but can be due to medical problems and thus can be considered as a symptom of an underlying disorder. The cause is almost universally emotional but it is important to rule out urinary tract infection in girls, a urinary concentrating defect, diabetes mellitus or undiagnosed spina bifida.

The management of enuresis is difficult but the high rate of spontaneous resolution offers hope. Drugs such as vasopressin nasal spray or tablets are useful for short-term control, for example during holidays, but do not provide a cure. Similarly, imipramine may be effective but tolerance may develop after a few weeks. A psychological approach with star charts and rewards to try to improve the number of dry nights is often helpful. Pad and bell systems change the pattern from wetting of the bed into waking up to urinate.

ENCOPRESIS

The passage of a stool in an inappropriate place is known as encopresis. The condition is not usually diagnosed until 4 years of age because control of defecation is dependent on developmental maturation. Fifty per cent of children have bowel control by 2 years and almost all children have control of their bowels by 30 months. However 3% of 5-year-olds occasionally soil their pants and 1% do this at least once a week. Some children have never gained control of their bowels and may have neurological disorders limiting bowel control such as spina bifida; others have been continent but regress under stress or illness; some others suffer from constipation and overflow soiling. A joint medical and psychological approach is most useful in solving these problems.

Enuresis

Primary—never dry at night, usually dry during the day
Secondary—previously dry at night

Incidence
- 15% of 5-year-olds
- 3% of 10-year-olds
- 1% of 14-year-olds

Causes
- Emotional/psychological
- Delayed maturation
- Urinary tract infection
- Familial
- Polyuria (hypercalcaemia, diabetes mellitus/insipidus, chronic renal failure)
- Urological (incontinence)
  —meatal stenosis
  —posterior urethral valves
  —ectopic ureter

History
- Change of routine, e.g. new school, new sibling, house move
- Enquire about family history of enuresis
- Check for UTI symptoms
- Consider spinal or urological cause

Examination
- Dipstick urine for sugar, protein, blood
- MSU for culture
- Consider renal function, serum calcium
- Check for renal enlargement/tenderness
- Check spine and scrotum

Management
- Explain the problem to both child and parents
- Star chart
- Consider pad and bell in a child under 6 years old
- Short-term treatment with DDAVP (avoid tricyclics because of cardiac side-effects)

PSYCHOTIC STATES IN CHILDHOOD

Psychotic states are extremely rare in early childhood. Children below the age of 7–8 years can be difficult to diagnose as having a psychosis as they have difficulty in communicating their hallucinations and abnormal thought patterns. Adolescents, however, do exhibit bipolar affective disorder and schizophrenia. Drug ingestion may also cause psychotic states in children.

Treatment of psychosis is along conventional lines with antipsychotic medication. Unfortunately less than 20% of children completely recover, half have relapses, and the rest remain ill.

AUTISM (INFANTILE PSYCHOSIS)

Autism is very rare and affects one in 5000 children. Boys are more commonly affected and the cause appears to be brain dysfunction which may have a genetic influence. Although the condition is present from birth the symptoms only become manifest when language and social interaction skills have developed sufficiently to allow abnormalities to be noticed. Coincidently, this is often at the time of MMR immunization.

In half of affected children no useful speech develops and in the remainder it is delayed in onset and abnormal in quality; there is abnormal grammatical development and inability to use abstract terms. There are also profound problems with social interaction, with lack of eye to eye contact and cooperative play. Stereotyped routines and rituals occur, and mental retardation and epilepsy are common accompaniments.

There is no cure for autism, but behavioural and drug treatments can produce symptomatic improvements. Only 10% of children will go on to be self-supporting adults and more than 60% will become severely handicapped adults in mental institutions.

Asperger's syndrome is an autistic-like syndrome; these children have high intelligence and normal speech, although non-verbal language and visual-spatial skills are dysfunctional.

ABSENCE FROM SCHOOL

Children who are chronically ill should have their education provided by the local education authority at home or in hospital. There are two situations in which children do not obtain education:

TRUANCY

Truancy occurs when a child is absent from school without the parents' knowledge. It usually involves children, especially boys, from inner city environments who find academic work unrewarding (Fig. 21.2). Truancy is usually an activity with groups of children spending time together and often being involved in petty crime or substance abuse.

It is difficult to motivate these children as they find the mainstream school curriculum unstimulating and their families may not see the need for schooling. The problem lies with the school as well as with the child, and the educational service has a responsibility to cater for the needs of different kinds of children.

SCHOOL REFUSAL

School refusal describes a child who stays at home with a parent's consent. Superficially the child is keen to attend school but is unable to. This may be because of a chronic illness such as asthma or because the child suffers non-specific symptoms such as headache, malaise or abdominal pain on going to school. There is often a history of neurosis in the mother and the child may be anxious about a parent's health or ability to cope. A positive attitude should be taken, with all the adults involved promoting a return to school. It is important to recognize that there may be hidden collusion between mother and child which may make this difficult.

Truancy and school refusal	
Truancy	**School refusal**
Boys more than girls	Same frequency in boys and girls
Poor academic record	Good academic record
Other behaviour problems	Emotional problems such as anxiety
Seldom physical symptoms	Commonly physical symptoms
Most common at end of period of compulsory education	Peaks at 5 and 11 years
Disorganized family background	

Fig. 21.2 *Truancy and school refusal.*

CHILDREN IN HOSPITAL

Hospitals are strange and frightening places for children. The presence of a parent, or at least an older sibling, is of vital importance in maintaining a degree of normality.

Children who are in hospital and isolated from their parents characteristically follow three stages of behaviour. They are initially distressed and inconsolable; they then become restless, continually searching for their parents; finally they withdraw and despair, often attaching to carers.

CHRONIC ILLNESS

Children usually cope with chronic illness remarkably well, especially if they have a secure and consistent home life. However, the demands of ongoing treatment and the feeling of being different can cause stresses and behavioural problems. Children should attend mainstream schools wherever possible with additional help if necessary. Teachers are also encouraged to help with children's treatment, for example use of asthma inhalers and recognition of diabetic problems.

Adolescence is a difficult time for all children and during this time children with chronic illness such as epilepsy, asthma or diabetes may exaggerate or provoke the symptoms of their illness. Managing adolescents can be difficult; direct confrontation is not a useful strategy.

Chronic illness also places strains on the rest of the family. Siblings may feel neglected. Parents may find difficulty in providing consistent discipline between children, and they may also have difficulty in maintaining their own marital relationship.

CONSENT

Children understand the concepts of illness and death to varying extents depending on their age. Even 5-year-olds may have views and should be consulted about their treatment, whether this is venesection or chemotherapy. This idea has found favour with the courts, and in the United Kingdom the age of 16 is no longer a lower limit for consent. If children are able to understand the issues involved, their views should be taken into account.

DYING

Children usually accept dying; this may be because they have not yet learnt to be afraid of death. Explanations are important and should be given in terms the child can understand which do not preclude honesty. It is often best for the parents to explain matters to the child as, although it is difficult for the parents, it is easier for the child to relate to a trusted carer. Even in emergency situations the benefit to the child from the presence of parents outweighs any distress or difficulty for doctors.

Distressing symptoms should be treated as they present. The child should be kept comfortable with analgesia and anti-emetics, which should be given regularly rather than as required, each symptom being tackled individually rather than with a standard cocktail.

chapter 22

Haematology

NORMAL HAEMATOLOGICAL FINDINGS IN INFANCY AND CHILDHOOD

Until the second trimester haemopoiesis occurs mainly in the liver and spleen. After this time haemopoiesis in the bone marrow becomes established and at term no longer occurs in extramedullary sites unless there are excessive demands, such as in haemolytic disease of the newborn. The blood cells originate from pluripotential stem cells which give rise to dedicated stem cells for the various cell lines (**Fig. 22.1**). This process is controlled by specific growth factors—erythropoietin (red cells), thrombopoietin (platelets) and granulocyte colony stimulating factor (GCSF; neutrophils)—which have found clinical use in stimulating the different cell populations.

Haemoglobin is a complex of two pairs of globulin chains that bind four oxygen molecules in a cooperative fashion. Fetal haemoglobin (haemoglobin F; α_2/γ_2) is the predominant form until around 36 weeks' gestation; then adult haemoglobin (α_2/β_2) begins to increase until at term it comprises 40% of the total (**Fig. 22.2**).

At birth, the polycythaemia and fetal haemoglobin required to strip maternal blood of oxygen become superfluous. There is a reduction in the circulating red cell mass. Bilirubin, the breakdown product of haemoglobin, is responsible for the common jaundice occurring during the first week of life, but the iron is stored and re-used. The haemoglobin level therefore falls to a minimum level at around 2 months postnatal age and then climbs through childhood (**Fig. 22.3**). Rapid growth means that term infants have exhausted their iron stores by around 6 months of age. This is less of a problem for breast-fed babies as, although breast milk contains little iron, it is more effectively absorbed and utilized than the iron in formula milks.

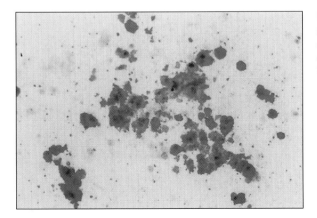

Fig. 22.1 *Stem cells responsible for producing megakaryocytes and other myeloid cell lines within the bone marrow.*

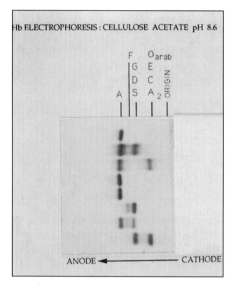

Fig. 22.2 *Electrophoresis of haemoglobin allows diagnosis of haemoglobinopathies. Either an abnormal haemoglobin is detected or there is persistence of haemoglobin F.*

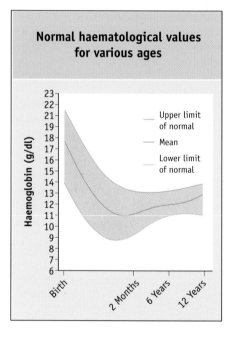

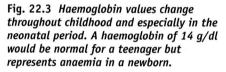

Fig. 22.3 *Haemoglobin values change throughout childhood and especially in the neonatal period. A haemoglobin of 14 g/dl would be normal for a teenager but represents anaemia in a newborn.*

Preterm infants are very likely to become iron deficient if fed solely with breast milk as they have high requirements and are also subject to frequent blood sampling. Preterm formulations contain extra iron.

IRON DEFICIENCY

Insufficient dietary intake of iron is the commonest cause of anaemia in childhood, especially at the end of the first year of life when neonatal stores are depleted and nutritional supplies inadequate due to delays in weaning. Gastrointestinal blood loss secondary to hookworm infestation is a common cause of anaemia in underdeveloped countries but other causes such as oesophagitis, gastritis, Meckel's diverticulum or vascular anomalies are rare. Gut losses can be excluded by faecal occult blood testing and microscopy for worms. Malabsorption of iron may be due to occult coeliac or Crohn's disease, but there are usually other symptoms such as growth failure.

Chronic anaemia is often well tolerated with few symptoms to remarkably low haemoglobin concentrations.

The common presenting symptoms of anaemia

Anaemia
- Pallor
- Irritability and listlessness
- Frequent infections
- Systolic apical murmur
- Rarely oedema and heart failure

Specific to iron
- Atrophic glossitis
- Koilonychia
- Pica
- Reduction in school performance

A full blood count and film (**Fig. 22.4**) showing microcytic and hypochromic cells is sufficient for diagnosis, and a ferritin level less than 10 µg/ml provides final confirmation. In continuing blood loss there is often a reactive thrombophilia and reticulocytosis.

Therapy

Transfusion is almost never warranted; oral iron supplements (ferrous sulphate) continued for 3 months after return to normal haemoglobin levels will replete body stores. The commonest cause of non-response is failure to comply with the medication. In African and Mediterranean populations thalassaemia minor or intermedia may be the explanation for a persisting anaemia (see below).

FOLATE AND B$_{12}$ DEFICIENCY

Folate and B$_{12}$ deficiency are rare in childhood, but malabsorption may cause anaemia. A mild and asymptomatic megaloblastic anaemia due to antagonism of folate by anticonvulsants such as phenytoin is commonly seen.

Children with other blood dyscrasias and high cell turnover are at risk of folic acid deficiency and are prophylactically supplemented with folic acid to avoid anaemia.

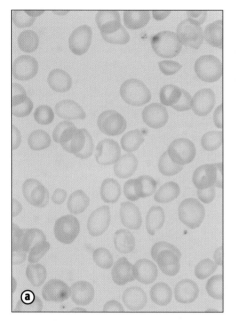

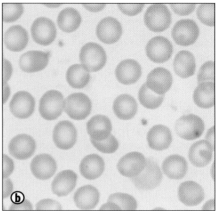

Fig. 22.4 *Blood smear showing (a) iron deficiency anaemia. The cells are small (microcytic) and pale (hypochromic). A normal film is shown for comparison (b).*

DYSFUNCTIONAL MARROW

In childhood, infection with parvovirus, hepatitis viruses, or Epstein–Barr virus can cause acquired aplastic anaemia. Drugs and toxins may rarely be responsible but most cases are idiopathic. It may be necessary to give blood products until spontaneous recovery.

Fanconi anaemia can present as a red blood cell aplasia but ultimately pancytopenia occurs. Children usually have dysmorphic features—skeletal, thumb (**Fig. 22.5**), renal and ear abnormalities, microcephaly and mental retardation. The inheritance is autosomal recessive and the diagnosis can be confirmed by finding typical chromosomal breaks in white cells after exposure to castogenic chemicals. The median survival is around 5 years and many such children develop secondary cancers such as myeloid leukaemia.

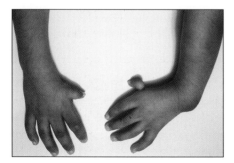

Fig. 22.5 *Thumb anomalies are characteristic of Fanconi anaemia.*

HAEMOLYTIC ANAEMIA

Haemolytic anaemias are a group of conditions characterized by an excessive rate of red cell destruction with markedly shortened red cell life span (**Fig. 22.6**). Excess unconjugated bilirubin and urobilinogen result, and if there is intravascular haemolysis the binding of free haemoglobin reduces the plasma haptoglobin concentration. The bone marrow is hypercellular and there are abundant reticulocytes. As well as symptoms of anaemia there is jaundice and an increased incidence of pigment gallstones. Folate deficiency, as well as viral infections (parvovirus), can arrest the marrow and cause temporary aplastic crises so prophylactic folate is given to all children.

Causes of haemolytic anaemia	
Red cell membrane	• Hereditary spherocytosis • Elliptocytosis
Red cell metabolism	• Glucose-6-phosphate dehydrogenase deficiency • Pyruvate kinase deficiency
Haemoglobin abnormality	• Sickle cell disease • Thalassaemias
Immune disorder	• Haemolytic disease of the newborn • Autoimmune disease • Drugs, e.g. methyldopa
External	• Trauma from prosthetic heart valves, infection, toxins, burns

Fig. 22.6 *Haemolytic anaemias are commonly diagnosed in the neonatal period because of excessive jaundice.*

HEREDITARY SPHEROCYTOSIS AND ELLIPTOCYTOSIS

Hereditary spherocytosis is an autosomal dominantly inherited disorder of spectrin—a red cell cytoskeletal protein. Cells released from the marrow are biconcave but they become small and spherical due to progressive loss of membrane, especially on passing through the spleen. The degree of anaemia and jaundice is variable but all children have splenomegaly and a tendency to cholelithiasis. The red cell appearances are characteristic (**Fig. 22.7**). In severe cases splenectomy is carried out, but this is usually deferred until at least 10 years of age. Pre-splenectomy pneumococcal vaccination and prophylactic penicillin for life protect against the increased risk of infection with capsulate bacteria.

Hereditary elliptocytosis (**Fig. 22.8**) is relatively common and causes a mild haemolytic anaemia due to abnormalities of the red cell cytoskeleton. No treatment is required.

GLUCOSE-6-PHOSPHATE DEHYDROGENASE (G6PD) DEFICIENCY

G6PD is a key enzyme involved in the maintenance of glutathione in its reduced state using glucose 6-phosphate as a substrate. Mutations of this gene, carried on the X chromosome, render the red cell membrane liable to damage by oxidant stress. Males of Oriental, Mediterranean, Asian or African descent are at risk. Neonates present with jaundice, and

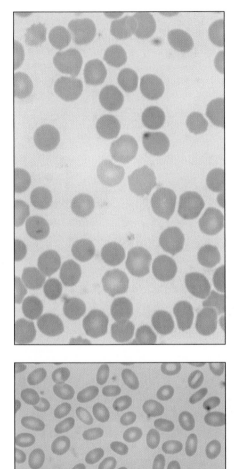

Fig. 22.7 *Spherocytes are red cells that have lost their doughnut shape. They are also excessively fragile in hypotonic solutions.*

Fig. 22.8 *The red cells in hereditary elliptocytosis are actually more oval in shape.*

in later life severe haemolytic crises can be provoked by drugs or eating fava beans in those individuals with severe deficiency of the enzyme (favism).

The diagnosis is easily made by assaying red cell levels of G6PD, but it must be remembered that reticulocytes have high enzyme levels and can be misleading. Avoidance of oxidant drugs is important, although vitamin K should be given due to the risks of haemorrhagic disease of the newborn. Infants with jaundice are treated conventionally, with phototherapy and exchange transfusion if necessary, as kernicterus is a risk. In haemolytic crises supportive care is all that can be given.

SICKLE CELL DISEASE

Disorders of haemoglobin chains are mainly due to mutations in the gene that codes for the two beta chains of the haemoglobin molecule. In the case of sickle haemoglobin there is a substitution of valine for glutamine in the beta chain and resultant deformation of the red cells (**Fig. 22.9**) at low oxygen tensions (sickling). Heterozygotes (sickle cell trait) have

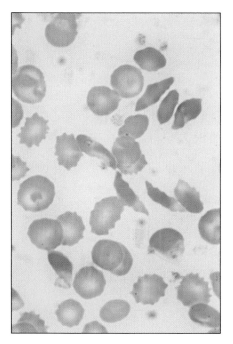

Fig. 22.9 *Blood film showing sickle cells.*

one normal gene and therefore some normal beta chain production. They sickle only during hypoxia, for example flying at altitude. Heterozygotes have the advantage of increased resistance to falciparum malaria. Homozygotes (sickle cell disease) have both abnormal genes affected and can only produce sickle haemoglobin. These individuals suffer severe anaemia and sickle crises.

Features of sickle cell disease

- Pallor and mild jaundice
- Splenomegaly in early childhood (under 4 years) and later splenic auto-infarction
- Susceptibility to pneumococcal and other capsulid bacterial infections
- Urinary concentrating defect and enuresis are common
- Crises (escalating episodes of sickling often precipitated by infection and worsened by dehydration, tissue hypoxia and acidosis):
  — Pulmonary
  — Abdominal
  — Neurological—stroke
  — Aseptic necrosis of head of femur and humerus
  — Hands and feet—often initial presentation in children

Management of sickle cell disease is dependent on early recognition of crises and compliance with regular long-term penicillin prophylaxis, because of the high risk of infection with capsulate bacteria. Crises are usually triggered by infections or dehydration. Treatment involves copious intravenous fluids, antibiotics if there is any possibility of infection, and effective analgesia. Blood transfusion may be necessary, and formal exchange transfusion can be performed for severe crises. Regular prophylactic exchange transfusions are given to children who have had cerebral (**Fig. 22.10**) or chest crises.

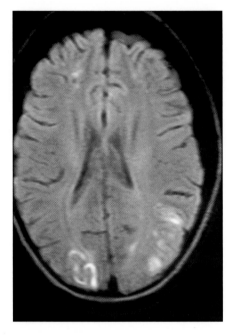

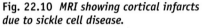

Fig. 22.10 *MRI showing cortical infarcts due to sickle cell disease.*

THALASSAEMIAS

Alpha and beta thalassaemias are due to a failure of production of one of the respective haemoglobin chains. In beta thalassaemia a homozygous genetic mutation produces a severe haemolytic anaemia with compensatory marrow hyperplasia. Diagnosis of thalassaemias is by haemoglobin electrophoresis (**Fig. 22.2**). Regular supportive blood transfusions are required, with accompanying chelation of excess iron stores with subcutaneous desferrioxamine. Iron overload eventually causes secondary haemochromatosis (cardiomyopathy, cirrhosis, endocrine failure and skin pigmentation). If there is an HLA-compatible sibling, bone marrow transplantation can be performed.

Beta thalassaemia trait is the heterozygotic condition; it is characterized by very mild anaemia and can be confused or co-exist with iron deficiency. Individuals are often asymptomatic but identification is important for genetic counselling.

PURPURAS

The clotting cascade, integrity of the blood vessels and presence of platelets are all involved in ensuring that clotting of the blood occurs when a vessel is breached (**Fig. 22.11**), but

Causes of bruising

Petechiae and mucosal bleeds	Thrombocytopenia	• Idiopathic thrombocytopenia • Haemolytic uraemic syndrome • Acute lymphoblastic leukaemia
Spontaneous bruising and bleeding on minor trauma	Coagulation defect	• Haemophilia • Haemorrhagic disease of the newborn
Spontaneous bruising or petechiae	Vasculitis	• Henoch–Schönlein purpura • Autoimmune vasculitis
Others	Physical causes	• Non-accidental injury • Whooping cough

Fig. 22.11 *An abnormal bleeding tendency is usually caused by disorders of the vessels, platelets or coagulation factors, but the possibility of non-accidental injury should be borne in mind.*

that clotting does not occur in the circulating blood. Purpura or bruising is due to leakage of blood into the tissues. This is usually due to trauma but may be due to disease.

A platelet count and coagulation tests allow diagnosis of the different bleeding diatheses (**Fig. 22.12**), but more specialized assays can be performed. The prothrombin time assays the intrinsic coagulation cascade which is dependent on the vitamin K dependent factors. Partial thromboplastin time measures the extrinsic factor VIII pathway and also the common final path shared between intrinsic and extrinsic cascades. The reptilase test excludes the effect of heparin which prolongs the PTT and thrombin time. Clotting of blood in the sample tube does not exclude a clotting disorder; this usually occurs due to tissue factors contaminating the sample and/or inadequate mixing of the tube.

Coagulation tests

	Platelet count	Prothrombin time	Partial thromboplastin time	Bleeding time
Idiopathic thrombo-cytopenic purpura	Reduced	Normal	Normal	Elevated
von Willebrand disease	Normal	Normal	Elevated	Elevated
Haemophilia A	Normal	Normal	Elevated	Normal
Haemorrhagic disease of the newborn	Normal	Elevated	Elevated	Normal
Disseminated intravascular coagulation	Reduced	Elevated	Elevated	Elevated

Fig. 22.12 *Coagulation tests in bleeding disorders.*

HAEMOPHILIA A AND B

Haemophilia A is an X-linked condition arising from a functional defect in the coagulation aspect of the factor VIII molecule. Haemophilia B (Christmas disease) is caused by deficiency of factor IX and is very similar to haemophilia A.

Spontaneous bleeding and marked bleeding after mild injury are the main problems but joint destruction after intra-articular bleeds can be disabling (**Fig. 22.13**).

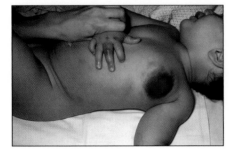

Fig. 22.13 *Severe bruise in haemophilia.*

Management of haemophilia

Sufferers with mild and moderate haemophilia may transiently increase factor VIII levels following injection with DDAVP (vasopressin), which is useful for minor surgery or tooth extraction. The mainstay of treatment, however, is prompt recognition and early treatment of bleeding episodes with factor VIII concentrate. In most instances enough factor VIII to raise blood levels to 30% of normal is sufficient, but for operations and severe bleeds this can be raised to 60%. Families are taught to carry out injections at home at the first indication of trouble. Haemarthroses require initial bed rest and analgesia followed by gentle mobilization to avoid contractures. Vaccinations are given subcutaneously or intradermally, and intramuscular injections and non-steroidal anti-inflammatory drugs are avoided. Similarly, good dental hygiene is important to avoid unnecessary dental extractions.

Support of children and families is important as there are often marked psychosocial problems in dealing with a chronic disabling disease that is disruptive for home and school life. Genetic counselling is also of great importance. It is possible to screen possible female carriers (reduced factor VIII activity) and to provide antenatal diagnosis using genetic probes.

VON WILLEBRAND DISEASE

Von Willebrand disease is an autosomal dominant disease with reduced factor VIII coagulation activity (compared to the level of VIII-related von Willebrand factor) and mild platelet dysfunction. Bleeding is mild in comparison with classical haemophilia. Tranexamic acid and desmopressin (causing release of stored factor VIII) are generally effective after bleeding.

HAEMORRHAGIC DISEASE OF THE NEWBORN

Newborn babies are deficient in vitamin K which is necessary for production of clotting factors II, VII, IX and X. Before the prophylactic administration of vitamin K many babies suffered serious gastrointestinal or umbilical bleeds. Intracranial bleeds also occurred which, if not fatal, produced great disability.

Oral vitamin K administration is probably as effective as intramuscular injection, but only if repeated doses are given until 6 weeks of age. There is no good evidence to suggest that vitamin K is linked with childhood leukaemia.

IDIOPATHIC THROMBOCYTOPENIC PURPURA

Idiopathic thrombocytopenic purpura is thought to be an immune-mediated disorder, occurring after viral infections or vaccinations. Platelets are coated with IgG and removed from the circulation primarily by the spleen. There are normal or increased numbers of megakaryocytes in the marrow (**Fig. 22.14**). Preschool children usually present acutely with unexplained petechiae and bruising and are otherwise well. Although they may have platelet counts below 10×10^9 they are functionally intact; serious bleeds, such as intracranial bleeds, are extremely rare. The platelet count is monitored and children are best kept at home as they are always too active in hospital. The course is self limiting and 75% have recovered after one month.

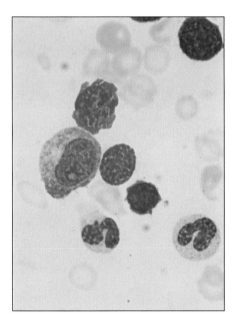

Fig. 22.14 *Megakaryocytes within the bone marrow.*

Intravenous immunoglobulin or corticosteroids are effective in raising counts. In atypical cases or if there is no spontaneous resolution, acute leukaemia or an aplastic anaemia should be excluded. It is important to exclude leukaemia before steroids are used to elevate platelet levels. Five per cent of children have chronic thrombocytopenia and may be helped by splenectomy.

HENOCH–SCHÖNLEIN PURPURA (HSP)

Henoch–Schönlein purpura is a self-limiting allergic vasculitis which commonly follows viral infections in young children. The clinical picture, when fully evolved, allows a clinical diagnosis but often abdominal pain or a swollen joint can cause initial diagnostic confusion.

The rash of HSP is petechial, non-blanching, and affects the extremities and buttocks. An arthritis affecting the large joints is common. Haematuria reflects a glomerulonephritis;

although this is usually of good prognosis, it can cause chronic renal impairment, later hypertension and, rarely, death. Abdominal pain may be caused by mucosal bleeding and oedema in the gut wall. Rarely intussusception may occur.

The condition is self limiting. Corticosteroids, although highly effective, are reserved for severe gastrointestinal symptoms. Analgesia and bed rest are required for the arthritis.

DISSEMINATED INTRAVASCULAR COAGULATION

Consumption of coagulation factors and platelets with production of fibrinogen degradation products occurs in seriously ill children. Sepsis, shock and acidosis are the usual causes. Acute haemolysis of red cells also occurs due to fibrin strands in the small blood vessels. Supportive measures with fresh frozen plasma, cryoprecipitate, red cells and platelets are required while the underlying cause is addressed; the outcome depends on the underlying condition.

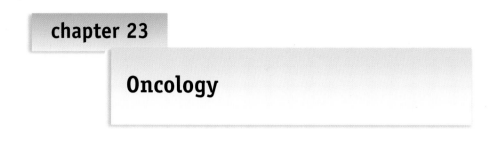

chapter 23

Oncology

Cancer is relatively uncommon in childhood and only affects about one child in 600 (**Fig. 23.1**). The treatment and prognosis for many tumours have improved considerably over the last 20 years. In general, the improvements in survival have been due to improved multi-agent chemotherapy, greater expertise in its administration, and better management

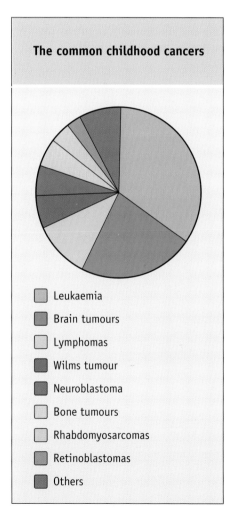

The common childhood cancers

- Leukaemia
- Brain tumours
- Lymphomas
- Wilms tumour
- Neuroblastoma
- Bone tumours
- Rhabdomyosarcomas
- Retinoblastomas
- Others

Fig. 23.1 *Pie chart showing the common childhood cancers. Acute lymphoblastic leukaemia is the commonest childhood cancer. Many cancers are inherited, and genetic counselling is needed for families and patients.*

of complications. Collaborative studies and strict treatment protocols have allowed variations in therapy to be quickly validated and then widely implemented.

AETIOLOGY OF CHILDHOOD CANCER

The factors responsible for causing cancer are becoming clearer (**Fig. 23.2**) and the molecular genetic controls of cell replication and cell death are beginning to be understood. Mutations of such genes (oncogenes) can result in uncontrolled proliferation of cells. One mutation may be found in apparently normal individuals but is generally insufficient to produce a cancer. If a second mutation occurs during normal cell replication this may be sufficient to allow uncontrolled proliferation to occur. In some tumours with a strong inheritance the second mutation may be already present as in, for example, neuroblastoma or retinoblastoma, or it may occur after exposure to environmental factors such as ionizing radiation. The finding of abnormal genes, chromosomal breaks and deletions in many tumours adds weight to this hypothesis. Chromosomal conditions are also frequently associated with an increased risk of cancer. Some viruses are able to activate genes within the cells of the host and have been implicated in tumours. For example, a retrovirus is known to cause lymphoma in adults, and Epstein–Barr virus is found in Burkitt lymphoma.

Aetiological factors in cancer	
Inherited factors	
Susceptibility genes	Retinoblastoma, nephroblastoma
Down syndrome	ALL is the commonest leukaemia in trisomy 21, but there is a high incidence of non-lymphoblastic leukaemias
Fanconi anaemia	Acute leukaemia and chromosomal breaks with ionizing radiation
Ataxia telangiectasia	Lymphoma and leukaemia and chromosomal breaks with ionizing radiation
Neurofibromatosis I	Brain tumours, optic glioma, sarcoma, neuroblastoma
Hemihypertrophy	Nephroblastoma
Familial polyposis coli	Gastrointestinal adenocarcinoma
Environmental factors	
Prenatal exposure to ionizing radiation	Suggested increase in childhood cancers
Survivors of the Hiroshima atomic bomb	Cancer—especially of the thyroid
Drugs	Maternal ingestion of diethylstilboestrol and vaginal carcinoma in female offspring
Immunosuppression	Increased risk of cancer with immunosuppression, e.g. for renal transplants

Fig. 23.2 *Aetiological factors in cancer.*

Immunodeficiency disorders are associated with lymphoid malignancy and it is postulated that this is because abnormally proliferating cells are allowed to survive.

ACUTE LYMPHOBLASTIC LEUKAEMIA (ALL)

Acute lymphoblastic leukaemia accounts for about 80% of leukaemia in childhood; the other 20% are mainly acute myeloid leukaemias. Other leukaemias, in particular the chronic forms, are rare in childhood.

ALL is the result of a malignant proliferation of a clone of immature lymphocytes. These cells crowd the bone marrow and suppress other blood cell lines producing typical clinical features (**Fig. 23.3**) and infiltrate other structures causing organomegaly and lymph node enlargement. As with other sporadic cancers the causes are still unknown.

Investigations

The clinical picture, together with the finding of lymphoblastic cells in the peripheral blood, suggests leukaemia (**Fig. 23.4**). Bone marrow examination is essential to confirm the diagnosis and the immunophenotype of the marrow cells has prognostic implications (**Fig. 23.5**).

Treatment

The aim of therapy is to reduce the number of leukaemic cells to a level that can be dealt with by the body's own defences. A general scheme is followed (**Fig. 23.6**) which is modified in the light of clinical trials.

Presenting features of acute leukaemia	
Suppression of blood cells	
Low platelet counts	Petechiae and skin purpura, nose bleeds
Suppression of red cell production	Pallor, lethargy, anorexia and breathlessness. Heart failure is very uncommon
Reduction in neutrophils and functional lymphocytes	Infection may disclose leukaemia. Pyrexia may occur in the absence of infection
Bone pain or arthralgia	
Marrow infiltration and osteoporotic changes	Two thirds of cases of ALL present with bone pain
Infiltration of other organs	
Hepatosplenomegaly	Asymptomatic
Lymphadenopathy	Commonly cervical nodes
Meningeal infiltration	Usually in relapse. Symptoms of raised intracranial pressure
Testicular infiltration	Common site of relapse

Fig. 23.3 *Presentation of acute leukaemias. Leukaemia may mimic many other conditions and present to a variety of specialists. The blood film is usually diagnostic.*

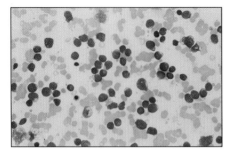

Fig. 23.4 *Blood film appearances of leukaemia.*

Prognostic indicators in acute lymphoblastic leukaemia

Good prognosis

- White cell count less than 20 × 10⁹/l
- Aged 2–5 years
- Common ALL phenotype

Poor prognosis

- White cell count more than 50 × 10⁹/l
- Aged less than 1 year
- B cell ALL phenotype
- Meningeal involvement
- Chromosomal translocations

Fig. 23.5 *Prognostic indicators in acute lymphoblastic leukaemia.*

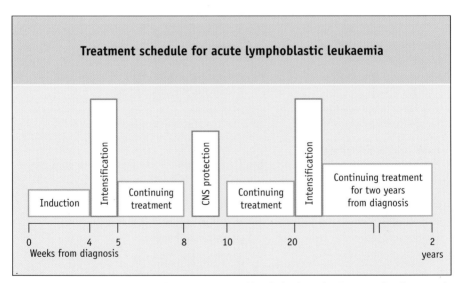

Fig. 23.6 *Treatment schedule for acute lymphoblastic leukaemia. See text for drugs and other therapy used at each stage.*

Treatment of ALL

- Induction of remission means eradication of the leukaemic cell population and restoration of normal bone marrow function. This is achieved with multiple cytotoxic drug therapy and intrathecal methotrexate lasting for 4 weeks; 97% of children will achieve remission. Those who are slow or who fail to respond have a poor prognosis. Prehydration and allopurinol are given as the rapid cell lysis can lead to uric acid crystals obstructing the kidney tubules.
- A block of intensification therapy is given following induction of remission and again at 20 weeks. These blocks aim to clear residual resistant leukaemic cells using cytotoxic drugs that were not used during the initial induction of remission.
- Continuation therapy is carried on for a total of two years. Daily 6-mercaptopurine or 6-thioguanine, weekly methotrexate, and monthly vincristine and steroids are given.
- Leukaemic cells in the central nervous system are a particular problem as drugs penetrate poorly into the CNS and neurodevelopmental problems occur after cranial irradiation. Children at low risk of CNS relapse are given intrathecal methotrexate only, whereas those at high risk may receive either intrathecal methotrexate with high dose intravenous methotrexate or cranial irradiation alone.

Relapse

Relapse (**Fig. 23.7**) can occur after stopping therapy and carries a poor prognosis. Although remission can be achieved a second time, the time to a further relapse is often quite short. Total body irradiation and high dose chemotherapy followed by bone marrow transplantation is an alternative to standard chemotherapy if a matching bone marrow donor is available.

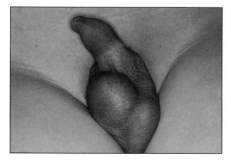

Fig. 23.7 *Testicular relapse of ALL.*

LYMPHOMA

Hodgkin lymphoma is rare in childhood and mainly occurs in young adults as isolated painless cervical lymphadenopathy (**Fig. 23.8**). It is unusual for there to be any systemic manifestations such as weight loss, itching or sweating. Localized disease is treated with radiotherapy and the more advanced stages with chemotherapy. The prognosis is good: 80% are cured.

Non-Hodgkin lymphoma is more common in childhood and some types probably represent a solid form of leukaemia. The usual sites of presentation are the gastrointestinal tract (with intussusception or obstruction) with B cell forms and the mediastinum (often with superior vena caval obstruction) with T cell forms (**Fig. 23.9**).

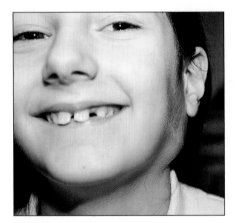

Fig. 23.8 *Cervical lymphadenopathy.*

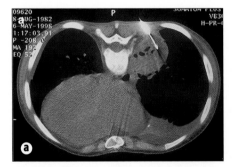
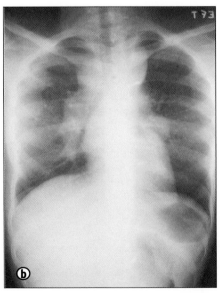

Fig. 23.9 *(a) CT-guided needle biopsy of an intrathoracic lymphoma. (b) X-ray showing mediastinal lymphadenopathy due to lymphoma.*

SOLID TUMOURS

CEREBRAL TUMOURS

Tumours of the central nervous system are the most common solid tumours in childhood. The classifications for such tumours are still not uniform but the commonest tumours are astrocytomas and medulloblastomas (**Fig. 23.10**). Secondary metastatic deposits are uncommon in children.

The symptoms of intracranial tumours fall into two groups: those due to raised intracranial pressure and those due to local disruption from the tumour mass (**Fig. 23.11**). Magnetic resonance imaging allows detailed three dimensional information on the tumour to be obtained (**Fig. 23.12**).

NEUROBLASTOMA

Neuroblastoma may arise at any point along the sympathetic chain or in the adrenal glands. It metastasizes early to lymph nodes and the bone marrow causing anaemia and thrombocytopenic bruising. The commonest presentation is as a large abdominal mass (**Fig. 23.13**). The ultrasound scan confirms a large mass which crosses the midline and is

Features of cerebral tumours			
Type of tumour	**Origin**	**Treatment**	**Survival**
Cerebellar astrocytoma	Areas of loose cellularity or cysts. The more solid forms have a worse prognosis	Up to 90% can be completely resected. If this is impossible or there is recurrence radiotherapy is useful. There is no place for chemotherapy	More than 90% of children with cystic/non-solid tumours are alive at 10 years; less than 35% of those with the more solid forms are alive at 10 years
Medulloblastoma	Tumour arising from the roof of the fourth ventricle	Surgical excision and CSF shunt. Radiotherapy and chemotherapy	About 50% at 10 years
Craniopharyngioma	The embryonic remnants of Rathke's pouch	Surgery with radiotherapy Hormone replacement therapy	70% at 10 years
Ependymoma	Lining of the ventricular system	Excision is difficult because of local infiltration of tumour. Radiotherapy needed as well	50% at 5 years

Fig. 23.10 *Features of cerebral tumours.*

Symptoms of intracranial tumours

Raised intracranial pressure

Children	• Morning headache • Vomiting • Visual disturbance • Lethargy • Personality change • Falling school performance
Infants	• Headache • Developmental delay or regression • Large head, sunsetting sign, widened sutures and prominent veins

Local effects

Craniopharyngioma	• Pressure on optic nerves—bitemporal hemianopia • Pressure on hypothalamus and pituitary—GH, TSH, ACTH or ADH deficiency
Brain stem and cerebellum	• Cranial nerve palsies • Ataxia
Cerebral cortex	• Headaches • Seizures • Long tract signs

Fig. 23.11 *Symptoms of intracranial tumours.*

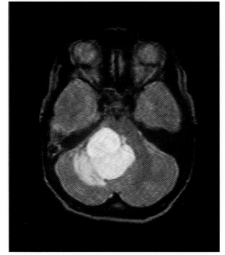

Fig. 23.12 *MRI of cerebellar astrocytoma.*

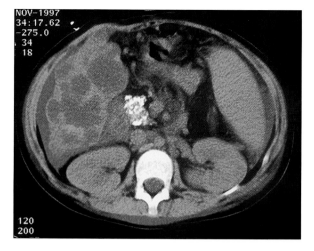

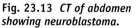

Fig. 23.13 *CT of abdomen showing neuroblastoma.*

distinct from the kidneys. Areas of signal drop-out indicate calcifications which are seen on the X-ray. Lethargy and pyrexia, local bone pain, and ptosis due to deposits behind the eye are common symptoms. Vanillyl mandelic acid (VMA) and homovanillic acid are produced by the tumour and their measurement in the urine can be used to aid diagnosis and assess the response to therapy.

Management

Radiological evaluation with computed tomography scans, bone marrow examination and biochemical markers are sufficient to reach a diagnosis of neuroblastoma.

Chemotherapy to shrink the tumour mass is often given before a surgical excision is undertaken. The resected tumour is carefully examined for antigen expression.

The outlook is good for localized disease in infants under 1 year of age, even if there is bone marrow involvement, as spontaneous remission is usual. The prognosis is worse for disseminated disease in older children; relapse is common even after an apparent good response to chemotherapy.

Screening

Screening programmes in Japan have shown that areas of neuroblastic tissue are common in healthy infants and usually regress. A concern of neonatal screening is that it may lead to many children being treated unnecessarily for tumours that would otherwise regress spontaneously.

NEPHROBLASTOMA—WILMS TUMOUR

Nephroblastoma is a tumour derived from embryonic kidney tissue and usually presents before 5 years of age. Most of the tumours in younger children, especially when bilateral, are inherited. The rare association with aniridia, which is caused by a known chromosomal deletion, led to the identification of Wilms tumour susceptibility genes on the short arm of chromosome 11.

Nephroblastoma usually presents with abdominal distension in an otherwise healthy child, although a few children are hypertensive, have haematuria, or feel generally unwell.

Ultrasound scanning or computed tomography shows the tumour to arise from the kidney (**Fig. 23.14**) and additional enlarged lymph nodes or involvement of the inferior

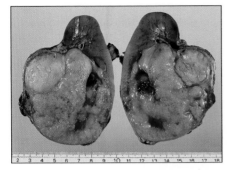

Fig. 23.14 *Nephroblastoma*.

vena cava can also be identified. It is important to assess the contralateral kidney for disease or abnormal development and function. The most common site of metastatic spread is to the chest, although the brain and bone may be affected.

Treatment

The treatment of choice for limited disease is removal of the tumour and the affected kidney. Chemotherapy may be used prior to surgery to shrink extensive tumours. After surgery, chemotherapy is given to all children and radiotherapy to those with more advanced disease.

The results of treatment are very good: up to 80% of children are cured, and children with less advanced disease can be offered less intensive treatment with no reduction in survival. Unfortunately, children who relapse have a very poor prognosis.

RETINOBLASTOMA

Retinoblastoma is a malignant embryonal tumour. Most cases present before 3 years of age. The susceptibility gene has now been linked to chromosome 13, and all bilateral tumours and about 20% of unilateral tumours are thought to be inherited as an autosomal dominant trait, but with incomplete penetrance.

The usual presenting feature is a white pupillary (in contrast to the usual red) reflex; if the macula is involved there may be a squint.

Treatment

The aim of treatment is to cure the disease but preserve eyesight wherever possible. Cryotherapy or photocoagulation is used for a single small deposit, but enucleation may be necessary if there is extensive disease. Although the tumour is very radiosensitive, chemotherapy is now preferred to avoid the cosmetic defects that follow radiotherapy. Tumours that have spread outside the eye into the orbit or skull have a worse prognosis, and surgery with high dose radiotherapy is given to include the whole central nervous system. For most children with limited disease there is a greater than 90% survival but an increased risk of secondary tumours in survivors, especially osteosarcoma.

Genetic counselling is important, especially in bilateral disease or if there is a family history. Recombinant DNA probes can also be used to detect carriers.

BONE TUMOURS

Osteosarcoma and Ewing's sarcoma (**Figs 23.15, 23.16**) tend to occur around puberty and are more frequent in boys. Metastatic spread is not uncommon at the time of diagnosis and has a very poor prognosis.

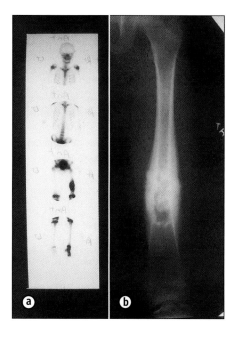

Fig. 23.15 *Bone scan (a) and X-ray (b) showing osteosarcoma of the right femur.*

Features of bone tumours

	Osteosarcoma	Ewing's sarcoma
Frequency	Commonest bone tumour at all ages	Commoner in younger children
Common sites	Distal femur, proximal tibia, proximal humerus and pelvis	Proximal femur, proximal humerus and pelvis
Presentation	Pain—mistaken for trauma	Pain, fever and tenderness—mistaken for osteomyelitis
X-ray appearances	Bone sclerosis and new periosteal bone formation	Often substantial soft tissue mass and bone destruction

Fig. 23.16 *Features of bone tumours.*

Treatment

Treatment of localized disease is by initial chemotherapy and radical surgery. Amputation of limbs is now avoided by resection of the tumour and insertion of an endoprosthesis which can be lengthened to match growth. Radiotherapy may be used for Ewing's sarcoma. Five year survival rates of 60–70% are achieved for non-metastatic disease.

LANGERHANS CELL HISTIOCYTOSIS

Langerhans cell histiocytosis was previously known as histiocytosis X; although it is not really a malignancy the abnormal proliferation of histiocytes can be destructive. Solitary deposits may be asymptomatic or cause pain or a pathological fracture; they are treated with curettage or injection of steroid. Multiple deposits may occur at any site in the body. Hypothalamic deposits cause diabetes insipidus and require lifelong replacement therapy with desmopressin. A more aggressive systemic disease tends to occur in infancy, often with a rash that resembles seborrhoeic dermatitis. All the organs of the body may be involved and the proliferation of histiocytes is usually progressive. Chemotherapy is curative in almost all cases.

PRINCIPLES OF CHEMOTHERAPY AND RADIOTHERAPY

CYTOTOXIC DRUGS

In general, cytotoxic drugs only affect proliferating cells as their action depends on interfering with synthesis or the division of cellular material. Some drugs act throughout the cell cycle whilst other drugs are specific to particular phases. Combinations of drugs that act in different ways can therefore increase cancer cell killing and reduce the damage to normal cells in the body (**Fig. 23.17**). Cells that are resting are not susceptible to

Some common cytotoxic drugs			
Drug	**Group**	**Mechanism of action**	**Side-effects**
Cyclophosphamide	Alkylating agent	Active metabolites permanently bind DNA strands together preventing transcription, and also disrupt the structure of DNA during cell division	Haemorrhagic cystitis is avoided by prehydration and Mesna
Methotrexate	Folic acid antagonist	Competes with folic acid and prevents formation of new DNA	Folinic acid displaces methotrexate and is used to prevent or speed recovery from myelosuppression
Vincristine	Vinca alkaloid	Interferes with the microtubules that are essential for mitosis	Neuropathy is common. Vinca alkaloids are lethal if given intrathecally
Daunorubicin	Antibiotic	Prevents synthesis of nucleic acids	Progressive cardiomyopathy
Prednisolone	Corticosteroid	Induces remission— mechanism not fully understood	Side-effects are rare as is only given for short periods

Fig. 23.17 *Some common cytotoxic drugs.*

cytotoxic drugs; long courses of treatment must therefore be given to eradicate these cells when they eventually divide. Intermittent high dose chemotherapy is often better than low dose continuous treatment. This kills the maximum number of cancer cells and, although normal tissues are severely affected, they can still recover (**Fig. 23.18**). The smaller the mass of cancer cells the better the results of treatment; this is due to many factors such as a higher proportion of cells in the resting phase in large tumours and ability of drugs to penetrate into tumours.

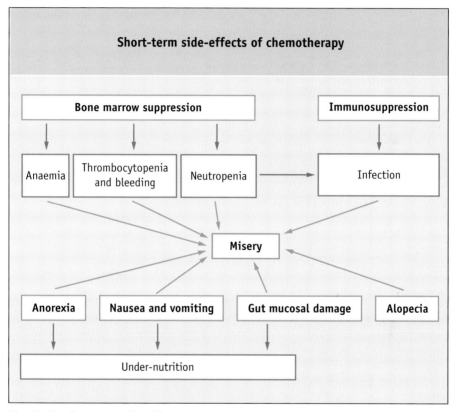

Fig. 23.18 *Short-term side-effects of chemotherapy.*

RADIOTHERAPY

Radiotherapy involves exposing a defined area of the body to a source of ionizing radiation which damages the DNA of the cells and prevents replication. The process is non-selective and the method of exposure aims to reduce the exposure of normal tissues.

Radiotherapy is highly effective for some tumours, but many are not radiosensitive.

The exact position of the area to be irradiated is first defined using scanning techniques and moulds to achieve reproducible positioning of the body. In children this often entails general anaesthesia. Beams of protons are directed from different directions to summate at the tumour site. Sensitive areas such as the eyes are shielded from the beams. Treatment is given in daily fractions to allow tissue recovery.

> **Problems with radiotherapy**
>
> - General side-effects of tiredness, anorexia, nausea and vomiting
> - Erythematous skin reactions are common
> - Brain irradiation leads to learning difficulties, especially in children under 3 years of age
> - Some syndromes with abnormal chromosomal fragility carry a high risk of cancer after exposure to ionizing radiation, for example ataxia telangiectasia and Fanconi anaemia (see Chapter 22)
> - Irradiation is particularly toxic to the bone marrow and is used for ablation before bone marrow transplantation

GENERAL CARE

GENERAL HAEMATOLOGICAL SUPPORT

At presentation, during treatment and during infection the circulating numbers of blood cells may be low. Transfusions of red cells and platelets are given, matched to the CMV status of the child. Irradiated blood products must be used in immunodeficient patients to prevent donated white cells attacking the patient (graft versus host disease). Haematopoietic stimulatory hormones such as GM-CSF may be used to elevate cell counts in neutropenic patients.

INFECTION

Neutropenia, secondary to marrow infiltration or due to the effects of cytotoxic therapy, is a common problem in oncology. Problems generally arise when the absolute neutrophil count is less than 1.0×10^9 and the risks can be grave when it is below 0.2×10^9. The organisms that cause infection in this situation are derived from the patient's own flora, either skin or bowel. General hygiene, hand washing and isolation procedures are essential at this time. An important focus of infection is the indwelling central venous access line. The organism is usually a coagulase negative staphylococcus but unusual organisms such as *Pseudomonas* spp. may occur.

Although many infections will be due to viruses, broad spectrum antibiotics are given after bacteriological samples have been obtained. They are continued until the neutrophil count rises again, and most bacterial infections come under control when the neutrophil count is greater than 0.5×10^9. If the pyrexia does not settle after 48 hours of antibiotics, antifungal agents, e.g. amphotericin or fluconazole, are added.

Prophylactic nystatin mouthwash or amphotericin lozenges are given to immunosuppressed children. Oral co-trimoxazole is used to prevent *Pneumocystis carinii* pneumonia (PCP). Chickenpox or re-activated herpes simplex lesions are treated with acyclovir, whilst ganciclovir is useful against cytomegalovirus.

Live vaccines should be avoided in the immunosuppressed child as they may cause disseminated infection.

NUTRITIONAL SUPPORT

Anorexia and nausea are common problems. It is important to try to maintain nutrition during therapy. If this is not successful parenteral nutrition may be started.

SOCIAL SUPPORT

Support of the family and child with cancer is one of the most difficult aspects of paediatric care. The discomfort of therapy together with the uncertainty of the outcome can have a lasting impact on the family. Counselling by the oncology team and practical help with travelling and finances are important aspects of care. Normality is difficult to achieve in this situation but children should be encouraged to continue with school, friends and family life. Behavioural problems in the child and in siblings are not unusual and may need specialist psychological help. At all stages of treatment the child should be involved in decision making and receive sensible and honest explanations.

LONG-TERM SURVIVAL

The improved outcome for childhood cancers is producing a growing population of young adults with residual difficulties. It appears that interruptions to education are generally overcome and social functioning is normal.

- Poor growth is not uncommon during therapy, and long-term growth impairment is a feature of cranial irradiation.
- Infertility may occur in males, but in general females are not affected.
- Genetic counselling is important for inherited cancers.
- Psychological problems are uncommon but some children continue to fear return of the cancer.
- Survivors may be at risk of secondary cancers, especially if they have inherited retinoblastoma or underlying conditions such as neurofibromatosis. Solid tumours occur within the field of previous radiotherapy.

TERMINAL CARE

Almost all children with cancer will receive some form of treatment; even if the cancer is incurable, the quality of remaining life can be improved. Children who relapse after treatment can be given further therapy but the chance of long-term survival diminishes. Palliative care encompasses pain relief and control of distressing symptoms for the child and family, as well as helping them to come to terms with death. Most families prefer to carry out this process at home and specialists in palliative care can facilitate this. After the child's death it is important to maintain contact with the family to help them during their bereavement.

chapter 24

Surgical Problems

CLEFT PALATE

The palate forms from two lateral shelves of tissue which fuse in the midline. Most cases of cleft palate are of unknown aetiology but cleft palate occurs in the Pierre–Robin sequence because the tongue prevents the shelves meeting in the midline (**Fig. 24.1**). Isolated cleft palate is common and may be limited to the posterior soft part of the palate (**Fig. 24.2**) or be covered with oral mucosa. Both these defects may be missed during the first-day check unless the palate is both inspected and palpated. Occasionally a posterior cleft palate will be detected because of regurgitation of fluids from the nose on swallowing.

Cleft palate is often associated with a cleft in the upper lip noticed at birth (**Fig. 24.3**). It is important for the paediatrician to see the parents immediately and reassure them of the excellent cosmetic outcome after surgery. Plastic surgical teams usually send a representative to see parents as a matter of urgency; they explain the surgery that will be needed and show pictures of postoperative results. There is no reason why feeding by breast or bottle cannot be accomplished. Special teats or palatal plates can be provided if necessary. The timing of palate surgery is a matter of debate: early closure allows speech to develop normally but can disturb midfacial growth. In general the lip defect is repaired first and the palate closed later at 3–4 months of age.

All children with cleft palate need careful audiological follow-up as glue ear due to Eustachian tube dysfunction is a universal finding. As with other midline defects there is also an association with growth hormone insufficiency.

In general the occurrence of cleft palate is sporadic and there is no increased risk to future children.

OESOPHAGEAL ATRESIA AND TRACHEO-OESOPHAGEAL FISTULA

The lungs develop as a bud from the ventral part of the foregut at 4 weeks' gestation. The most common congenital abnormality in this region is a blind-ending oesophagus which is usually accompanied by a communication with the trachea (**Fig. 24.4**). Problems may be obvious at birth because the blind-ending oesophagus presents with inability to swallow saliva or milk or because of the abnormal communication causing air to be blown into the stomach or acid to reflux into the lungs. Tracheo-oesophageal fistula is diagnosed by failure to pass a nasogastric tube which coils in the blind-ending oesophagus (**Fig. 24.5**). Prior to surgery a drainage tube is left in the pouch to remove swallowed saliva that would otherwise be aspirated. Small H-type fistulae can be responsible for chronic cough or recurrent chest infections due to aspiration. These can be difficult to diagnose and

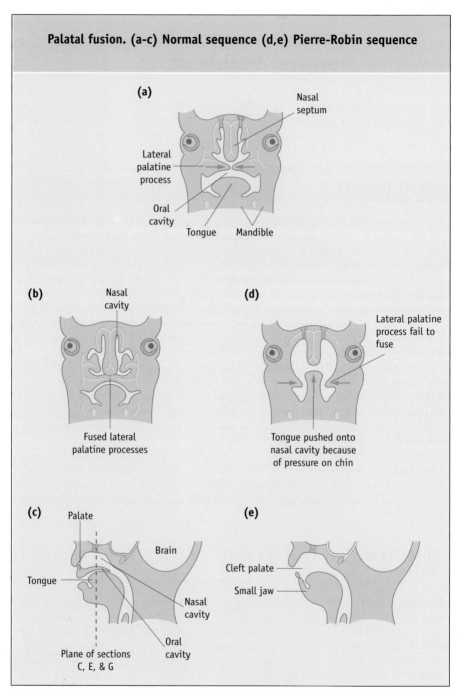

Palatal fusion. (a–c) Normal sequence (d,e) Pierre-Robin sequence

(a)

Nasal septum

Lateral palatine process

Oral cavity

Tongue   Mandible

(b)

Nasal cavity

Fused lateral palatine processes

(d)

Lateral palatine process fail to fuse

Tongue pushed onto nasal cavity because of pressure on chin

(c)

Palate

Brain

Tongue

Nasal cavity

Oral cavity

Plane of sections C, E, & G

(e)

Cleft palate

Small jaw

Fig. 24.1 *Palatal fusion. (a–c) Normal sequence; (d,e) Pierre–Robin sequence.*

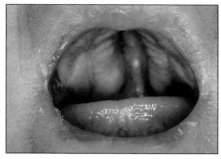

Fig. 24.2 *Posterior cleft soft palate.*

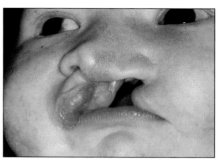

Fig. 24.3 *Cleft lip and cleft palate.*

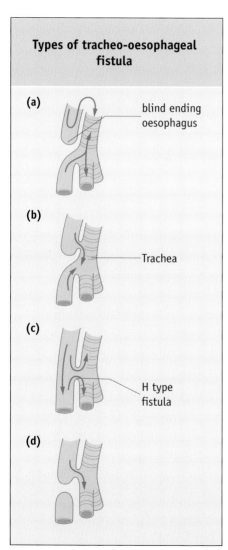

Fig. 24.4 *Types of tracheo-oesophageal fistula.*

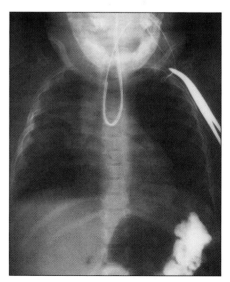

Fig. 24.5 *Blind ending oesophagus.*

endoscopy may be required to detect them. Problems with oesophageal motility often persist after surgical repair of these fistulae.

VOLVULUS OF THE STOMACH

Volvulus of the stomach is important as, unlike the other abdominal catastrophes, there may be no bile-stained vomiting and the baby often remains well until ischaemic damage has occurred and shock begins. Vomiting of sudden onset in a baby needs an abdominal X-ray (**Fig. 24.6**) to exclude this possibility, as the mass may be difficult to palpate.

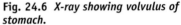

Fig. 24.6 *X-ray showing volvulus of stomach.*

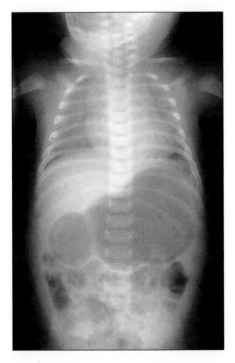

PYLORIC STENOSIS

Obstruction to the outflow of the stomach is a common surgical problem in early infancy. It occurs most frequently in firstborn males between the ages of 4 and 14 weeks and there is often a family history. Studies have shown that hypertrophy of the pyloric muscle is present often before birth and is a progressive disorder. Initially the stomach is able to empty normally but with time there is intermittent and then complete obstruction to the passage of milk. Vomiting is forceful and described as projectile. With time the infant loses weight and becomes dehydrated. The loss of hydrochloric acid as vomited stomach acid leads to hypokalaemic hypochloraemic alkalosis. As potassium ion depletion becomes more severe, hydrogen ions are exchanged instead of potassium ions in order to facilitate sodium absorption in the kidney and the urine becomes paradoxically acidic.

The traditional way of diagnosing pyloric stenosis is by palpation during a feed. As the stomach fills, the olive-shaped pyloric muscle or tumour is felt under the fingers. The usual method of diagnosis is now ultrasound examination (**Fig. 24.7**) and, if necessary, a contrast examination (**Fig. 24.8**).

Although therapy with anticholinergic drugs and balloon dilatation has been successful, the usual treatment is surgical release of the hypertrophied muscle (**Fig. 24.9**).

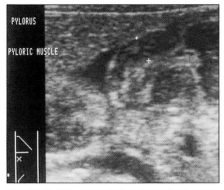

Fig. 24.7 *Ultrasound showing pyloric tumour.*

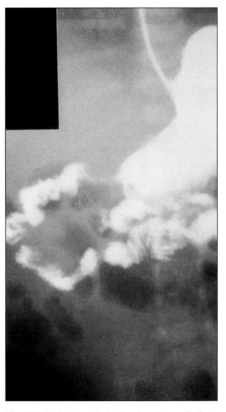

Fig. 24.8 *Contrast study showing pyloric stenosis.*

Fig. 24.9 *Ramstedt procedure for pyloric stenosis.*

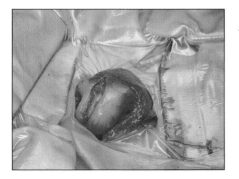

INTESTINAL ATRESIA

The origins of duodenal atresia and the lower atresias seem to be different. Duodenal atresia is often associated with oesophageal atresia or rectal anomalies, cardiac and renal defects and, in a third of babies, Down's syndrome. The presentation is with early non-bilious vomiting and the X-ray characteristically shows a double-bubble appearance (**Fig. 24.10**). At surgery there is often a thin membrane responsible for the duodenal atresia. In contrast, the other lower atresias are complete interruptions to the bowel (**Fig. 24.11**), probably caused by interruptions in blood supply during embryonic life. The proximal segment is distended and hypertrophied while the distal portion seems thin and unused (**Fig. 24.12**). The symptoms and signs of high gastrointestinal obstructions differ

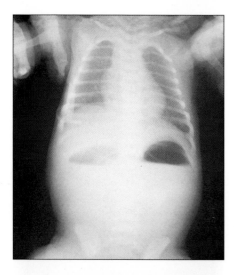

Fig. 24.10 *X-ray showing double bubble in duodenal atresia.*

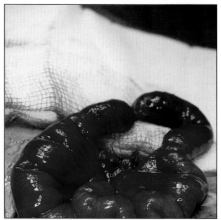

Fig. 24.11 *Interruption of bowel in jejunal atresia.*

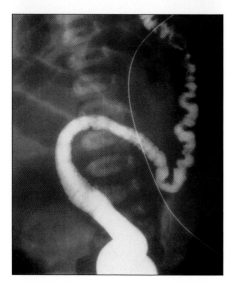

Fig. 24.12 *Microcolon, which occurs distal to midgut atresias.*

from those of low obstruction (**Figs 24.13, 24.14**). Perforation or ischaemic damage is associated with abdominal rigidity and shock.

It is essential to examine the hernial orifices in children as the commonest cause of intestinal obstruction in children is an incarcerated inguinal hernia (*see* page 342). The other causes of obstruction are mainly due to congenital abnormalities. Hirschsprung's disease involving only the rectum, rectosigmoid or long segments may present in the neonatal period or beyond with bowel obstruction. Meconium ileus is an important presentation of cystic fibrosis, and occasionally milk curd can obstruct preterm infants.

Clinical signs of high and low obstruction

Feature	High obstruction, e.g. duodenal or high intestinal	Low obstruction, e.g. distal ileal or rectal atresia
Vomiting	Early	Late—after abdominal distension
Bile	Absent if obstruction proximal to ampulla of Vater	Important sign
Abdominal distension	Not prominent	Marked feature
Constipation/passage of meconium	Continues often apparently normally	Small passage if any, e.g. rectal atresia

Fig. 24.13 *Symptoms and signs of high and low intestinal obstruction.*

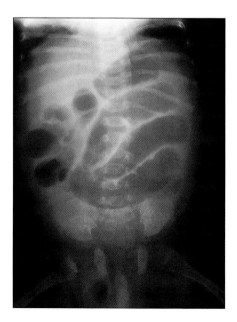

Fig. 24.14 *Dilated loops of gas-filled bowel in intestinal obstruction.*

MALROTATION, SMALL BOWEL VOLVULUS, GASTROSCHISIS AND EXOMPHALOS

The embryonic bowel lies outside the abdomen and within the developing umbilical cord until 14 weeks' gestation when it returns to the peritoneal cavity by coiling in an anticlockwise fashion (**Fig. 24.15**). Malrotation is in fact incomplete rotation of the bowel such that the caecum lies high and close to the liver. Two main problems result from

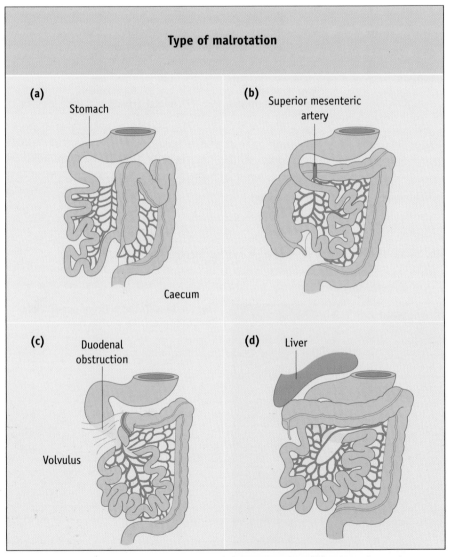

Fig. 24.15 *The mechanism of malrotation. (a) Non-rotation; (b) reversed rotation; (c) mixed rotation and volvulus; (d) subhepatic caecum and appendix.*

malrotation: firstly, the duodenum can be partially or totally obstructed because of a peritoneal (Ladd's) band; secondly, it is possible for the bowel to twist on its pedicle because the mesentery has an abnormally narrow base. This can cause intermittent abdominal pain and vomiting or, if complete, can lead to volvulus and complete infarction of the small bowel.

The diagnosis is confirmed by ultrasound which can show the abnormal relationships between the mesenteric artery and vein or by a contrast study showing the abnormal appearances of the duodenum (**Fig. 24.16**). Surgical correction (Ladd's procedure) is always required.

Gastroschisis and exomphalos are conditions in which there is herniation of the intra-abdominal organs through the anterior abdominal wall. In gastroschisis (**Fig. 24.17**) the defect is lateral and separate from the umbilical cord, but in exomphalos (**Fig. 24.18**) there is herniation through the base of the umbilical cord. The principles of repair are the same in both cases. Initially, if the bowel is exposed it should be wrapped and fluid losses

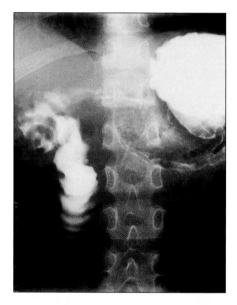

Fig. 24.16 *Contrast study showing malposition of the duodeno-jejunal flexure in malrotation.*

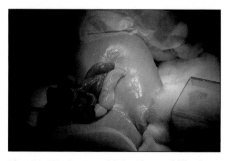

Fig. 24.17 *Gastroschisis. The umbilical cord lies separate and to the left of the abdominal wall defect.*

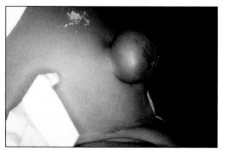

Fig. 24.18 *Exomphalos.*

replaced intravenously. In large defects it is not always possible to return the intra-abdominal contents immediately and a silo is created. As the bowel becomes less swollen it can be returned to the abdominal cavity.

INTUSSUSCEPTION

Intussusception should be borne in mind when seeing any child with vomiting or episodic crying, although it generally occurs in infants under 1 year of age. In this group the lead point is usually an enlarged Peyer's patch (intestinal lymphoid tissue). Less commonly intussusception occurs in older children and the lead point may be a Meckel's diverticulum, a polyp (**Fig. 24.19**), or a haemorrhage into the bowel wall as with Henoch–Schönlein purpura.

Typically there are intermittent episodes of colic with drawing up of the knees and vomiting. In between the child lies still and is often remarkably pale; the mass of the intussusception may often be felt as a large sausage in the area of the ascending or transverse colon. The typical sign of redcurrant jelly stool is a late sign (**Fig. 24.20**) and suggests that the bowel is already compromised. Rarely the intussusception may present at the anus.

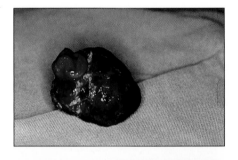

Fig. 24.19 *Polyp acting as a lead point in intussusception.*

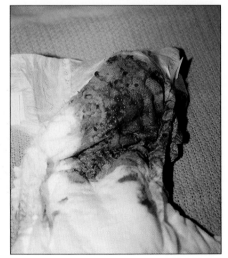

Fig. 24.20 *This nappy shows the typical but late appearance of the stool in intussusception. The blood from ischaemic damage to the bowel gives it the appearance of redcurrant jelly.*

Management

A plain X-ray may suggest the diagnosis (**Fig. 24.21**) but confirmation by ultrasound scan or radiographic enema is needed. Sixty to eighty per cent of cases are successfully reduced by insufflating air into the rectum under ultrasound screening (air enema). If reduction fails then an operation is carried out (**Fig. 24.22**). There is a recurrence rate of about 10% by either method.

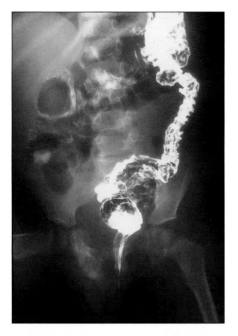

Fig. 24.21 *X-ray of intussusception.*

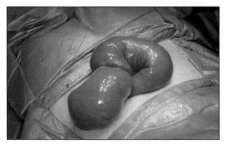

Fig. 24.22 *Intussusception at surgical reduction.*

MESENTERIC ADENITIS AND APPENDICITIS

The commonest reason for emergency abdominal surgery in childhood is appendicitis. Delay in diagnosis occurs with a worrying frequency and still leads to avoidable deaths and morbidity from peritonitis and appendix masses. The diagnosis remains a clinical one, which is confirmed on histological analysis when the appendix is surgically removed. Surgeons expect to remove a proportion of normal appendices to ensure that all diseased ones are removed. There is no such entity as grumbling appendicitis.

There is a classical progression of symptoms and signs in appendicitis (**Fig. 24.23**) but because variations are common the differential diagnosis includes all causes of acute abdominal pain. Pus cells in the urine may suggest a urinary tract infection (UTI), or diarrhoea suggest gastroenteritis; However, these symptoms may also be produced by an inflamed appendix irritating the bladder or bowel respectively.

It is important to review the diagnosis if symptoms do not settle, but repeat examinations of a clearly painful abdomen should not be carried out on children. Similarly, if all the features of appendicitis are present and surgery is unavoidable, a rectal examination is not a necessary part of the examination.

Once the diagnosis has been made intravenous antibiotics are given and an appendicectomy performed. If the appendix has burst and there is an appendix mass then antibiotics are initially given and the appendix is removed later when the symptoms have settled.

The symptoms of appendicitis occur almost without exception in the following order	
1 Vague abdominal discomfort or loose bowel motions	A few hours before pain—often missed in children
2 Umbilical pain	Like indigestion or needing to pass stool
3 Anorexia, nausea and vomiting	All degrees of the same sensation. Children may say they are hungry but feel ill when food is described
4 Tenderness over the appendix on deep palpation	Palpation of an inflamed appendix
5 Rigidity of the abdomen and pain in the right iliac fossa	As peritoneal irritation occurs
6 Fever and then leukocytosis	

Fig. 24.23 *Symptoms and signs of appendicitis.*

The differential diagnosis of appendicitis

- Meckel's diverticulitis
- Urinary tract infection
- Basal pneumonia
- Diabetic ketoacidosis related abdominal pain
- Sickle cell disease
- Henoch–Schönlein purpura
- Gastroenteritis
- Terminal ileitis (Crohn's disease)
- Ovarian cysts and salpingitis

MESENTERIC ADENITIS

The commonest condition confused with appendicitis is a viral infection causing enlargement of the mesenteric lymph nodes and consequent stretching of the small bowel. The presence of red eardrums, pharyngitis and cervical lymphadenopathy points to a viral infection, but the symptoms of nausea, vomiting abdominal pain and pyrexia can be very similar to appendicitis. Children are often admitted for observation; if they are allowed home, clear instructions should be given to return if there is any progression of symptoms.

ANORECTAL ANOMALIES

Anorectal anomalies are rare (**Fig. 24.24**). They are divided into high anomalies, which end above the levator ani muscle, and low anomalies that end below the levator ani muscle. There may be a fistula into the female external genitalia or into the bladder in the male. Treatment involves an initial defunctioning colostomy (**Fig. 24.25**) and then a later operation to create an anus.

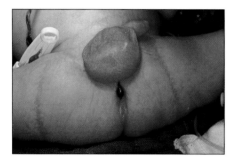

Fig. 24.24 *Absent anus.*

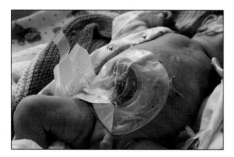

Fig. 24.25 *Ileostomy and pull-through colostomy.*

TESTES AND PENIS

TESTICULAR DESCENT AND THE PROCESSUS VAGINALIS

The testes develop from the urogenital ridges and, because of differential growth in the embryo, appear to migrate towards the pelvis. The gubernaculum under androgenic stimulation guides the testes towards the scrotal sac. The gubernaculum inserts not only into the scrotal sac, but also into the perineum, pubic tubercle and fascia lata (in the femoral triangle). This explains how a testis may end up in an ectopic site. The processus vaginalis is a pouch of peritoneum that is drawn down during testicular descent and lines the scrotum. The communicating neck is usually obliterated but if it persists fluid may collect (hydrocele) or bowel may pass into it (inguino-scrotal hernia) (**Fig. 24.26**).

HYDROCELE AND INGUINAL HERNIA

The difference between a hydrocele and a hernia is that a hernia has a wide processus vaginalis that allows the passage of bowel into the scrotum, whilst in a hydrocele the passage is only large enough to allow fluid to pass. Hydroceles are very common in all newborn male infants and usually settle in the first year of life with no intervention. Rarely, if they persist after this time they may need to be surgically ligated.

Inguinal hernias always require closure as there is a risk of incarceration with compromise of both the trapped bowel and the testis. The mother commonly gives a history of a lump appearing during crying, and then disappearing during sleep. This should always be presumed to be an inguinal hernia and surgery performed as soon as possible. The surgical procedure is a herniotomy—removal of the hernial sac—and is different from the usual adult operation (a herniorrhaphy) which involves strengthening the tissues. If bowel becomes stuck in the hernial orifice (an irreducible hernia) it can often be reduced by sedation. If it does not reduce then surgery should be performed immediately rather than later. Inguinal hernias are very common in preterm infants (**Figs 24.27, 24.28**) but it is usual to wait until their other medical problems have settled before undertaking the risk of an anaesthetic.

UNDESCENDED TESTES

Preterm infants often have testes palpable in the inguinal region as the testes finish their migration into the scrotum during the last trimester of pregnancy, (**Fig. 24.29**). At term, for every 100 boys, 2 will have bilateral and another 3 will have unilateral undescended testes. Two thirds of these boys will be found to have both testes in the scrotum at the 6-week check.

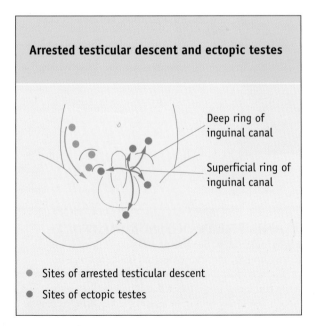

Arrested testicular descent and ectopic testes

Deep ring of inguinal canal

Superficial ring of inguinal canal

● Sites of arrested testicular descent
● Sites of ectopic testes

Fig. 24.26 *Arrested testicular descent and ectopic testes.*

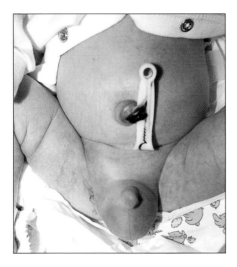

Fig. 24.27 *Right inguinal hernia in a preterm infant.*

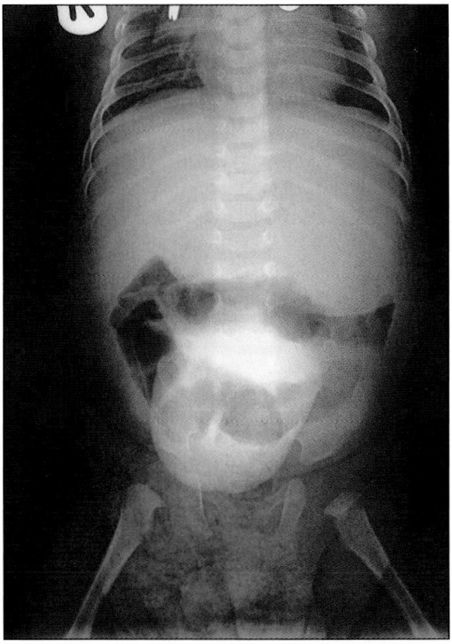

Fig. 24.28 *X-ray showing bowel within the scrotal sac.*

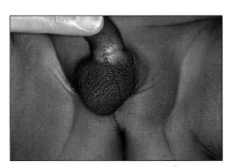

Fig. 24.29 *Inguinal testis.*

When examining for the testes it is important to have warm hands and to use a warm room as many testes at this time lie high in the scrotal sac and easily retract. These are known as retractile testes. True undescended testes, however, stop in the line of normal descent, often in the inguinal region; ectopic testes are usually found in the superficial inguinal, perineal, femoral or suprapubic sites.

Occasionally one or both testes are absent. Anorchia is assumed to have occurred after normal testicular formation because of normal androgenic development of the external genitalia. Abnormal tubular development and reduced numbers of spermatogonia occur if the testis remains within the abdomen after the second year of life. Undescended and ectopic testes are therefore placed in the scrotal sac before this time. If a testis cannot be found, by clinical examination or ultrasound scan, human chorionic gonadotrophin injections can be used to stimulate the testicular tissue to produce measurable quantities of

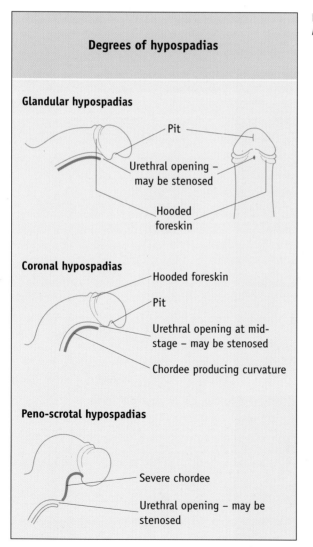

Degrees of hypospadias

Glandular hypospadias

Pit

Urethral opening – may be stenosed

Hooded foreskin

Coronal hypospadias

Hooded foreskin

Pit

Urethral opening at mid-stage – may be stenosed

Chordee producing curvature

Peno-scrotal hypospadias

Severe chordee

Urethral opening – may be stenosed

Fig. 24.30 *Degrees of hypospadias.*

testosterone. The testis usually needs to be localized at surgery and this is now often done by laparoscopy.

There is an increased risk of malignancy in undescended and ectopic testes. Placing them in the scrotum does not reduce this risk but does allow for easy examination. There is also a reduced level of fertility with undescended and ectopic testes.

TORSION OF TESTES

Sudden swelling, erythema and pain in the scrotum suggest testicular torsion or torsion of the testicular appendages. This occurs mainly in the neonatal period and then at the time of puberty. The main differential diagnosis is epididymo-orchitis, or a testicular tumour which is uncommon. Surgical exploration is usually needed.

HYPOSPADIAS

Hypospadias refers to an abnormal exit to the penile urethra; it occurs in up to one in 400 boys. There is a spectrum of severity (**Fig. 24.30**) ranging from minor displacement of the meatus to the ventral tip of the glans, to perineal hypospadias, with a shawl scrotum and chordee (**Fig. 24.31**). The minor deviations of the meatus do not usually need surgery but the more severe examples are corrected at a few months of age. Fistula formation is unfortunately a common complication.

BALANITIS AND PHIMOSIS AND PARAPHIMOSIS
Physiological and pathological phimosis

In infants the foreskin is adherent to the glans and protects it from the irritation of urine. By the age of 5 years, in 90% of cases, there is a normal separation of this physiological phimosis as the epithelium under the foreskin becomes keratinized.

Forced retraction of the foreskin with bleeding and scarring or repeated infection can lead to an inability to retract the foreskin normally. This is pathological phimosis and requires circumcision.

Features of hypospadias	
Anatomical feature	**Clinical importance**
The urethral meatus lies on the ventral part of the penis or, in severe cases, on the perineum	Check where urine appears from
The urinary meatus may be narrowed	Ensure good stream
There may be ventral flexion of the penis due to tight fibrous bands—chordee	Check whether a spontaneous erection is straight
The foreskin is often deficient and appears like a shawl	Do not perform circumcision—skin is needed for repair
The genital appearance may be of indeterminate sex	Check for congenital adrenal hyperplasia

Fig. 24.31 *Features of hypospadias.*

Paraphimosis occurs when the foreskin is pulled behind the glans and cannot be returned. There may be occlusion of venous return with swelling of the glans. Return is usually accomplished with anaesthetic cream and gentle pressure.

Balanoposthitis, inflammation or infection occurring under the foreskin, usually settles with regular cleansing and antibiotics. If persisting adhesions under the foreskin are felt to be responsible, these can be divided under anaesthesia to permit proper hygiene.

Lichen sclerosus may affect the tip of the foreskin following infancy. This is known as balanitis xerotica (**Fig. 24.32**). The treatment is circumcision.

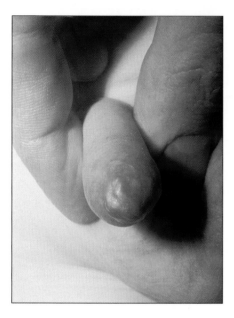

Fig. 24.32 *Balanitis xerotica.*

CIRCUMCISION

Circumcision, the removal of the foreskin, is usually carried out for cosmetic reasons in the neonatal period, often without anaesthesia. Another common reason is religious grounds in the Muslim and Jewish communities. There are very few medical indications for removal of the foreskin.

LABIAL ADHESIONS

Adhesion of the labia minora is a common problem in young girls. It is assumed that the adhesions occur because of mild intertrigo; often there is only a small orifice for passage of urine. Although the labia can be mechanically separated, a simple alternative is a weak oestrogen cream (0.01% dienoestrol cream) which temporarily keratinizes the epithelium to allow separation.

chapter 25

Orthopaedic Problems in Childhood

One of the main roles of the paediatrician is to differentiate a normal variation from a pathological condition. This is particularly true when dealing with the skeleton. In practice, most serious conditions are congenital and rare, but common conditions cause concern to many parents.

TALIPES

In talipes equinovarus, or club foot, the heel is held high and rotated inwards and the forefoot is twisted medially. It is not possible to return the foot to a normal posture because of soft tissue contractures and bony abnormalities (**Figs 25.1, 25.2**). The condition occurs in about one in 500 births. The cause is often not clear but it is often associated

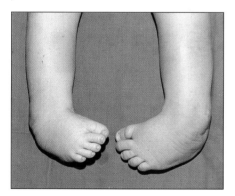

Fig. 25.1 *The typical appearance of talipes equinovarus.*

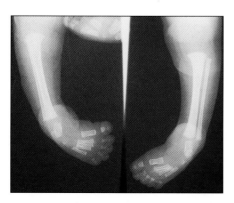

Fig. 25.2 *X-ray of talipes equinovarus.*

351

with a family history, lack of amniotic fluid causing intrauterine moulding and, in some cases, with neuromuscular imbalance as in spina bifida and congenital muscular dystrophy. It must be differentiated from the commonly seen positional talipes (**Fig. 25.3**) in which, although held in an unusual position, the foot has a normal range of movement. Positional talipes resolves spontaneously or with gentle passive stretching whilst talipes equinovarus usually needs strapping or serial plaster casts (**Fig. 25.4**).

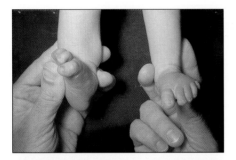

Fig. 25.3 *The right foot has positional talipes but the left foot shows correctable talipes equinovarus.*

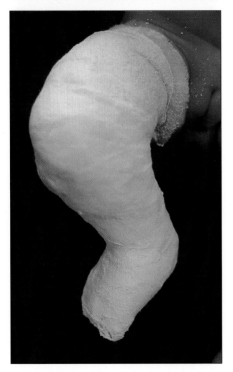

Fig. 25.4 *Plaster cast for congenital talipes equinovarus.*

THE HIP

CONGENITAL DISLOCATION OF THE HIP (CDH)

All babies in the United Kingdom and in other developed countries are examined soon after birth to ensure stability of the femoral head in the acetabular socket. It has been

Predisposing factors for unstable hips

- Family history
- Breech presentation
- Female sex
- Other orthopaedic anomalies of the spine or lower limbs
- First-born baby

estimated that for every 1000 births there will be about 10 babies who demonstrate some degree of hip instability. In 80% of these infants the hips will stabilize spontaneously, the majority within the first week of life. The other 20% will require treatment, but the outcome is good with almost all achieving normal hips with simple measures. Some babies are at increased risk for unstable hips.

Unfortunately, even with screening at birth, CDH is sometimes discovered later when the child may be noticed to have a waddling gait and asymmetrical skin creases (**Fig. 25.5**).

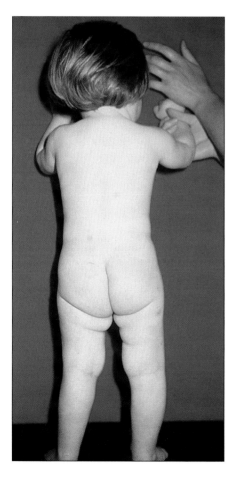

Fig. 25.5 *Late detection of right congenital dislocation of the hip.*

Examination for dislocatable and dislocated hips at birth

The examiner's fingers are placed over the outer aspect of the greater trochanter and the thumbs on the medial aspect of the thigh. The hips are fully abducted and adducted; a dislocated head may relocate or a dislocatable head dislocate posteriorly on full adduction.

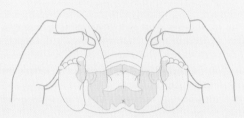

Barlow manoeuvre

Pressure to the inner part of the thigh will reveal a dislocatable head as it is pushed posteriorly out of the socket.

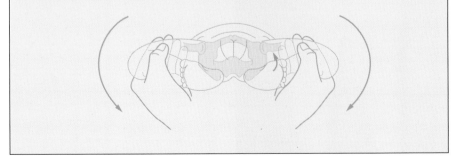

Ortolani manoeuvre

By applying pressure to the greater trochanter with the fingers, as the hips are adducted, a dislocated hip can be pushed back into the socket.

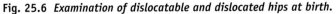

Fig. 25.6 *Examination of dislocatable and dislocated hips at birth.*

Examining for unstable hips

The neonatal hip examination (**Fig. 25.6**) is usually performed by a junior member of staff and it is vital that he or she understands the manoeuvres employed. The test should be carried out on a firm surface. Clicks originating from the ligaments are common, whilst dislocation produces a juddering and sometimes a clunk. If a problem is detected an ultrasound scan (**Fig. 25.7**) should be performed, even if a more experienced member of staff cannot reproduce the finding. All babies born after a breech presentation or with a family history are usually screened by ultrasound as well.

Treatment

Most cases will resolve without any treatment but careful management is required for those that do not. Hips that are dislocatable but otherwise stable within the socket are observed. Others that are unstable require a device to hold the hip in abduction (**Fig. 25.8**); if this fails or the hip is irreducible, gallows traction is tried. If, despite all measures, the hip is still not reduced and stable at 1 year a hip spica is tried before open reduction and osteotomy. The main danger in trying to reduce a dislocation in the first year of life is disruption to the growth plate of the femoral head with consequent avascular necrosis.

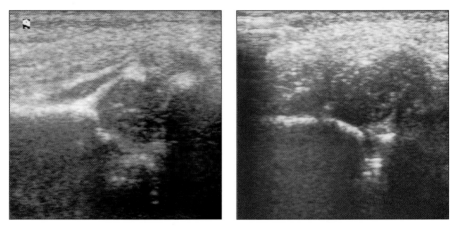

Fig. 25.7 *Ultrasound showing (a) normal and (b) shallow acetabulum in CDH.*

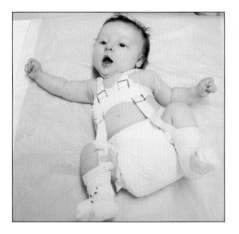

Fig. 25.8 *Pavlik harness for congenital dislocation of the hip.*

Causes of limping and knee pain	
Primary hip conditions	• Congenital dislocation of the hip • Irritable hip syndrome • Perthes disease • Slipped upper femoral epiphyses
Inflammatory arthritis	• Septic arthritis • Juvenile chronic arthritis
Trauma	• Fractures, dislocations and ligamentous injuries • Foreign bodies, e.g. glass
Neurological	• Spinal cord abnormalities • Neuromuscular disease
Psychological	

Fig. 25.9 *Causes of limping and knee pain.*

PAINFUL KNEE AND LIMP

Older children may present with a limp or pain in the knee. In either case the cause may originate in the knee or hip and even in the spine or foot, and it is imperative to take a full history and examine the child thoroughly (**Fig. 25.9**).

IRRITABLE HIP SYNDROME

Irritable hip syndrome is a transient synovitis of the hip which may follow a viral upper respiratory tract infection. There is a limp because movements at the hip are restricted and painful. It is important to check for infection in the hip, and although the C reactive protein may be elevated it rapidly becomes normal. X-ray of the hip is normal and ultrasound shows a small effusion. The management is supportive: bed rest and traction for a short period allows the pain to settle.

PERTHES DISEASE

Perthes disease is a rare condition which is often confused with irritable hip syndrome. There is ischaemic necrosis of the femoral head followed by revascularization. The condition occurs most commonly in children between the ages of 4 and 9 years and occurs four times more often in boys than girls. In 10% of cases it is bilateral. The presentation is with the insidious onset of limp, knee or hip pain. Movements are limited on examination, particularly when the flexed hip is abducted or rotated. Although initial X-rays may appear normal, the femoral head shows increased densities and then fragmentation and collapse (**Fig. 25.10**).

Prognosis and treatment

The prognosis depends on age and the degree of involvement of the femoral head. Children under 6 years, who tend to have less than half of the femoral head involved, have a good outlook and they often recover without any intervention. However, older children with involvement of most of the femoral head generally have a poor outcome and require active treatment. The aim of treatment is to keep the affected part of the femoral head completely enclosed in the acetabulum while revascularization occurs. This can be done with splinting and bed rest, but a femoral osteotomy (**Fig. 25.11**) has the advantage of avoiding splinting and prolonged bed rest.

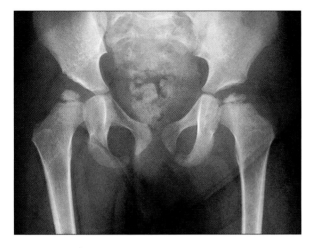

Fig. 25.10 *X-ray of Perthes disease.*

Fig. 25.11 *X-ray of femoral osteotomy.*

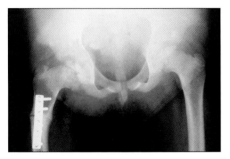

SLIPPED UPPER FEMORAL EPIPHYSES

Slipped upper femoral epiphysis is a common cause of limp in adolescents and must always be considered if there is a limp or pain in the knee. It occurs during the pubertal growth spurt. Many of the children are obese and have evidence of skeletal immaturity. The condition is often associated with minimal trauma.

In the early stages the slipped epiphysis can be difficult to detect on routine X-rays as the femoral head literally slips back down and behind the shaft of the femur (**Fig. 25.12**). In 20% of cases there is bilateral involvement.

Treatment is surgical. In the early stages pinning or screwing the femoral head to the femoral neck may be sufficient. In more severe cases an osteotomy of the femoral neck may be needed to realign the femoral head (**Fig. 25.13**).

SCOLIOSIS

The vertebral bodies sit on each other such that they form a stable weight-bearing column. The lower spine normally has a backward-facing curve (lumbar lordosis) and the upper spine a forward curve (thoracic kyphosis). Curving sideways (scoliosis) is abnormal. There are two general types of scoliosis: those that can be eradicated by changing posture (postural scoliosis) and those that remain (structural scoliosis) (**Fig. 25.14**). In addition,

357

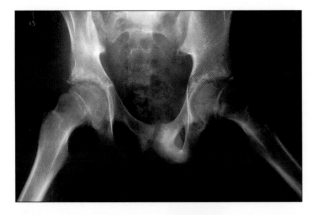

Fig. 25.12 *X-ray of slipped capital epiphysis.*

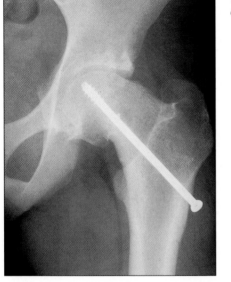

Fig. 25.13 *X-ray of slipped capital epiphysis treated by osteotomy and screw.*

Causes of scoliosis		
Postural		
Compensatory	• Differing leg lengths	
	• Generalized hypotonia in developmental delay	
Structural		
Vertebral anomaly	• Hemivertebrae and vertebral fusion	
	• Dumbbell tumours in neurofibromatosis	
Neuromuscular imbalance	• Cerebral palsy, muscular dystrophy, poliomyelitis	
Idiopathic	• Commonest group	

Fig. 25.14 *Causes of scoliosis.*

structural scoliosis also has an element of rotation which produces a rib hump on the convex side of the vertebral curve (**Fig. 25.15**).

Management

Scoliosis often progresses, especially during periods of rapid growth, for example during mid childhood and puberty. Initial observation and serial measurements by X-rays (**Fig. 25.16**) will determine whether the curvature is progressing. If this is the case, a

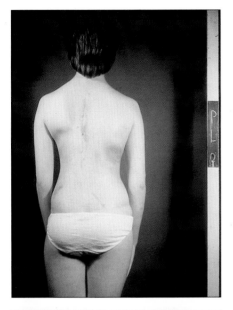

Fig. 25.15 *Scoliosis.*

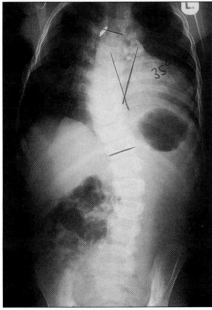

Fig. 25.16 *X-ray showing scoliosis and measurement of Cobb's angle.*

lightweight plastic brace (**Fig. 25.17**) may provide sufficient support to prevent further progression. In some children the progress cannot be controlled by conservative means and internal fixation by metal rods is necessary (**Fig. 25.18**). The aim of therapy, as well as to

Fig. 25.17 *Plastic brace for scoliosis.*

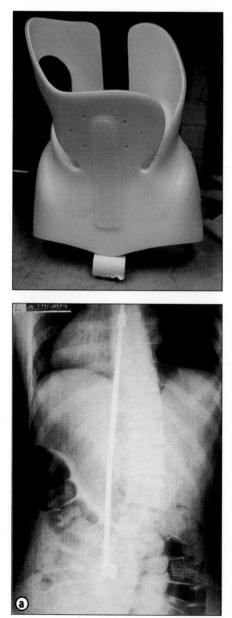

Fig. 25.18 (a,b) *Harrington rods for correction of scoliosis.*

improve the appearance, is to prevent the cardiorespiratory complications of severe scoliosis.

NORMAL DEVELOPMENTAL VARIANTS

One of the commonest reasons for an orthopaedic consultation is that parents are concerned because their child's legs or feet are not straight. Provided that underlying rickets is not the cause, many of the problems are developmental variants that resolve with time.

FLAT FEET

Many toddlers appear to have flat feet due to fat pads and lax arch ligaments. Older children may have physiological flat feet; although they appear flat footed (**Fig. 25.19a**), standing on tip toe will demonstrate a normal arch (**Fig. 25.19b**). True pes planus is uncommon (**Fig. 25.20**).

Toe walking may be a developmental variant but it is important to exclude tightness of the Achilles tendon which is seen in cerebral palsy and in Duchenne muscular dystrophy.

ANGULAR DEFORMITIES

Genu varum, or bow legs, is defined as inability to bring the knees together when standing with the feet together. Genu valgum (knock knees) is the opposite; when the knees are together the feet cannot be brought together (**Fig. 25.21**). These conditions are often normal developmental variants in early childhood, and only very gross degrees need surgery.

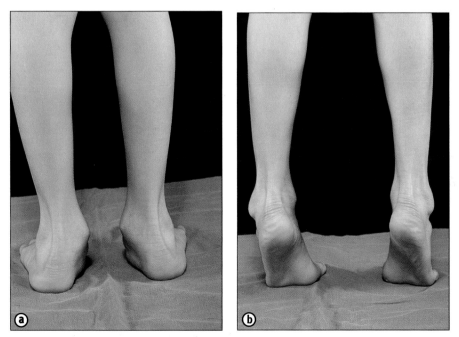

Fig. 25.19 *Physiological flat feet (a) and normal arch when on tip toe (b).*

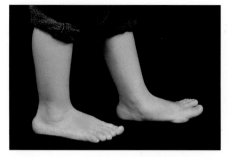

Fig. 25.20 *Pes planus—true flat feet.*

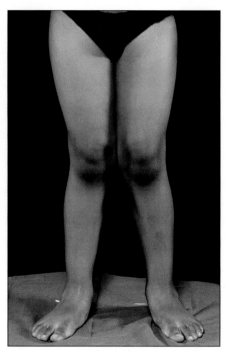

Fig. 25.21 *Knock knees.*

ROTATIONAL DEFORMITIES

The normal child below about 3 years of age tends to have no rotation to the lower limb; after this time about 20° of outward rotation develops. However, it is very common to see children of all ages with in-toeing of one or both legs.

Femoral anteversion

In femoral anteversion the neck of the femur is twisted more than normal such that the knees and feet point inwards (**Fig. 25.22**). This may be associated with lax ligaments and improves by later childhood. These children are more comfortable sitting in the W position than cross legged.

Tibial torsion

Tibial torsion is an abnormal position of the tibia on the femur such that the lower leg and foot are rotated—usually inwards (**Fig. 25.23**). This is common in toddlers and corrects spontaneously.

METATARSUS VARUS

Metatarsus varus is in-toeing that originates from the forefoot. As long as the heel sits normally, the condition corrects spontaneously (**Fig. 25.24**).

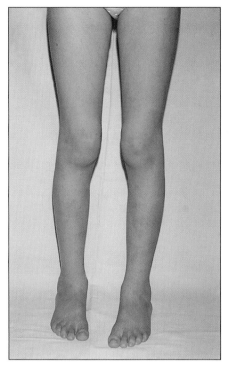

Fig. 25.22 *Persistent femoral anteversion.*

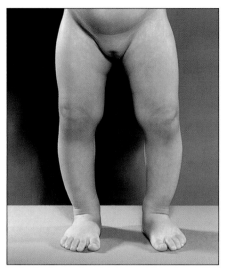

Fig. 25.23 *Tibial bowing and internal tibial torsion.*

Fig. 25.24 *Metatarsus varus.*

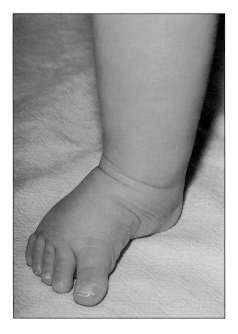

FRACTURES

Children often break bones. A spiral fracture along the length of a long bone suggests a twisting force, whilst a transverse injury suggests a bending force (**Fig. 25.25**). In childhood, the greater plasticity of bone is more likely to produce a bend in the bone which is known as a greenstick fracture. Fractures across the epiphyseal (growth) plate need to be carefully aligned to facilitate good healing and reduce the risk of later osteoarthritis. Compression injuries to the plate, however, can lead to death of the germinal cells of the epiphyseal cartilage and growth arrest. This crushing injury often affects the lower fibula. The bones usually appear normal on the X-ray but there is soft tissue swelling. The principles of treatment are reduction, immobilization until the bone is united (**Fig. 25.26**) and protection until consolidated.

As in any traumatic injury, the possibility of a non-accidental cause must be excluded. The story of the injury must be plausible and fit in with the nature of the injury. Unexplained multiple fractures of differing ages suggest a bone condition such as osteogenesis imperfecta or non-accidental injury.

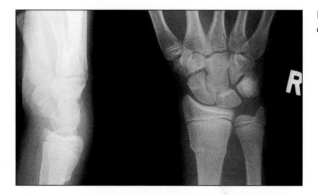

Fig. 25.25 *Fracture to distal radius.*

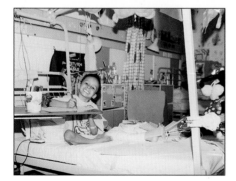

Fig. 25.26 *Immobilization by traction.*

chapter 26

Dental Health

TEETHING

Newborn babies often have small incisors present at birth which are the separated apical portions of the primary dentition (**Fig. 26.1**). If they are loose they should be removed to prevent aspiration, but more commonly they are removed because of discomfort during breast feeding. The first true teeth to appear are the lower incisors at around the age of 6 months. There is a regular order of emergence but a wide variation in the age at which each tooth appears (**Fig. 26.2**).

Toddlers with febrile illness or rashes are often said 'to be teething' but there is no clear evidence for this statement. Certainly tooth eruption may be uncomfortable but serious systemic illness must always be excluded in any sick febrile child, regardless of the state of the teeth.

DENTAL DISEASE

The two major causes of tooth loss are periodontal (gum) disease, which occurs mainly in older people, and decay (caries) which is a problem at all ages. Both diseases are preventable and in the early stages are asymptomatic. As children do not complain, surveillance by the dentist should begin ideally at birth or at the eruption of the first teeth. At this stage advice on brushing and fluoride can be given.

CARIES

Brushing of teeth removes not only food debris but also plaque which is a mixture of bacteria and glycosaminoglycans. In the presence of refined sugars (sucrose, glucose) cariogenic bacteria predominate within plaque and produce acids which dissolve tooth enamel. After a meal containing sugar the pH of the mouth also becomes more acidic and

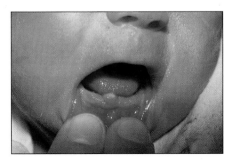

Fig. 26.1 *Neonatal teeth. If loose they should be removed to prevent aspiration, but are usually removed because of discomfort during breast feeding.*

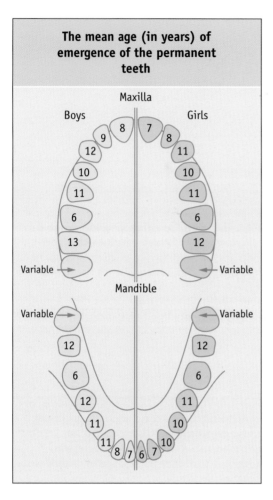

The mean age (in years) of emergence of the permanent teeth

Maxilla

Boys   Girls

Mandible

Variable   Variable

Fig. 26.2 *The mean age (in years) of emergence of the permanent teeth.*

removal of calcium from the tooth enamel is enhanced. It takes about 20 minutes for the flow of saliva to restore an alkaline pH and establish net remineralization. Frequent ingestion of sugars causes prolonged acidity and accelerates decay. Without dental surveillance and correct tooth brushing, 15% of children will have caries by 3 years of age (**Fig. 26.3**). Progression of damage to the enclosed nerve eventually produces infection, pain and loss of the tooth.

PERIODONTAL DISEASE

In periodontal disease the gums become inflamed, bleed and are painful due to poor oral hygiene. This makes brushing difficult and exacerbates the disease process (**Fig. 26.4**). Chronic inflammation of the gum margins leads to destruction of tissue and bone and loosening of teeth.

PREVENTION OF DENTAL DISEASE

The key to preventing dental disease is regular brushing with a fluoride toothpaste, once or preferably twice a day, and the avoidance of refined sugars.

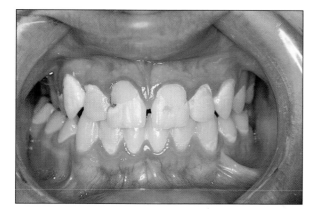

Fig. 26.3 *Caries. Without dental surveillance and correct tooth brushing, 15% of children will have caries by 3 years of age.*

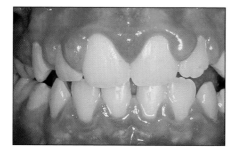

Fig. 26.4 *Periodontal disease. The inflamed gums in periodontal disease bleed and are painful, making brushing difficult and exacerbating the disease process.*

Fluoride is provided in some water supplies, in toothpaste, and also can be taken as supplements. It complexes with the tooth enamel and makes it more resistant to the effects of acid. High concentrations of fluoride can produce discoloration of teeth but this is rarely a problem compared to the dangers of decay itself. Since the advent of fluoridation there has been a reduction in the general incidence of tooth decay by around 50%. However, the preventive measures of tooth brushing, a non-sugar-based diet, and avoidance of sweets are mainly the province of middle and upper class families. Children in social classes IV and V, and especially those who are immigrants, still have high rates of dental disease. All children should receive regular surveillance by the dentist to reinforce preventive measures and to treat decay early before there is severe damage. Preventive applications of fluoride can be provided, as well as measures to seal the grinding surfaces of the teeth and protect them from plaque action.

Children with chronic medical problems may have abnormalities of their teeth (**Figs 26.5–26.7**) and should receive regular dental check-ups.

MALOCCLUSION

Minor degrees of malocclusion are very common. In severe examples where there is difficulty eating or problems with the temporomandibular joint the malocclusion can be corrected by a brace.

Thumb sucking leads to protrusion of the front teeth, but this remains permanent only if the habit is carried on after the age of 9 or 10 years.

Abnormalities of the tooth

Abnormality	Cause	Features
Discoloured enamel	Tetracycline antibiotics	Use of tetracycline antibiotics when the dentition is forming produces discoloration of the enamel
Abnormally soft enamel	Osteogenesis imperfecta and hypothyroidism	In the absence of major malnutrition or rickets, soft teeth do not exist in otherwise healthy individuals
Pitting of the teeth due to demineralization from contact with gastric acid	Bulimia nervosa	Tooth marks seen on knuckles
Gum hypertrophy	Phenytoin	If there are cosmetic or hygiene problems the hypertrophy associated with phenytoin resolves on changing to another anticonvulsant
Difficulty in hygiene	Developmental delay or cerebral palsy	Malocclusion often seen
Increased caries	Regular sugar-containing medication, e.g. antibiotics in cystic fibrosis	Sugar-free formulations available
Risk of bacterial endocarditis	Congenital heart disease	Scrupulous attention to dental health and antibiotic prophylaxis

Fig. 26.5 *Abnormalities of the tooth.*

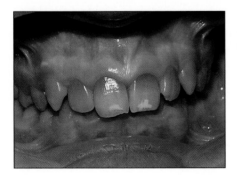

Fig. 26.6 *Tetracycline staining of teeth is now seen only in parts of the world where parents can buy the cheap tetracyclines without a prescription.*

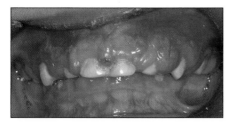

Fig. 26.7 *Gum hypertrophy is a well recognized side-effect of the anticonvulsant drug phenytoin.*

TRAUMA

It is not unusual for a child to lose a tooth as a result of a playground accident. It is only really of importance if the permanent dentition is affected. An avulsed tooth can survive if placed back in its socket immediately after being dislodged. If dirty the tooth should be rinsed, but re-implantation should not wait for professional help.

When assessing such children in casualty it is vital to consider if the story of trauma is plausible and if there are any other physical signs if child abuse is not to be missed.

Older children who participate in contact sports should be fitted with gum shields.

chapter 27

Health Promotion

The principal role of the paediatrician is to promote health in children. This intervention can be delivered at three stages in the disease process:

- Primary prevention aims to avoid the occurrence of a disease; for example, maternal ingestion of multivitamins with folic acid has been shown to reduce the incidence of spina bifida.
- Secondary prevention aims to detect a disease at an early, even asymptomatic stage, with a view to halting or reversing the process.
- Tertiary prevention aims to limit the complications of an established disease.

PRIMARY PREVENTION

The form taken by primary prevention of ill-health is largely related to the economic wealth of a country. Although the risks of diseases associated with poverty, such as malnutrition, respiratory infection and diarrhoea, fall with increasing wealth, the problems linked with an affluent lifestyle such as obesity and atherosclerotic heart disease increase. Thus, in the industrialized world, dietary improvements and the avoidance of smoking are important national targets, but in underdeveloped countries, measures to provide a clean water supply, safe disposal of sewage and adequate housing have the greatest impact on health.

Prevention of infectious disease is based on four classic principles which can essentially be achieved by improved social conditions, nutrition and immunization:

- isolation of infected individuals
- eradication of disease vectors
- elimination of the infecting organism
- increasing the resistance of the host.

IMMUNIZATION AGAINST INFECTIOUS DISEASE

The primary prevention of infectious disease by immunization depends on generating a long-lasting and strong immune response. Those children who are immunosuppressed, or infants under a few months of age may not reliably generate an immune response (Fig. 27.1). The diseases that can be best prevented are those that produce lifelong immunity after natural infection, for example the childhood diseases of mumps, rubella and measles. It is difficult to produce vaccines against agents with many different serotypes (rhinovirus and the common cold), or with changing antigenic profiles (malaria). It is possible to eradicate an infectious agent completely, as was achieved with smallpox. More importantly, when the level of immunity is raised in the population at large, the proportion of susceptible individuals that can support the natural contagion of disease becomes too low. This is known as herd immunity. Thus, if the level of immunization in the population

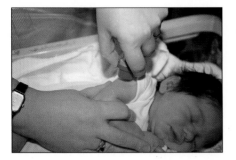

Fig. 27.1 *Neonatal BCG vaccination is a form of primary prevention.*

can be raised above a certain threshold, those who are unable to receive the vaccine will be protected. Similarly, it is possible to treat epidemics of infection by mass immunization programmes.

Vaccines are fragile and must be kept at the correct temperature if they are not to become ineffective. The maintenance of the correct temperature from manufacture to the point of injection is known as the cold chain.

As with all medical treatments, there is a risk of adverse reactions to vaccines and this frightens many parents (**Fig. 27.2**). However, the side-effects after vaccination are generally slight and transient whereas the risks of complications of the natural disease are usually much higher and of greater severity.

There are few contraindications to immunization. Children are not immunized during a pyrexial illness, but can be if they have a mild cold. Children with immune deficiency, for example those taking corticosteroids or those with a primary immunodeficiency or HIV, should be reviewed by their specialists as live attenuated vaccines can produce disseminated disease. If there has been a previous severe local or general reaction the

Major and minor adverse reactions to vaccines

Vaccine	Major reaction	Minor reaction
Measles, mumps and rubella (MMR)	Encephalopathy (rare), thrombocytopenia	Local inflammation
Diphtheria/tetanus	Neurological (rare)	Local inflammation
Pertussis	Convulsions (1:300 000), encephalopathy (rare)	Fever, crying
Polio	Vaccine-associated polio (1:2 000 000)	—
BCG	Adenitis	Local abscess
Hepatitis B	—	Fever, local inflammation
Haemophilus influenzae type b (Hib)	—	Fever, local inflammation

Fig. 27.2 *Major and minor adverse reactions to vaccines.*

benefits of further doses should be discussed. It is possible to perform a skin test to exclude hypersensitivity before immunization but this should be done in hospital where full resuscitation facilities are available. Children with progressive neurological disorders should probably not be given pertussis vaccine, but other children with non-progressive neurological disorders, for example cerebral palsy, should be vaccinated. Children with epilepsy or febrile convulsions can be immunized in hospital if parents are worried that immunization may cause a convulsion. The schedule of vaccination varies around the world and is related to the economic wealth of the country (**Fig. 27.3**). In some countries, for example the USA, vaccinations are compulsory before school attendance.

SUDDEN INFANT DEATH SYNDROME (SIDS)

SIDS is not a disease but a diagnostic category for those deaths in infants for which no cause can be found after a thorough post-mortem examination. It is the commonest cause of death in this age group. Epidemiological studies have been important in the understanding and prevention of SIDS.

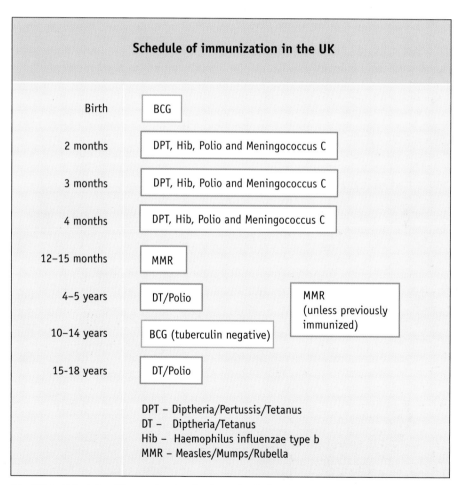

Fig. 27.3 *Schedule of immunization in the United Kingdom.*

Risk factors for SIDS

- Occurs most commonly at around 2 months of age
- Slightly more common in boys
- Prone position
- Excessive bedclothes in a warm environment, typically in winter when additional heating and blankets are provided
- Maternal smoking
- Young mothers
- Ex-preterm infants
- There is a *reduction* in risk for breast-fed babies

It is suggested that babies rely on the face for heat loss during the first months of life, and if this heat loss is prevented their immature autonomic nervous systems are unable to cope with overheating. Although the process is not understood, a reduction in deaths has occurred following publicity aimed at placing infants on their back or sides to sleep.

Some babies have life-threatening episodes in which they appear to stop breathing and need resuscitation by the parents. These babies are at high risk of further events and require careful evaluation for at least 48 hours in hospital with oxygen saturation monitoring. Although a cause will be found in some cases, such as infection, gastrointestinal reflux or convulsions, no diagnosis is usually made.

SECONDARY PREVENTION—SCREENING

Secondary prevention is the detection of disease at a presymptomatic stage and therefore necessitates effective screening of an at-risk population.

The best established screening test is the biochemical Guthrie test for phenylketonuria. Blood taken at the same time can be tested for hypothyroidism. Both these diseases have an asymptomatic phase and the mental handicap that results can be completely prevented by dietary manipulation or thyroxine supplementation respectively. Screening for

Criteria for an effective screening programme

- The untreated disease must have serious consequences
- There must be a diagnostic test which can be carried out early in the disease, before symptoms are obvious
- The test must be cheap, sensitive and specific, and acceptable to the population
- Effective treatment must be easily and economically available

haemoglobinopathies such as thalassaemia and sickle cell disease is often offered in communities where there is a high non-Caucasian population. The same racial groups should be screened for haemoglobinopathies in early pregnancy and also before surgery is performed.

TERTIARY PREVENTION—DEVELOPMENTAL SURVEILLANCE

In the past a great emphasis was placed on formal hearing and vision tests. Currently, although such tests are still carried out, there is a broader approach to surveillance to ensure that developmental progress and health in general are satisfactory. It is well recognized that parental worries that a baby cannot hear or see, or concerns over general health are often more sensitive than screening tests. Child health surveillance is a set of activities that includes supervision of the physical, social and emotional needs of children and includes the provision of immunizations. Parents, paediatricians, health visitors, school nurses and general practitioners are all involved in this process.

INTERNATIONAL CHILD HEALTH

Three quarters of the population of the world live in developing countries, where children comprise up to 50% of the population. The majority live in rural areas rather than cities. In these circumstances poverty is the major determinant of health. Simple infections such as diarrhoea and pneumonia are commonly life threatening where there is malnutrition. There are also strong associations between the decline in infant mortality and the provision of basic sanitation and health resources. The major causes of death in the preschool age groups are still preventable infections such as neonatal tetanus, polio and pertussis. Community health worker schemes have been set up in many countries to improve local basic health care. Health workers are trained to provide advice on contraception, feeding and weaning of babies and use of oral rehydration solutions and to diagnose and treat common conditions.

There are no statistics on children with disabilities in developing countries because these problems have a low priority. Mental handicap is four times as common as in developed countries; although it may be genetic in origin, much is due to treatable conditions such as meningitis. Physical disability is also common as a result of polio, accidents and war. Blindness due to vitamin A deficiency is common, as is trachoma. Deafness is rarely noted as there are no physical signs.

Malaria is a major problem of international child health: almost half the world's population lives in areas where the Anopheles mosquito is found (**Fig. 27.4**). The clinical features of malaria may progress rapidly in children, with a flu-like illness leading to anaemia, jaundice and often death, especially if there is cerebral involvement. The diagnosis should be suspected in anyone who has been to an endemic area and it should be remembered that serious infections can occur many months after inoculation. Prevention has been attempted by spraying houses with insecticides but it has proved difficult to eradicate the mosquito vector. Treatment is with quinine as there is considerable resistance to other drugs. It is important to give malarial prophylaxis for children from the UK visiting malarial areas.

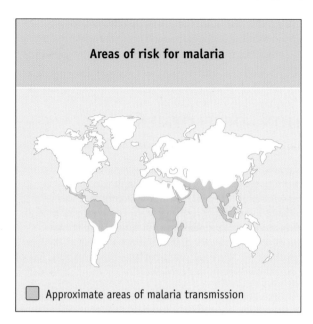

Fig. 27.4 *Areas of risk for malaria.*

chapter 28

Accidents

Accidents are the most common cause of death in children above the age of 1 year. Ninety five per cent of all accidents in children occur in the home and are generally of a minor nature with the exception of scalds. The accidents that occur often mirror the child's developmental progress. For example, objects placed in the mouth by toddlers are often swallowed or aspirated. If swallowed, they will pass through the gastrointestinal tract unless they lodge in one of three narrow areas: below the cricopharyngeal muscle (**Fig. 28.1**), at the level of the aortic arch, or at the level of the diaphragm. Batteries are particularly harmful as they can cause a corrosive injury to the mucosa; if needles are swallowed the child should be closely observed for evidence of perforation.

The commonest serious accidents that occur are road traffic accidents; these have a mortality rate greater than 50% (**Fig. 28.2**). The types of accident depend on the environment. For example, falls from tower blocks and road accidents are more common in inner city areas whilst those involving machinery are very common on farms.

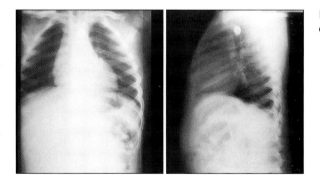

Fig. 28.1 *Coin lodged in oesophagus.*

POISONING

Accidental poisoning is a common problem and mainly affects the preschool age group (**Fig. 28.3**). Children at this age frequently confuse pills for sweets and chemicals for drinks. The use of child-resistant tops on medicine bottles and household products has been an important preventive measure. Small children often ingest tricyclic antidepressants or digoxin found in the handbags of elderly visitors.

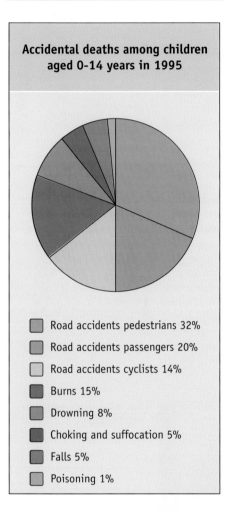

Fig. 28.2 *Accidental deaths among children aged 0–14 years in 1995.*

Accidental deaths among children aged 0-14 years in 1995

- Road accidents pedestrians 32%
- Road accidents passengers 20%
- Road accidents cyclists 14%
- Burns 15%
- Drowning 8%
- Choking and suffocation 5%
- Falls 5%
- Poisoning 1%

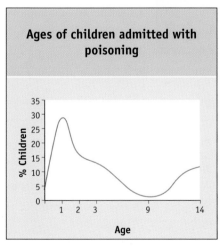

Fig. 28.3 *Ages of children admitted with poisoning.*

Ages of children admitted with poisoning

SPECIFIC POISONS

Aspirin

Aspirin (salicylate) is found in tablet form and also in oil of wintergreen. In excess it is a metabolic poison which produces metabolic acidosis and hyperglycaemia. Tinnitus (ringing in the ears), nausea and vomiting are other symptoms but unconsciousness is a late finding. Respiratory alkalosis is uncommon in children.

Plasma salicylate levels should be measured and, as with paracetamol poisoning, a nomogram consulted. Treatment is dependent on alkalization of urine: if the urinary pH is greater than 8.0, the aspirin is readily excreted. Electrolyte imbalances should be sought and vitamin K given if the prothrombin time is prolonged. Forced diuresis is no longer advocated because of the dangers of cerebral and pulmonary oedema.

Paracetamol

The sweet nature of paediatric formulations means that most children vomit before they ingest enough paracetamol to cause harm. Similarly, the adult tablets are too large and unpleasant for many to be taken. Despite this, blood levels should always be measured as there is a specific antidote, N-acetylcysteine, which prevents liver damage if given early (**Fig. 28.4**). The symptoms of overdose only appear a few days after the ingestion with the onset of acute hepatic failure. If hepatic function does not recover, liver transplantation is needed.

Tricyclic antidepressants

Tricyclic antidepressants are widely prescribed to adults and frequently ingested by children. The main symptoms are loss of consciousness, due to sedative effects, and anticholinergic (atropine-like) effects of dry mouth, dilated pupils, urinary retention and tachycardia. Cardiac arrhythmias may occur but it is best to avoid anti-arrhythmic drugs.

Sedatives

Loss of consciousness and respiratory depression are common features following ingestion of all sedatives, for example the benzodiazepines or opioid drugs. Naloxone is a competitive inhibitor for opioids such as morphine and methadone. It acts immediately but has a short half-life and re-sedation may occur. To overcome this an infusion may be used. Flumazenil reverses the effects of the benzodiazepines; as with naloxone this is a short-lived effect. It is useful in confirming that the reduction in level of consciousness is due to benzodiazepines. In general, treatment for sedative ingestion is symptomatic and ventilatory support may be necessary.

Iron

Iron tablets look like sweets (**Fig. 28.5**) and are extremely toxic. Initially there may be gastrointestinal bleeding and vomiting; this is followed by a symptom-free period, but after 24 hours collapse with encephalopathy and hepatic failure occurs. Early treatment consists of emptying the stomach and the use of desferrioxamine both enterally and intravenously. Late presentation necessitates supportive intensive care.

Alcohol

Alcohol is often taken by older children. Hypoglycaemia is more common in children than in adults; after inducing emesis, the blood glucose level should be monitored.

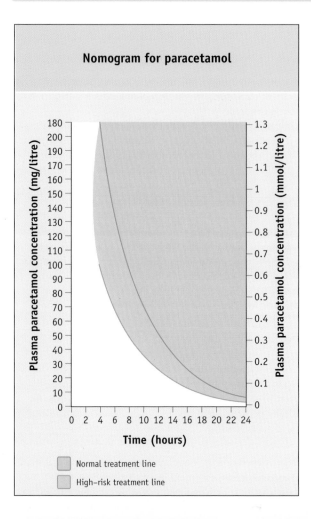

Fig. 28.4 *Nomogram for paracetamol. Patients whose plasma paracetamol concentrations are above the normal treatment line require N-acetylcysteine by intravenous infusion or, if the dose has been taken within 10–12 hours, methionine by mouth. Patients on enzyme-inducing drugs require treatment if the plasma paracetamol concentration is above the high-risk treatment line.*

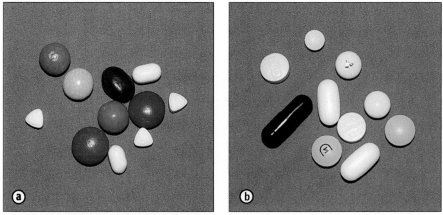

Fig. 28.5 *Medicines and sweets look very similar.*

Household products

Bleach and other corrosive chemicals may be tasted by children and sometimes drunk. Painful mucosal burns can occur which may lead to later oesophageal stricture formation.

Plants

Some plants, such as deadly nightshade, the laburnum pod (**Fig. 28.6**) and fungi, are toxic.

MANAGEMENT OF POISONING

The commonest presentation of possible poisoning is when a child is found playing with a bottle that contains a poison. It is, however, important to think of drug ingestion in any ill child, especially where there is a reduction in the level of consciousness, neurological or cardiorespiratory symptoms (**Fig. 28.7**).

- An attempt is made to assess what has been taken, how much, and when. If there is doubt, it is safest to assume ingestion and take appropriate measures. In the UK there

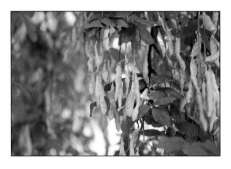

Fig. 28.6 *The seed pods of the laburnum are poisonous.*

Signs suggesting ingestion of specific poisons

Sign	Poison
Dilated pupils	Atropine, tricyclic antidepressants
Pinpoint pupils	Opioids, organophosphates
Confusion, excitability, ataxia	Alcohol, tricyclic antidepressants, solvent abuse, antihistamines
Drowsiness	Sedatives, opioids, hypnotics, tricyclic antidepressants
Cardiac arrhythmias	Tricyclic antidepressants, theophylline, digoxin
Convulsions	Alcohol, tricyclic antidepressants, theophylline, lithium
Dystonic reactions	Phenothiazines, metoclopramide
Tachypnoea	Salicylates
Hypotension	Sedatives, hypnotics, iron
Haematemesis	Iron, salicylates

Fig. 28.7 *Signs suggesting ingestion of specific poisons.*

are regional drug information centres from which advice on the management of ingestion can be sought.

- In general, if the substance is harmful and has been ingested within the last 4 hours, it is reasonable to try and remove it from the stomach by stimulating vomiting with ipecacuanha syrup. Aspirin, tricyclic antidepressants and Lomotil all delay gastric emptying and so can be removed much later than this.
- Volatile or corrosive agents should be diluted by drinking milk, as if they are vomited they may cause further oesophageal burns or be aspirated and cause pulmonary damage.
- If the child is not conscious and able to protect the airway, then induced vomiting is not safe; an anaesthetist should be asked to intubate the child with a cuffed endotracheal tube and pass a large bore tube for gastric lavage.
- Activated charcoal is often given to children but it is unpalatable and may merely chase the poison through the gut rather than reducing its absorption.
- Many children are seen a long time after ingestion. The child can be allowed home if the expected symptoms or signs of the drug have not occurred.

SPORTS AND PLAYGROUND INJURIES

Children tend to become preoccupied while playing and do not think about their own safety. It is therefore important that they are properly supervised when playing sport. For example, cervical injury can occur in rugby if the scrum is not performed correctly. Other sports can be dangerous: many children have suffered head injuries from golf clubs (Fig. 28.8). Crash helmets and lifejackets are essential pieces of safety equipment in sailing and canoeing.

Children's playgrounds can be dangerous places. In recent years they have become much safer, primarily due to better design of apparatus and cushioned floors. Adventure playgrounds have a particularly good safety record. This is probably because they are designed with safety in mind and children are usually supervised.

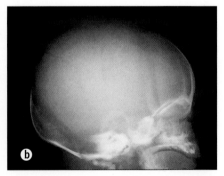

Fig. 28.8 Anteroposterior (a) and lateral (b) X-rays of skull fracture caused by golf club.

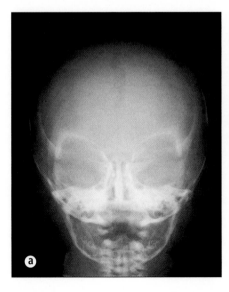

DROWNING

Accidental drowning is more common in warm countries because of the abundance of ornamental ponds and outdoor swimming pools. The risk can be reduced by erecting a fence around the pond or by covering the surface with a strong net. Teaching children to swim at an early age is also a good principle. Toddlers may easily drown in a few inches of water, for example if left unsupervised or in the care of an older sibling during bath time. Drowning is rare in public swimming pools because of the level of supervision and resuscitation available. Older boys often drown in ponds or canals. In winter, children of all ages can drown after misjudging the thickness of ice covering lakes and ponds.

In most cases of drowning, water is aspirated into the lungs. If this occurs in the sea, the hypertonic saline draws water into the alveolar spaces causing hypoxia. Freshwater drowning fills the lungs with a hypotonic solution which is then drawn into the body; this causes electrolyte disturbances and also renders the alveoli unstable and liable to atelectasis. Freshwater drowning may also be complicated by pneumonia because of micro-organisms in the water. The cooling effect of cold water has a protective effect on the body; although arrhythmias may occur and all seems hopeless, resuscitation should not be abandoned until body temperature has been restored to normal.

ROAD TRAFFIC ACCIDENTS

Road traffic accidents (RTAs) are the most common cause of death due to accidents. Children in the lower income groups are most affected, probably because they are more likely to live by a busy road and play on the pavement (**Fig. 28.9**). There is also an excess of teenage boys because they are generally more adventurous as a group and more likely to ride cycles and motorcycles on the road.

Children who are passengers in a car should be appropriately restrained otherwise they may distract the driver, leading to an accident, or, if the car does stop suddenly, are in danger of being thrown through the windscreen. The compulsory use of seatbelts in the

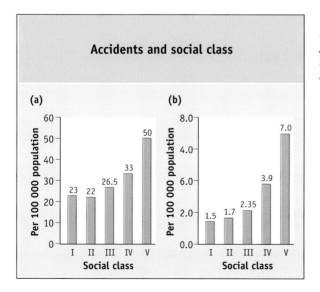

Fig. 28.9 *Accidents and social class: (a) deaths from traffic collisions with pedestrians aged 1–14 years; (b) mortality (all causes) in children aged 1–14 years. Data from OPCS DS 8.*

front seats of cars for adults has had a major effect on the incidence of serious injury during a crash. Small children should be strapped in proper child seats in the back of the car and small babies should be facing rearward.

Teaching children to cross the road safely has not been as successful as hoped because children forget to use kerb drill when they are preoccupied and their perception of speed and distance is not good enough to judge whether it is safe to cross the road. Changing the environment rather than the child's behaviour has been more successful. Creation of enclosed playing areas to keep children away from roads, speed bumps and road islands to reduce the speed of cars are effective measures.

The use of helmets when riding bicycles is an important measure that is still not compulsory.

MANAGEMENT OF RTA VICTIMS

The initial management of major trauma involves initial resuscitation with attention to patency of the airway and adequacy of breathing and the circulation. The cervical spine must be stabilized with a collar until the vertebrae have been X-rayed and shown to be stable. A full examination and skeletal survey (**Fig. 28.10**) should be carried out and if necessary the child admitted for a period of observation. The possibility of internal injuries should be suspected from surface bruising and the circumstances of the accident.

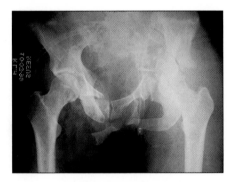

Fig. 28.10 *X-ray of fractured pelvis.*

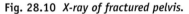

BURNS AND SCALDS

Thermal injury is the second commonest cause of death from accidents in childhood. The physical and psychological scars that remain in survivors often last throughout life.

The main group affected by scalds are young children. Injury commonly results from pulling on the lead of an electric kettle that is hanging down from a work surface or tipping teapots or saucepans on themselves. In older children, burns predominate. In the past many were due to fireworks. Most deaths from house fires are due to asphyxiating and toxic fumes from burning furniture rather than from the fire itself.

TREATMENT OF THERMAL INJURY

First aid for a burn or scald consists of dissipating the heat with large amounts of cold water. This limits the tissue damage and relieves pain. All burns require adequate analgesia which may vary from paracetamol to opiates.

The raw surface of the burn weeps protein-containing fluid. In burns affecting more than 10% of the body's surface area (**Fig. 28.11**) this will necessitate intravenous

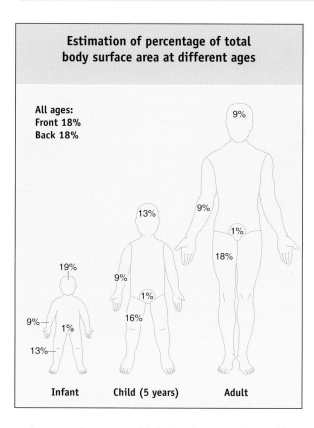

Estimation of percentage of total body surface area at different ages

All ages:
Front 18%
Back 18%

9%

13%

9%

1%

18%

19%

9%

1%

9%

1%

16%

13%

Infant   Child (5 years)   Adult

Fig. 28.11 *Estimation of percentage of total body surface area at different ages.*

replacement. Streptococcal infection is a particular problem and prophylactic antibiotics are given. Skin grafting may be required at a later stage.

PREVENTION

General education of parents or attempts to change social attitudes are less effective in preventing accidents than is often supposed. The reasons for this are not clear but it may be that parents do not consider their home dangerous or that accidents occur when parents are distracted or suffering from stress. There is some benefit in one-to-one discussions with health professionals, such as a health visitor. This approach targets potential problems and provides specific remedies.

After a child has suffered an accident there is an appreciable rate of re-occurrence of a similar type of accident. For example, it has been estimated that 7% of children who present after ingestion of a harmful product have been seen before with the same problem. In these circumstances it is important to consider whether a child may have come to harm as a result of neglect.

Legislation has had the greatest effect in reducing the occurrence of accidents. An important example is the accidental ingestion of drugs and household chemicals by young children. Rather than attempting to change parental behaviour and ensure that these substances are locked away from children, the containers themselves have been made childproof (**Fig. 28.12**).

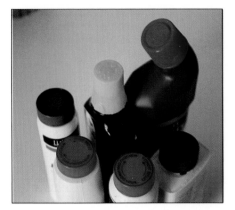

Fig. 28.12 *Childproof packaging.*

Fire-retardant nightwear and furniture coverings and fillings that do not produce toxic gases in a fire are now universally available. Poorer families cannot afford new furniture and there is still a lot of dangerous furniture in use. Cigarette smoking and the use of open electric or gas fires are also more common in this population.

Unfortunately, accidents are more likely to occur in poor families which tend to have higher stress levels and more difficulty in supervising children's play. This, together with the lack of facilities for safe play in the inner cities, places their children at increased risk of suffering an accident. It is argued that, because accidents occur as a result as poverty, improving social circumstances would have the greatest effect on the problem.

NON-ACCIDENTAL INJURY (NAI) AND ABUSE

Unfortunately, some children are harmed by their carers. This may be through direct physical injury or sexual or emotional mistreatment. It is important to recognize that the neglect of a child's needs which impairs his or her well-being is also a form of abuse.

It is the duty of a paediatrician to identify abused children and to arrange for such children to be protected (**Fig. 28.13**). Often this can be managed within the home environment. Paediatricians work closely with social services and child protection teams, and there are local guidelines indicating how suspected abuse should be managed.

PHYSICAL ABUSE
Physical abuse was first recognized in babies—the battered baby syndrome—and in general it is confined to the preschool child. Although all children and infants can have genuine injuries, NAI must be considered if a reasonable explanation cannot be given, if the injury suggests an unusual magnitude or application of force, or if there are multiple unexplained injuries that may vary in age. Careful clinical judgement is required and the opinion of another experienced paediatrician is always useful, particularly when sexual abuse is suspected.

Fractures
Fractures are uncommon in children below the age of 2 years and very suspicious of NAI below the age of 1 year. Some types of fracture are particularly worrying (**Fig. 28.14**). When a fracture is suspicious it is important to carry out a radiographic skeletal survey. This is a complete set of X-rays of the whole body to detect evidence of unreported bony

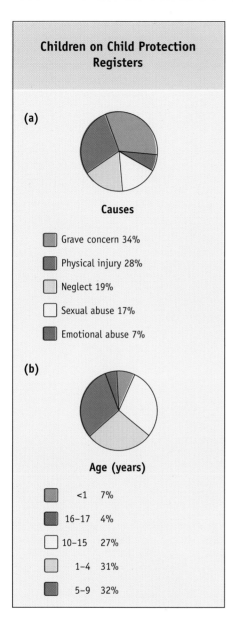

Children on Child Protection Registers

(a)

Causes

Grave concern 34%

Physical injury 28%

Neglect 19%

Sexual abuse 17%

Emotional abuse 7%

(b)

Age (years)

<1   7%

16–17   4%

10–15 27%

1–4   31%

5–9   32%

Fig. 28.13 *Children on Child Protection Registers in England, 31st March 1992. (a) Cause; (b) age.*

injuries or demonstrate fractures that are in different stages of healing. Sometimes medical disorders that allow fractures to occur easily are discovered. Osteogenesis imperfecta is an example of this (Figs 28.15, 28.16).

Bruising

Once infants can crawl, they usually have bruises. These are found in obvious areas of contact such as knees, shins, elbows and forehead. Bruises on other parts of the body are more suspicious. Sometimes the pattern of the marks is clearly not accidental. Finger marks

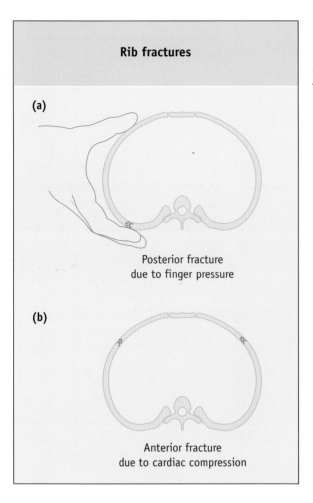

Fig. 28.14 *Rib fractures. Posterior fractures occur because of finger tip pressure (a), anterior fractures from cardiac massage (b).*

Rib fractures

(a)

Posterior fracture
due to finger pressure

(b)

Anterior fracture
due to cardiac compression

on the face suggest slapping, and gripping marks around the chest are seen in shaking injuries. Straight edges to the bruises are seen when children have been beaten with belts or sticks. The ageing of bruises and fractures is very inaccurate (**Fig. 28.17**).

Scalds and burns

Scalds and burns can occur by accident, but may occur as a result of neglect of the child or as a form of punishment. Scalds to the buttocks can only occur if a child is placed in hot water (**Fig. 28.18a**); scalds on the feet are also suspicious. Accidental burns to the hands usually involve the fingers and palm whereas non-accidental burns occur on the back of the hand. Circular cigarette burns and linear burns from contact with an iron are easily recognized (**Fig. 28.18b**).

EMOTIONAL ABUSE AND FAILURE TO THRIVE

Emotional abuse may take the form of neglect, for example not recognizing the child's needs for love, consistency of care, and security. It may also take the form of open hostility and scapegoating. It is important to recognize that parents may abuse in this way because

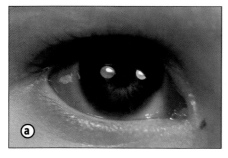

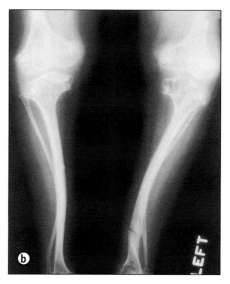

Fig. 28.15 *(a) Blue sclera in osteogenesis imperfecta; (b) fracture in osteogenesis imperfecta.*

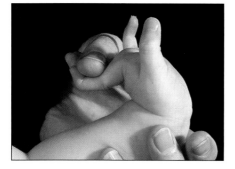

Fig. 28.16 *Ligamentous laxity in osteogenesis imperfecta.*

The ages and appearances of bruises and fractures

Age	Appearance of bruise	Age	Appearance of fracture
Less than 24 hours	Red or purple and swollen	2–10 days	Soft tissue swelling
1–2 days	Purple and swollen	More than 10 days	Periosteal reaction
3–5 days	Starting to become yellow	More than 14 days	Loss of definition at fracture line
5–7 days	Yellow and fading	More than 14 days	Soft callus
More than a week	Yellow, brown or faded	More than 21 days	Hard callus
		More than 3 months	Remodelling of callus

Fig. 28.17 *Ageing of bruising and fractures.*

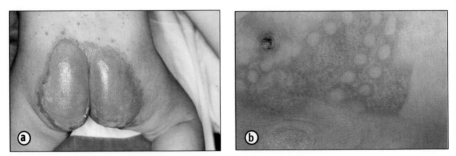

Fig. 28.18 *(a) Scald on buttocks; (b) burn marks from an iron.*

they lack parenting skills, having themselves been raised in this way by their own parents. These children may come to attention because of behavioural problems at school, but emotional abuse can also cause failure to thrive (*see* Chapter 4).

MUNCHAUSEN SYNDROME BY PROXY

Munchausen syndrome by proxy is a rare and bizarre form of abuse in which a carer fabricates symptoms or signs of illness. The child may become ill as a result of this or be subjected to unnecessary investigation and treatment. Examples include repeated suffocation and laxative abuse producing diarrhoea. Diagnosis can be difficult.

SEXUAL ABUSE

Sexual abuse occurs when children are involved in sexual activities that they do not understand or that are not in keeping with our society's expectations. Although it may be carried out by strangers, it is much more commonly perpetrated by members of the family, including the mother, or close friends. Sometimes injuries to the genitalia can have simple explanations (**Fig. 28.19**).

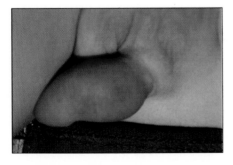

Fig. 28.19 *Bruised penis after bicycle accident.*

Management of abuse

- If abuse is suspected the paediatrician has a duty to act in the interests of the child and it is always correct to involve a senior colleague at this stage.
- A full history and detailed examination should be made of the child by an experienced paediatrician. This is particularly important if sexual abuse is suspected.
- The first issue is the immediate safety of the child. The social services department may already be aware of the family and should be contacted for information. Social workers may allow a relative to look after the child or arrange temporary foster care.
- If physical harm is suspected, admission to hospital may be appropriate while exclusion of blood abnormalities that produce bruising, skeletal surveys or other tests are carried out.
- Honest explanations should always be given to the parents and every effort should be made by hospital staff to be non-judgemental.
- Once investigations and inquiries by social workers and police child protection teams are complete, a case conference is held. All information regarding the case is discussed by the involved agencies, including the parents.
- Many children are allowed home under careful supervision and support.

chapter 29

Therapeutics

The decision to use a specific medical therapy is based on the balance between the beneficial effects and the risks of the treatment. This is known as the therapeutic index. For example, evacuation of haematoma following plastic surgery can be performed with leeches (**Fig. 29.1**) which are effective and safe and have a high therapeutic index. Chemotherapeutic agents, which have major side-effects such as bone marrow toxicity associated with them, have low therapeutic indices (**Fig. 29.2**).

Children are exposed to drugs at all ages: before birth drugs cross the placenta, in the neonatal period vitamin K is administered, and throughout childhood antibiotics and

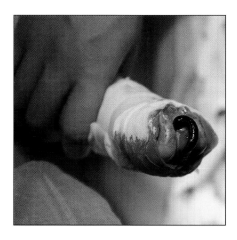

Fig. 29.1 *Evacuation of haematoma by leeches.*

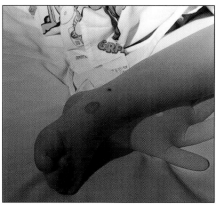

Fig. 29.2 *Extravasation burn from chemotherapy.*

antipyretics are given intermittently. Prescribing for children and babies differs from that for adults because of the child's continuing physical growth, changing body composition and maturing excretory systems.

Pharmacokinetics is the study of what the body does to a drug in terms of absorption, availability at different sites and excretion. Pharmacokinetic studies of new drugs are usually performed in the adult population before being used in children. Less is known about the pharmacokinetics of most drugs in children and neonates than in adults.

Pharmacodynamics is the study of what a drug does to the body in respect to its mode of action and the relationship between concentration in body fluids and effect.

FETAL EXPOSURE TO DRUGS

Drug therapy is essential for some conditions during pregnancy. Unfortunately, if a drug can be absorbed across the maternal gut mucosa, then it is also likely to be freely passed into the feto-placental circulation. Many drugs have no apparent effects but some can cause abortion in the early part of pregnancy and others can disrupt normal morphogenesis. Drugs such as opioids readily cross the placenta, and babies can suffer from their effects following birth. Long-term exposure leads to the occurrence of withdrawal symptoms that may need opioids or sedatives to control them; acute use prior to delivery can cause sedation in the baby. Another example is indomethacin, which is used by obstetricians to prevent preterm labour and reduce the accumulation of amniotic fluid. These important actions must be balanced against the potential for causing constriction of the arterial duct. Regular ultrasound examinations of the fetal circulation must be carried out to ensure that no harm is being done.

BREAST FEEDING

Breast milk provides ideal nutrition for babies and infants; however, drugs ingested by the mother can be passed into the milk. In general, most drugs are present in small amounts and the effects are clinically insignificant. The presence of other infrequently used drugs may warrant the stopping of breast feeding.

It is always important to obtain specialist advice as breast feeding is stopped more commonly than is absolutely necessary. There is a real danger that if breast milk is not expressed its production will diminish or stop. It is often possible to choose alternative drugs that are not passed into breast milk or even to discard breast milk immediately after a drug dose is taken and then allow breast feeding later when levels in the mother's body are lower.

Symptoms of opioid withdrawal

- Irritability, tremors, crying, inconsolable
- Seizures
- Temperature instability
- Tachypnoea or apnoea, sneezing
- Poor feeding, vomiting, diarrhoea
- Failure to gain weight

> **Drugs contraindicated in breast feeding**
>
> - Lithium
> - Cytotoxic drugs
> - Immunosuppressants
> - Iodine and radiopharmaceuticals
> - Bromocriptine and oestrogens
> - Ergotamine

DRUG ABSORPTION

In general, the same principles of drug delivery apply in childhood as in adults. Oral administration is preferred for children where possible—in a sugar-free formulation to avoid caries. However, the intravenous route is preferred if a high blood level of a drug, for example an antibiotic, is required quickly. Intramuscular injection is generally reserved for immunizations but can be used for other drugs although the injection of large volumes is painful. Insulin is injected subcutaneously; deeper injection into fat can produce erratic absorption.

Gastrointestinal

Although the neonatal stomach produces very little acid for several days after birth and the bacteriological flora of the gut is sparse, oral absorption of drugs in babies is very similar to that in adults. Small children prefer liquids to tablets and although there are theoretical differences in the absorption these are not borne out in practice.

Absorption of glucose gel across the gums is used in diabetic children who are unconscious because of hypoglycaemia (Hypostop).

The rectal route is not used routinely as parents and probably children find it unpleasant. However, metronidazole, paracetamol and sodium diclofenac suppositories are well absorbed and this route is preferable when the oral route is unavailable such as following gastrointestinal surgery.

Skin

The skin in infants and preterm babies is thin and lacks the keratinized stratum corneum. Drugs are easily absorbed across this barrier and can have systemic effects. Thus topical steroids should be used cautiously, and lignocaine-based topical anaesthetics are not used at all (**Fig. 29.3**). Topical applications are applied for skin conditions such as eczema in older children but again the minimum dose of steroid is used, as sparingly as possible.

Inhaled therapy

Inhaled therapy is preferred in respiratory disease as high concentrations of drugs can be applied to the airways with fewer systemic effects. Aminoglycosides such as tobramycin or colomycin are often used in cystic fibrosis, and pentamidine for *Pneumocystis carinii* prophylaxis (**Fig. 29.4**). The particle size is very important; although nebulizers appear to be effective they are in fact quite inefficient as most of the drug droplets are too large to pass into the smaller airways. Aerosols used in conjunction with spacer devices are much better and allow a greater proportion of the drug dose into the small airways (*see* Chapter 13, Respiratory Disorders).

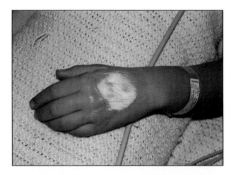

Fig. 29.3 *Occlusive dressing enhancing absorption of topical local anaesthetic cream into skin.*

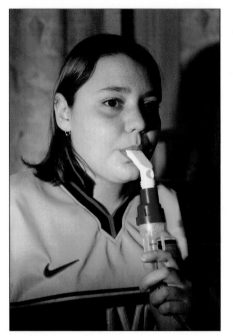

Fig. 29.4 *Inhaled antibiotics in cystic fibrosis.*

DISTRIBUTION AND ELIMINATION OF DRUGS

The chemical structure of a drug determines its solubility in water and fat. Most drugs are bound to proteins in the blood but also circulate freely in the body's aqueous phase. This is important as there are great differences in the relative proportions of water at different ages and thus the drug's apparent distribution volume. Drugs do not pass readily from the blood into the CSF during health but in meningitis the permeability of the CSF–brain barrier is altered, allowing antibiotics to penetrate readily.

Drugs are generally cleared by breakdown and conjugation in the liver and excretion by the kidneys. The hepatic metabolism of drugs is slower in the neonatal period but probably reaches adult rates for most drugs at between 1 and 3 months of life. For example, in neonates the half-life of caffeine, which is used to treat apnoea, is about 4 days whilst in adults it is about 4 hours.

The glomerular filtration rate (GFR) is lower in newborns compared to adults and thus the dosage of drugs with a principally renal excretion such as gentamicin must be reduced. The GFR often falls during systemic illness which complicates therapy and requires frequent drug level determinations.

ADVERSE REACTIONS

Drug reactions are either dose related (a blood level is important to prove the association), idiosyncratic (**Fig. 29.5**) or allergic. The most common dose-related side-effects occur with anticonvulsants where it is usual to increase dosage until control of convulsions or side-effects occur. Side-effects are almost universal when systemic corticosteroids are used (*see* Chapter 15). Idiosyncratic reactions are unwanted reactions that occur on exposure to a drug but which are not related to dose; for example, carbimazole may rarely cause agranulocytosis and suxamethonium may produce malignant hyperpyrexia. Drug allergies are reactions that occur with an immunological basis; antibiotics such as penicillins are frequently, though wrongly, blamed. In many cases a viral rash may be mistaken for an allergy (**Fig. 29.6**). To investigate this a test dose, with safety precautions, may be given to the child on another occasion.

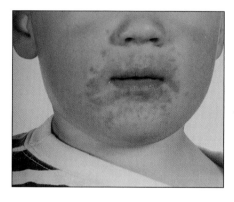

Fig. 29.5 *Skin reaction from inhaled steroids delivered via mask and spacer.*

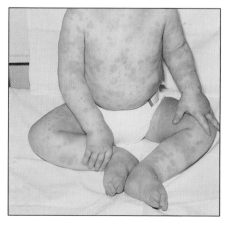

Fig. 29.6 *Red rash of possible drug reaction.*

Tetracyclines stain developing teeth (*see* Fig. 26.6) and should not be used in children. Aspirin is avoided in childhood because of the association with Reye syndrome unless it is specifically indicated for Kawasaki disease or its anti-platelet activity.

DRUG INTERACTIONS

Some drugs interfere with each other. This is particularly important when anticonvulsants are used as toxic blood levels or subtherapeutic levels may result. For example, rifampicin, carbamazepine and phenobarbitone induce hepatic enzymes and increase elimination of other drugs, whilst erythromycin and cimetidine reduce hepatic elimination and can lead to increased plasma levels of other drugs such as cisapride and terfenadine. Both these drugs can cause dangerous arrhythmias in this situation.

THERAPEUTIC MONITORING

Monitoring of drug levels is not routinely necessary, however they should be measured in certain circumstances. This may be because a drug is highly toxic or its elimination is impaired and accumulation is a danger. The other common reasons for measuring the level of a drug are to check compliance if the expected effect has not been produced at a conventional dose or to confirm toxic levels when apparent dose-related side-effects occur. Unless a loading dose is given, five times the half-life of the drug must have passed before a steady state blood level is achieved (**Fig. 29.7**).

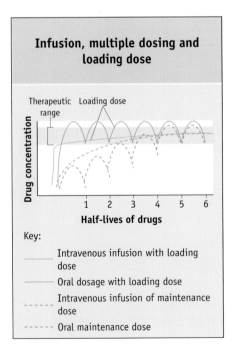

Fig. 29.7 *Infusion, multiple dosing and loading dose. Oral dosage with initial loading dose and intravenous infusion with loading dose rapidly achieve therapeutic range. Initiation of treatment with maintenance dose (either intravenously or orally) requires five half-lives of the drug to achieve steady state.*

PRACTICAL ASPECTS OF PRESCRIBING

When drugs need to be prescribed it is important to use an appropriate agent. Antibiotic usage should be guided by the sensitivities of the likely or known organisms. Broad spectrum antibiotics should be reserved for serious illness to prevent drug resistance.

In childhood it is generally possible to prescribe for most drugs in relation to a child's weight. Where the therapeutic index (benefit versus side-effects) is high, approximate doses based on age band are often given, for oral antibiotics for example. For more toxic drugs, especially those given to neonates, more precise doses are calculated and often monitored by drug levels. For other drugs the dose is titrated against the effect; for example, the minimum effective dose of an anticonvulsant is given and then increased until control of seizures or side-effects occur. It is important to realize that although precise doses can be calculated, depending on the preparation and its concentration it is only possible to physically measure to a reasonable degree of accuracy.

Doses should be given at fixed times but this is rarely possible and convenient times are chosen around school time or sleep periods. This adjustment improves compliance. It is very clear that medication given once or twice a day is more likely to be taken regularly than medicines that need to be taken three or four times in the day. Duration of therapy should also be kept to a minimum; for example, 5–7 days is usually sufficient for most antibiotics.

Index

Note: Page references in *italics* refer to Figures